Linda Johnsen

Alpha
Teach Yourself
Yoga

in **24** hours

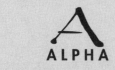

ALPHA

A Pearson Education Company

Alpha Teach Yourself Yoga in 24 Hours

International Standard Book Number: 0-02-864412-3
Library of Congress Catalog Card Number: 2002111658

Printed in the United States of America

First printing: 2002

04 03 02   4 3 2 1

Trademarks

For marketing and publicity, please call: 317-581-3722

The publisher offers discounts on this book when ordered in quantity for bulk purchases and special sales.

For sales within the United States, please contact: Corporate and Government Sales, 1-800-382-3419 or corpsales@pearsontechgroup.com

Outside the United States, please contact: International Sales, 317-581-3793 or international@pearsontechgroup.com

SENIOR ACQUISITIONS EDITOR
Randy Ladenheim-Gil

DEVELOPMENT EDITOR
Lynn Northrup

SENIOR PRODUCTION EDITOR
Christy Wagner

COPY EDITOR
Cari Luna

INDEXER
Angie Bess

PRODUCTION
Angela Calvert
Brad Lenser

COVER DESIGNERS
Charis Santillie
Douglas Wilkins

BOOK DESIGNER
Gary Adair

MANAGING EDITOR
Jennifer Chisholm

PRODUCT MANAGER
Phil Kitchel

PUBLISHER
Marie Butler-Knight

To the yogi from Garhwal who taught me.

Overview

Introduction xxvii

Part I Stretch, Breathe, Focus

Hour 1 Understanding Yoga 3

Hour 2 Stretch and Release 15

Hour 3 Relax and Focus 29

Hour 4 Ride Your Breath 47

Part II Basic Hatha Yoga Postures

Hour 5 Beginning Hatha Yoga 63

Hour 6 More Basic Postures 77

Hour 7 Beginning Bends 91

Hour 8 Basic Twisting Poses 105

Hour 9 Strengthen Your Abdomen 119

Part III More Challenging Yoga Poses

Hour 10 Intermediate Hatha Yoga 131

Hour 11 Advanced Hatha Yoga 143

Hour 12 Flowing Postures 159

Hour 13 Your Hatha Routine 175

PART IV Mastering Meditation

    Hour 14 Introduction to Meditation   189

    Hour 15 Learn to Meditate   203

    Hour 16 Create Inner Focus   217

    Hour 17 Overcome Obstacles   229

    Hour 18 Ignite Inner Energies   239

    Hour 19 Awaken Your Awareness   253

PART V Live Your Yoga

    Hour 20 The Yoga Lifestyle   269

    Hour 21 Yoga Psychology   281

    Hour 22 Yoga Ethics   295

    Hour 23 Types of Yoga   307

    Hour 24 The Yoga Universe   317

Appendixes

    Appendix A Twenty-Minute Recap   329

    Appendix B Glossary   335

    Appendix C Resources   345

    Appendix D Further Reading   349

    Appendix E Quiz Answers   355

    Index   361

Contents

Introduction   **xvii**

PART I Stretch, Breathe, Focus

HOUR 1 Understanding Yoga   **3**

The Evolution of Yoga 3

    How Yoga Came West 4

    Influential Yoga Teachers 5

    Different Styles of Yoga 6

Identifying Your Inner Body 7

    Discover Your Five Levels 8

    Uncover the Bliss Within 10

Your Three Energy States 11

Realize Your Higher Self 12

    A Deeper Reality 12

    The Play of Spirit 13

    Yoga and Religion 13

HOUR 2 Stretch and Release   **15**

Play It Safe 16

    Check with Your Doctor 16

    Special Rules for Women 16

    Dress for Movement 17

    Eat Later 17

    Breathe Through Your Nose 18

    Avoid Force 18

Loosen Up 19

    Head Roll 19

    Shoulder Roll 20

    Wrist Roll 21

    Hip Roll 21

    Knee Roll 22

    Ankle Roll 22

Mastering the Stretching Poses 23

    Standing Stretch 23

    Reclining Stretch 23

    Cat Stretch 24

    Lunge Stretch 27

HOUR 3 Relax and Focus   **29**

Mastering Relaxation Poses 29
    Mountain Posture 31
    Child's Posture 32
    Knees-to-Chest Posture 34
    Crocodile Posture 34
    Corpse Posture 35
Travel the Body 37
    Visit the 31 Points 38
    Visit the 61 Points 41
Mastering Your Balance 42
    Tip Toe Stretch 43
    Tree Posture 44

HOUR 4 Ride Your Breath   **47**

The Link Between Body and Mind 47
Mastering the Basics of Breath 48
    Diaphragmatic Breathing 49
    Complete Breath 51
    Alternate Nostril Breathing 52
Energize Your Awareness 56
    Glowing Face Breathing 56
    Bellows Breathing 57
    Humming Breath 57
    A Few Words of Caution 58
Recognizing Life Force 59

PART II Basic Hatha Yoga Postures

HOUR 5 Beginning Hatha Yoga   **63**

Mastering the Basic Postures 63
    Cobra Posture 64
    Locust Posture 66
    Boat Posture 68
    Bow Posture 70
    Half Fish Posture 71
    Arch Posture 72
    Bridge Posture 73
Know Your Limits 75

HOUR 6 More Basic Postures **77**

Mastering More Floor Postures 77
Staff Posture 77
Shoulder Stand 79
Plow Posture 81
Pigeon Posture 83
Down Facing Dog Posture 85
Mastering More Standing Postures 86
Warrior Posture 86
Horse Riding Posture 88

HOUR 7 Beginning Bends **91**

Mastering the Bending Poses 91
Standing Side Bend 92
Standing Backward Bend 93
Standing Forward Bend 95
Sitting Forward Bend 97
Churn 99
Symbol of Yoga 100
Butterfly 102
Bend Without Breaking 104

HOUR 8 Basic Twisting Poses **105**

Mastering the Twisting Postures 105
Angle Pose 106
Triangle Pose 107
Revolving Triangle 109
Torso Twist 111
Half Spinal Twist 112
Reclining Twist 115
Straighten Your Back 116
Rocking Chair Roll 116
Respect Your Spine 117

HOUR 9 Strengthen Your Abdomen **119**

Maintain Your Center 119
Mastering the Abdominal Poses 120
Stomach Lift 121
Stomach Roll 123
Leg Lift 124
Balance Pose 125

PART III More Challenging Yoga Poses

HOUR 10 Intermediate Hatha Yoga 131

Expand Your Limits 131
Mastering the Intermediate Postures 132
   Inclined Plane Posture 133
   Camel Posture 134
   Eagle Posture 135
   King Dancer Posture 136
   Archer Posture 138
   Back Bending Monkey Posture 140

HOUR 11 Advanced Hatha Yoga 143

Reach Beyond Your Limits 143
Mastering the More Challenging Postures 144
   Dolphin Posture 144
   Headstand 146
   Crow Posture 150
   Peacock Posture 152
   Full Spinal Twist 153
   Wheel Posture 155
   Scorpion Posture 156

HOUR 12 Flowing Postures 159

Make the Postures Flow 159
Mastering the Sun Salutation 160
Learn the Sun Series 160
   Sun Salutation Pose 1 161
   Sun Salutation Pose 2 162
   Sun Salutation Pose 3 163
   Sun Salutation Pose 4 164
   Sun Salutation Pose 5 165
   Sun Salutation Pose 6 166
   Sun Salutation Pose 7 167
   Sun Salutation Pose 8 168
   Sun Salutation Pose 9 168
   Sun Salutation Pose 10 169
   Sun Salutation Pose 11 170
   Sun Salutation Pose 12 171

Hour 13 Your Hatha Routine **175**

Design Your Session 175
    Design Your Gentle Routine 177
    Design Your First Beginning Routine 178
    Design Your Second Beginning Routine 180
    Design Your Intermediate Routine 181
    Design Your Advanced Routine 182
Creating an Atmosphere 183
Aids to Hatha Practice 184
Yoga Retreat Centers, Classes, and Events 185

Part IV Mastering Meditation

Hour 14 Introduction to Meditation **189**

Go Beyond Your Body 189
    Benefits of Meditation 190
    A Natural High 191
    Mood- and Mind-Altering Drugs 192
Mastering the Meditation Postures 192
    Easy Posture 194
    Auspicious Posture 196
    Accomplished Posture 197
    Lotus Posture 199
    Chair Posture 200
    Comfortable but Steady 201

Hour 15 Learn to Meditate **203**

Enter the Inner World 203
    Checking Your Breathing Cycle 204
    Focus on Your Breath 206
    Regulate Your Nervous System 208
Chant Your Mantra 208
    Control the Genie 209
    Choose a Mantra 210
    Work with Inner Sound 211
Mastering Your Mind 212
    Use a Mala 213
    Practice Japa 215

HOUR 16 Create Inner Focus   **217**

Establishing a Meditation Routine 218
    Prepare to Sit 218
    Begin Your Meditation Routine 219
Visualize an Object 221
    Meditating on an Image 221
    Visualizing a Cosmic Pattern 222
Contemplation of an Ideal 224
    Find Your Inner Core 224
    Expand Your Sense of Self 225
Connect with Inner Guidance 226
Guidance or Garbage? 227

HOUR 17 Overcome Obstacles   **229**

Inner Roadblocks 229
    Doubt 231
    Sloth 231
    Poor Health 231
    Delusion 232
    Craving 232
    Misunderstanding 233
    Failure 234
    Inconsistency 234
Western Concerns 235
    Stilling the Mind 236
    Facing Fear 236
Group Meditation 237

HOUR 18 Ignite Inner Energies   **239**

The Power Within 240
    Your Degree of Awareness 241
    The Energy of Consciousness 242
Experience Your Chakras 242
The Seven Centers 245
    Your Sacral Center 245
    Your Sex Center 246
    Your Navel Center 247
    Your Heart Center 248
    Your Throat Center 249
    Your Eyebrow Center 250
    Your Brain Centers 251

Hour 19 Awaken Your Awareness **253**

Latent Mental Powers 253
  Special Yogic Abilities 254
  Beware of Psychic Powers! 255
  Inner Messages 255
Yogic Sleep 257
  Prepare for Lucid Sleep 258
  Practice Lucid Sleep 259
  Reduce Your Need for Sleep 261
Higher States of Consciousness 262
  The Experience of Samadhi 263
  Recognize Your Own Presence 264
Evaluating Your Progress 265

Part V Live Your Yoga

Hour 20 The Yoga Lifestyle **269**

Yoga and Nutrition 269
  Eat Like a Yogi 270
  Easy Yoga Recipes 271
Cleaning Out Your Body 275
  Nasal Wash 275
  Stomach Wash 277
Ayurveda: Yoga Therapy 278
  What's Your Ayurvedic Type? 279
  Finding Balance 280

Hour 21 Yoga Psychology **281**

Understand Yourself 282
  Analyze Your Mind 282
  Analyze Your Intellect 283
  Analyze Your Memory 284
  Analyze Your Self-Identity 285
From Life to Life: Reincarnation 286
Understand the Karmic Process 288
  Action and Its Consequences 288
  Watch What You Think 289
  Erase Bad Karma 290
  Banish Negativity 291
Calculate Your Karma: Yoga Astrology 292
Get Off the Karmic Wheel 293

HOUR 22 Yoga Ethics **295**

The Ten Commitments 295
Yoga's Do's and Don'ts 296
　Don't Harm Anyone 297
　Don't Lie 297
　Don't Steal 298
　Don't Overindulge 298
　Don't Be Greedy 299
　Keep Clean 299
　Stay Content 300
　Be Self-Disciplined 300
　Study Yourself 301
　Surrender to a Higher Force 301
Take Stock of the Day 302
The Guru-Disciple Relationship 302
　Recognize the Guru 303
　The Levels of Enlightenment 304
　Crazy Wisdom 304
　Test the Teacher 305

HOUR 23 Types of Yoga **307**

Raja Yoga 307
Karma Yoga 309
　Work Without Worry 309
　Serve Selflessly 310
Bhakti Yoga 311
　Empower Your Practice 311
　Express Your Emotions 313
Jnana Yoga 313
　Study, Contemplate, Realize 314
　Experience Truth 315

HOUR 24 The Yoga Universe **317**

Tantra Yoga 318
　Mental Mechanics 319
　The Value of Symbols 320
　Invoke Blessing Force 320
　Meditate on Blessings 322
Read the Classics 323
　The *Yoga Sutras* 324
　The *Bhagavad Gita* 325
　Hatha Yoga Texts 325
　Texts on Inner Awareness 325

Reach for Enlightenment 326
Live Consciously 327

Appendixes

APPENDIX A Twenty-Minute Recap   329

APPENDIX B Glossary   335

APPENDIX C Resources   345

APPENDIX D Further Reading   349

APPENDIX E Quiz Answers   355

Index   361

Introduction

Several years ago I developed a horrendous case of sciatica. I was in constant pain; my legs hurt so much I could barely walk or even sleep. Multiple visits to the doctor didn't help much. I took high doses of pain killers and anti-inflammatory drugs for months to no avail.

Then a friend recommended I try yoga. "I used to have sciatica too," Debra said. "Yoga cleared it right up." I had never been attracted to the complicated looking postures of yoga myself, but I was desperate enough to try anything. With deep reservations, I signed up for my first class.

Incredibly, after only four days of doing yoga exercises the pain in my legs vanished completely. I know it was the postures that did the trick because whenever I get lazy and stop doing my yoga routine, the sciatica comes back!

Hatha Yoga has been used in India for at least a thousand years to promote health and vitality and to increase longevity. Old texts note the "luster" of the hatha yogis; today we would call it beauty. Radiant good health is always beautiful.

But I soon learned yoga had a lot more to offer than physical postures. Yoga is a complete system that works at all levels, aiming not only at physical well-being but at emotional balance, mental clarity, and spiritual growth. It teaches you how to eat and even how to breathe in order to generate the energy you need to live life to the fullest. It even comes with its own set of ethics, because the yogis recognized that no one who hurts other people is completely healthy.

I can't guarantee that yoga will cure your sciatica, or any other medical problems you may have, within a matter of days—although it sure did help me! But I will say that I've never met anyone who took up the practice of yoga who didn't benefit from it. Yoga is not a substitute for a visit to the doctor; in fact, if you have a medical condition you should check with a physician before beginning a yoga program. But people who do these practices regularly may find themselves needing to visit their doctor less often because they look and feel better and better.

Yoga is an excellent addition to any lifestyle. Good luck with your new yoga routine!

What You'll Find in This Book

Part I, "Stretch, Breathe, Focus," explains how yoga incorporates hatha postures, breathing exercises, and meditation techniques to achieve a state of physical health and emotional balance. You'll learn the most essential beginning-level yoga practices, including stretches, relaxation, and concentration exercises, as well as diaphragmatic breathing. You'll begin working toward physical poise, flexibility, and vitality.

Part II, "Basic Hatha Yoga Postures," introduces you to some bending and twisting postures that will strengthen and tone your muscles. You'll also start practicing classical yoga poses such as the Cobra and the Shoulder Stand. One full hour will be devoted to yoga exercises that tone the abdominal muscles, to help you keep looking as good as you feel.

Part III, "More Challenging Yoga Poses," focuses on more advanced yoga postures, as well as the Sun Salutation, the famous series of yoga poses that gracefully flow into one another like a dance. Then you'll design your own yoga session, based on your unique needs and level of fitness.

Part IV, "Mastering Meditation," introduces you to yoga exercises for the mind: basic meditation and visualization practices. You'll begin experiencing both the physical and mental benefits of meditation practice right away. You'll learn how to deal with any obstacles that might arise and how to recognize higher states of consciousness.

Part V, "Live Your Yoga," highlights the vast expanse of the yoga tradition. You'll discover how you can benefit from a yogic diet, internal cleansing techniques, and yoga therapy and psychology. You'll learn how yogis understand the universe and the different branches of yoga that are designed for different personality types.

Extras

At the end of each hour, you'll find a quick quiz that will help you test your newfound knowledge of the most important points taught in that hour. Every quiz includes 10 true or false statements for you to consider.

There are 5 appendixes at the end of the 24 one-hour lessons. There is a 20-minute recap to help you organize the mass of information you've found in this book in your mind. A glossary of Sanskrit terms will help you with foreign words commonly used in yoga. A resources section will guide you to organizations that teach Hatha Yoga and yoga-related topics. The lengthy bibliography lets you know some of the very best books on important aspects of the yoga tradition. And finally, you'll find the answers to the quizzes you took at the end of each hour.

There's another important extra you'll find useful. Throughout the book you'll find cross-references, tips, cautions, and definitions to enhance your understanding of the material. Here's how they stack up:

GO TO ▷
This sidebar directs you to other hours in this book where there is more information about a topic you're studying.

JUST A MINUTE

This sidebar offers advice and further guidance about yoga techniques and concepts you've just learned.

PROCEED WITH CAUTION

This sidebar warns you of pitfalls you may encounter as you begin practicing some of the exercises explained in the text.

FYI This sidebar directs you to other books and websites where you can learn more about the topic under consideration.

TIME SAVER

This sidebar offers a faster or more convenient way to do something.

STRICTLY DEFINED

This sidebar helps you keep track of the new terminology you're learning in each hour.

About the Author

LINDA JOHNSEN, M.S., is author of *Daughters of the Goddess: The Women Saints of India* (winner of the 1995 Midwest Book Association award for "Best New Age Book of the Year"), *The Living Goddess* (a book about the Hindu Goddess tradition, assigned reading in several college courses), and *The Complete Idiot's Guide to Hinduism*. Her fourth book, *Meditation Is Boring?* garnered rave reviews for its frank discussion of typical problems beginners encounter when they start practicing yoga and meditation.

Linda is one of the most familiar writers in the American yoga community. She is a contributing editor and columnist for *Yoga International* magazine, and has often written for *Yoga Journal*. Her books and many feature articles cover all aspects of the yoga tradition, and some have been translated into European languages. Over the years, the list of figures she has interviewed reads like a Who's Who of the yoga universe. In addition, her essays have appeared in a nearly a dozen anthologies, among them *The Divine Mosaic, Uncoiling the Snake: Ancient Patterns in Contemporary Women's Lives,* and *Yoga Abenteuer Meditation* (in German).

Linda has lectured throughout the United States on yoga-related topics, and has been featured on numerous radio programs and on cable television. She graduated first in her class from the University of Scranton's innovative Program in Eastern Studies, and from 1983 through 1986 served as the program's administrator. This fully accredited Master's degree program focused on the many facets of the yoga tradition: Hatha Yoga postures, stress reduction and breathing exercises, diet, physiology, ethics, philosophy, Sanskrit studies, meditation, and research.

Acknowledgments

Many thanks to the staff at Alpha Books who transform writers' thoughts and ideas into actual, practical series of books. Special thanks to Lynn Northrup, my skilled and gracious editor, who shaped and crafted this book; to Christy Wagner, who juggled the mass of photos and artwork I tossed at her and made sure they all landed in the right place; to Steve Adams for supplying the illustrations, and to Randy Ladenheim-Gil, who got the ball rolling in the first place.

My terrific agent, Jacky Sach from BookEnds, went way beyond the call of duty, organizing a massive photo shoot for the book. I'm deeply grateful to Jacky for all her support! I want to especially acknowledge Delia Quigley, Director of StillPoint Schoolhouse, the brilliant yoga teacher who posed for most of the pictures; and Ramaiah Collins of the Yoga Company in Sonoma, California, who posed for the rest. Thanks also to Johnathan Brown, my computer technician, backup photographer, and husband, who wrestled with my computer equipment and made it behave.

Finally, let me express my deepest gratitude to Swami Rama and the teachers of the Himalayan tradition, who made sure we students knew our yoga inside and out.

PART I

Stretch, Breathe, Focus

HOUR 1 Understanding Yoga

HOUR 2 Stretch and Release

HOUR 3 Relax and Focus

HOUR 4 Ride Your Breath

HOUR 1
Understanding Yoga

CHAPTER SUMMARY

LESSON PLAN:

In this hour you will learn ...

- Yoga is a holistic system devoted to physical and spiritual well-being, which evolved in India over thousands of years.

- The wisdom of the yoga masters has been legendary in the West since at least the time of the ancient Greeks.

- Yogis believe people are more than simply physical beings and that there are subtler dimensions to the human personality.

- Of active, passive, or balanced personality types, yoga aims for balance.

- The ultimate goal of traditional yoga practices is to put you in touch with the center of consciousness within you.

Yoga is a complete system of physical and mental exercises designed to help you become healthy, emotionally balanced, mentally clear, and spiritually illumined. The Sanskrit word *yoga* actually means "link" (think of a "yoke"). A successful yogi is a person whose body, emotions, and intellect are linked in a positive way, working together instead of conflicting with each other, to achieve a goal such as prosperity, harmonious relationships, service to humanity, or inner peace.

Traditionally, the ultimate goal of yoga was the most important link-up of all, the union of the mind with the Higher Self within. By connecting with his or her innermost spirit, the yogi gained access to hidden reserves of creative energy, healing power, and intuitive guidance.

THE EVOLUTION OF YOGA

The yoga tradition evolved over thousands of years in the Himalayan mountains (including parts of Nepal and Tibet) and throughout the Indian subcontinent. Yogic meditations are described in the *Rig Veda*, a holy text composed in northwestern India and Pakistan some five thousand or so years ago. In one of the most famous verses of the *Rig Veda*, a priest prays, "With loving reverence, we bow to the divine inner sun, the most splendid light in all the worlds. Please illumine our minds!" This shows that even at an early date, yogis in India were searching for the inner light.

Today in the West most people think of yoga primarily as a system of physical exercises, the famous postures of Hatha Yoga. These were developed by yoga teachers called *siddhas*, which means "accomplished masters." Some of the most famous siddhas hailed from Bengal, which is in the northeastern section of the subcontinent, but others came from as far away as China and south India. Two of the most renowned siddhas, Gorakh Nath and Matsyendra Nath, probably lived somewhere between 1,000 to 1,300 years ago. Traditional Indian yogis believe the original source of the hatha postures was God himself, who taught them to enlightened masters for the benefit of humanity.

STRICTLY DEFINED

Yoga literally means "linked" or "yoked." It refers to the physical and mental exercises that help "yoke" the different parts of the human personality together in a harmonious unity, as well as linking the mind with the higher awareness within oneself. A **siddha** is an accomplished yoga master who has achieved perfection in his or her yoga practice.

HOW YOGA CAME WEST

Tales of the extraordinary abilities of India's yogis have circulated in the West for millennia. When Alexander the Great reached India in 327 B.C.E., he met a yogi named Dandamis who impressed him so deeply he declared that while he had conquered the world, Dandamis had conquered *him*. At least one Greek philosopher who traveled with Alexander to India appears to have been deeply influenced by the yogis. This remarkable sage, named Pyrrho, introduced components of the yoga tradition to his students when he returned home, greatly influencing the course of Greek thought.

In the first century C.E., a physician from Turkey named Apollonius of Tyana visited both India and Egypt. Apollonius reported back to the Western world that the yogis of India were the wisest men he had met anywhere in his extensive travels. He also felt that the mystical tradition of Egypt had been deeply affected by yogic teaching. Since the Egyptian writer Manetho confirms that the immigration of a large number of Indians to Egypt around 1400 B.C.E. was one of the great events of Egyptian history, it's quite possible they may have brought knowledge of yogic philosophy and practices with them. Incidentally, Apollonius's students included several Roman emperors, so his high opinion of the yoga masters was widely reported.

Hints that yoga may have been better known in the West than modern historians have previously thought recur in Western literature. For example, the *Enneads* was one of the most influential books in Western history. It was written by a philosopher named Plotinus who lived in Rome in the third century C.E. It describes the process of meditation and the different states of consciousness you experience as your meditation deepens in a manner completely identical to that of Indian yoga texts. We know that Plotinus set out to visit India, though he was stopped in Persia. It's not unlikely a strong desire to learn more about yoga was the reason he risked his life trying to reach the Himalayas.

INFLUENTIAL YOGA TEACHERS

Yoga was first brought to the modern Western world in 1893 by a very famous Hindu monk named Swami Vivekananda. When Vivekananda spoke at the World Parliament of Religions in Chicago that year, he caused a sensation. The swami's teachings about practical techniques ordinary people could practice to attain well-being and peace of mind were exciting news to open-minded people of the time. Vivekananda was invited to lecture throughout North America and Europe. He established numerous centers where people could come to learn the fundamental teachings of yoga.

Many teachers came over from India in the following years. The best known was Paramahansa Yogananda, who arrived in the United States in 1920. His book, *Autobiography of a Yogi,* was filled with stories of the yoga adepts' miraculous-seeming powers. It inspired tens of thousands of Westerners to take up yoga practice. This classic remains popular even today. In the mid- to late 1960s, there was an explosion of interest in yoga in the Western world. Swami Rama demonstrated, under rigorous laboratory conditions, that at least some of the claims about the powers you can develop through yoga were true. He had spent much of his childhood in the cave monasteries of Uttara Pradesh, mastering advanced physical and mental techniques of the yoga tradition.

Swami Rama was the first yoga adept to be thoroughly tested by American scientists. Through the pure power of his directed will, he could make his heart appear to stop beating, raise and lower the temperature in particular cells in his hands, and even remain fully conscious while monitoring equipment showed his brain was supposed to be asleep. After Swami Rama, Western scientists could no longer brush off as pure myth stories about yoga's amazing value.

FYI An excellent introduction to the yoga tradition is *The Royal Path: Practical Lessons on Yoga* by Swami Rama. Or check out one of the great Hatha Yoga manuals of all time, *Integral Yoga*. It was written by Swami Satchidananda in the 1970s and may have turned more people in the West on to yoga postures than any other single book.

Other important yoga teachers from this period included Maharishi Mahesh Yogi, who also inspired Western scientists to further research the benefits of yoga. Swami Vishnudevananda published a thick illustrated volume of yoga postures, which included a number of very advanced poses. These stunned many new students in the West, who could scarcely believe the human body could bend and fold and lift itself in such impossible-looking ways! Meanwhile, bushy-bearded Swami Satchidananda was so popular that he was invited to preside over the legendary music festival at Woodstock in 1969.

Western-born yoga teachers also began to appear. In the 1960s, Richard Hittleman helped popularize Hatha Yoga, explaining it in terms that were easy for non-Indians to understand. In 1970, Ram Dass (Richard Alpert, Ph.D.) published a classic account of his own encounter with yoga called *Be Here Now,* which excited a whole generation of readers. Meanwhile, Lilias Folan's syndicated Hatha Yoga television program beamed basic yoga techniques into homes across America.

Today there isn't a city in North America without several yoga centers. Yoga is taught at the YMCA, in physical education programs in many schools, and at hospitals and medical clinics across the country. Magazines like *Yoga Journal* and *Yoga International* grace the magazine racks in supermarkets. Yoga has established itself as a valued part of American life.

FYI Want to learn more about America's two leading yoga magazines? Find out what *Yoga International* has to offer by logging on to www.YogaInternational.com. You can check into *Yoga Journal* at www.YogaJournal.com.

DIFFERENT STYLES OF YOGA

Many different styles of yoga are being taught in the West today. Gentle Yoga classes are most appropriate for beginners who are not particularly agile. In Hour 2, you'll learn some of the introductory-level yoga stretches appropriate for inflexible beginners. Gentle Yoga may also be appropriate for the elderly and for those recovering from illness or surgery.

Classical Indian Hatha Yoga tends to take it slow and easy, so you can progress as rapidly in your practice as possible without injuring yourself. *Alpha Teach Yourself Yoga in 24 Hours* takes a classical approach.

Some students prefer a dynamic approach to yoga. Power Yoga is a more aggressive form of hatha exercise that may include aerobic elements. You'll get your heart rate up and work in some aerobic conditioning, which most yoga classes de-emphasize.

The world-renowned Hatha Yoga instructor B.K.S. Iyengar teaches another demanding form of yoga. Iyengar asks you to hold each posture perfectly for some length of time, focusing on exact alignment. Viniyoga, inspired by T.K.V. Desikachar, is quite different. It builds to the perfect posture gradually, allowing every student to mature into the pose at his or her own pace, and making adjustments depending on each student's individual needs.

Ashtanga Yoga, as formulated by K. Pattabhi Jois, synchronizes yogic breathing techniques with a progressive series of postures designed to heat your body and make you sweat. This detoxifies your body and creates a sense of lightness, energy, and strength.

Anusara Yoga, developed by John Friend, is a holistic system that treats not only the physical but the emotional and spiritual aspects of Hatha Yoga. You are asked to focus not just on your physical alignment in a posture, but on your attitude toward the pose and the actions that arise out of your practice.

Yin Yoga is the most passive type of yoga, in which you relax into a posture and allow gravity and the natural traction created by the pose to stretch and tone your muscle groups.

Today, there are numerous forms of Hatha Yoga, with more developing all the time. Modern teachers strive to accommodate the needs and capacities of today's students, but still base their training on the insights of yoga's ancient adepts—the masters who formulated the yoga system in the first place.

IDENTIFYING YOUR INNER BODY

Hatha Yoga is just one small part of the yoga tradition as a whole, however. The ancient yoga masters saw life in a radically different way than most people do today in the more materially oriented West. They saw the entire universe as pervaded by consciousness and energy. Energy was not a blind force in their view, but was directed by an inconceivably vast intelligence. All living beings were linked to each other through their union with this inner network of intelligence.

The ancient adepts also believed that individual souls cycle through different planes of existence until they reach a state of perfection. Practicing yoga helps students achieve greater states of health, longer lives, and deeper self-understanding during this process. For the yogi, self-knowledge comes through exploring the many different levels of your being. This includes not only the physical body, but more subtle inner dimensions of your personality.

JUST A MINUTE

 Western psychology focuses on unhealthy people, and directs most of its treatment modalities to those suffering from neuroses and psychoses. Yoga psychology, on the other hand, was developed to explore the positive potentials of the personality. It offers modalities to help people become more physically fit, self-aware, and fulfilled.

DISCOVER YOUR FIVE LEVELS

In the multidimensional universe of the siddhas, you are not just a material being. In addition to your physical body, you have four other increasingly subtle bodies, one layered over the next. Yoga was designed to work with all five levels, or dimensions, of your being:

- *Anna Maya Kosha*—the body made of food (*anna*)
- *Prana Maya Kosha*—the body made of life force (*prana*)
- *Mano Maya Kosha*—the body made of your sensory awareness and everyday thoughts (*manas*)
- *Vijnana Maya Kosha*—the body made of higher intelligence and will (*vijnana*)
- *Ananda Maya Kosha*—the body made of inner joy (*ananda*)

You can actually experience these five levels by directing your awareness inward and carefully observing your inner states.

1. Sit comfortably with your head, neck, and trunk straight. Close your eyes. Be aware of your physical body. Feel your head, torso, arms, abdomen, and legs. This is the most dense or physically gross aspect of your being, the "overcoat" of your soul.

2. Bring your attention to your breath. Breathe slowly and smoothly through your nose, not your mouth. Be aware of the energy pulsing through your physical body, making your heart beat, your lungs inhale and exhale, your stomach gurgle. This life energy is called *prana* in the yoga tradition. It is the "jacket" your soul has on under its overcoat.

GO TO ▶
In Hour 22, you'll learn more about yoga psychology. The yogis offer a wealth of sound advice on how to deal with psychological complexes so you can free yourself from the mental limitations that block your vision and restrict your growth.

3. Shift your attention to the thoughts passing through your mind. Be aware of yourself thinking and feeling, planning or remembering. Yogis do not believe these thoughts are actually you. Instead they call this layer of mental activity another drape of your soul, the "vest" your soul is wearing under its jacket.

4. Pull your attention up inside your skull to a point about three inches behind your eyebrows. Notice how mentally energized you feel, how sharp your concentration becomes. You are now focused at the level of your higher intellect, the part of your personality that evaluates things rationally, makes concrete decisions, and wills yourself into action. This is the "shirt" your soul wears under its vest.

5. Now move your attention to a point just inside your chest, between your breasts. Let go of all thoughts for a moment, and just allow yourself to be. In the perfect stillness of the present moment lies a profound sense of contentment, tranquility and inner peace. This is the body of bliss, the "undershirt" the soul has on beneath its shirt.

The soul itself is none of these bodies, traditional yogis believe, but is the pure witnessing consciousness that experiences these five levels of selfhood. In the yoga tradition the soul is called *purusha*, which means "the inner person."

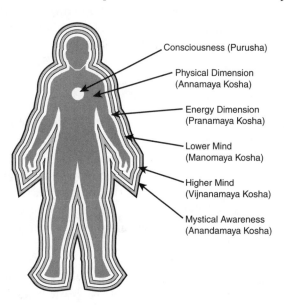

Consciousness (Purusha)

Physical Dimension
(Annamaya Kosha)

Energy Dimension
(Pranamaya Kosha)

Lower Mind
(Manomaya Kosha)

Higher Mind
(Vijnanamaya Kosha)

Mystical Awareness
(Anandamaya Kosha)

Five dimensions of the soul.

STRICTLY DEFINED

Prana is the life force active in your body. Its most physical manifestation is your breath. **Purusha** literally means "person." It refers to the immortal spirit at the core of your being.

UNCOVER THE BLISS WITHIN

To further understand the five components of your being, all of which you will be working with in the following hours, try this visualization:

1. Imagine a human corpse. This is the physical body alone, with none of the other four components activating it.

2. Imagine a man in a coma. His body is alive because prana, or life energy, keeps it functioning. However, he doesn't think or feel or respond to others because the higher three components are not active.

3. Imagine a man who is senile. He moves around, is aware of objects around himself, and instinctively responds to other people who walk into the room. He doesn't think logically or communicate rationally, however, because his higher two components are in a dormant state.

4. Imagine a man preparing his tax return. In addition to his awareness of events around him, his intellect is now engaged as he fills out his tax form, decides which deductions he's eligible for, and calculates how much he owes. Still, he doesn't feel happy or at peace because the highest component of his personality is not engaged.

5. Imagine a man talking with a woman he loves deeply. He feels profoundly joyful and satisfied with life. He thinks his deep sense of pleasure comes from the woman sitting near him, but according to yoga, this sense of happiness actually comes from the highest part of his personality, his body of inner bliss. He feels as if he's in heaven but actually it's a heaven of his own making, as he experiences the love emanating from the center of his being.

According to the yoga tradition, the first two bodies dissolve at the time of death, but the other three components of the human personality continue to exist. At the moment of reincarnation, the next body (which holds our thoughts and memories) dissolves, which is why most people don't remember their past lives. Only the innermost two bodies are reborn, carrying with them the karma from past lives. At the time of spiritual liberation, even these last layers fall away, and only the purusha or innermost consciousness continues on.

JUST A MINUTE

Yogis in India believe the four "subtle bodies" really exist, though you may be more inclined to think of them as aspects of the personality. Western scientists are puzzled how acupuncture and homeopathy could really work since they don't affect any obvious physical structures. Yogis say they affect the Prana Maya Kosha, the body of life force.

This is how the yoga tradition engages each of these layers of your being:

- Hatha postures work with the physical body.
- Breathing exercises work with the pranic level, the life energy.
- Concentration exercises work with the mind.
- Meditation, visualization, and ethical practices work with the higher intelligence.
- Deep states of meditative absorption work with the most subtle level, helping you to "follow your bliss."

In this manner yoga is said to strengthen and tone all five "bodies" the soul is "wearing" at once.

YOUR THREE ENERGY STATES

There are three ways in which energy can manifest both in the universe and in our personalities:

- *Rajas*—active, dynamic
- *Tamas*—inert, dull
- *Sattva*—balanced, harmonious

A woman who spends her evening out jogging or playing tennis has chosen a rajasic or active way to spend her time. One who sits in front of her television watching reruns while sipping a martini has placed herself in a comparatively tamasic state that may leave her feeling relaxed but also lethargic. A woman who's doing yoga, however, is moving into a sattvic state, and will probably end the evening feeling relaxed, but also refreshed and mentally composed.

Rajas impels you to action, but can also cause agitation and instability of mind. Tamas slows you down, but also grounds you. Both qualities are necessary in our day-to-day lives. While practicing yoga, however, students aspire for sattva, for tranquility, even-mindedness, and calm lucidity.

In Hour 4, you'll learn more about yogic breathing and how it affects the two hemispheres of your brain. Yogis breathe through their left nostril to stimulate tamas, through their right nostril to stimulate rajas, and through both nostrils at once to experience sattva. This only sounds silly until you try it. Once you experiment with these principles, you'll be amazed at how dramatically the breathing exercises affect your energy state.

GO TO ▶
The vigorous yogic breathing exercises taught in Hour 4 can help you become more rajasic by filling your body with energizing oxygen. The calming and balancing breathing exercises in Hour 4, however, increase the quality of sattva in your energy state. They leave you feeling alert but relaxed and refreshed.

REALIZE YOUR HIGHER SELF

From time to time, life pitches everyone into an emergency situation. It may be a life-threatening accident, falling victim to a crime, or being caught in a fire or earthquake. Some people panic. Others report that, perhaps to their own surprise, instead of feeling terrified they experienced a deep sense of calmness and clearheadedness. They suddenly understood exactly what they needed to do to save themselves or others, and quickly and effectively took steps to deal with the emergency.

Yogis say that certain events can trigger the mind to become still. During an emergency, for example, the work-a-day mind might temporarily go into shock. Then the clear light of pure consciousness shines through your awareness and instinctively you know precisely what you have to do. When you connect with your Higher Self, or purusha, inner guidance instantly directs your actions in a spontaneous and completely natural way. Yogis aspire to live in the light of this higher knowledge as much as possible.

A DEEPER REALITY

Reading about a Higher Self might seem abstract and far-fetched. Yet the yoga masters insisted that learning to connect with higher aspects of your personality is not actually that hard. All you need to do is still the mind enough so that you can concentrate deeply, and then pay close attention to your own inner state. Try the following exercise and you'll see how easy the journey within actually is.

PROCEED WITH CAUTION

Classic yoga texts specify that concentration and meditation exercises should only be performed by students who are inwardly prepared. These techniques were not designed to be practiced by mentally or emotionally unstable individuals, and can actually aggravate mental problems in particularly fearful or delusional individuals.

1. Sit comfortably with your head, neck, and trunk straight. Close your eyes.
2. Breathe slowly and smoothly. Spend a minute or so allowing your body to relax.
3. Bring your full awareness to a point inside your brain about three inches behind your eyebrows.
4. Now lift your awareness upward an inch farther, as high within the center of your brain as you feel comfortable.

5. Don't pay attention to your thoughts and feelings. Instead, for just a moment, be aware of awareness. Simply be conscious of your own consciousness.

6. Lower your focus of attention back down to the point behind your eyebrows. Open your eyes and relax.

Beginners sometimes find it difficult to hold their attention in the higher brain centers, as some yoga concentration exercises require them to do. If you have this problem, you might find it easier if you look upward, though you should still keep your eyes closed. Your brain, after all, is used to following the direction of your gaze.

THE PLAY OF SPIRIT

The yoga tradition says that the world we experience around us, which seems so real and tangible to our senses, is in fact an infinite ocean of energy called prakriti. This limitless energy has three modes, which you've already learned: rajas, tamas, and sattva. These three qualities correspond to the kinetic energy, potential energy, and dynamic equilibrium of Western physics.

The energies of our five bodies can work together or against each other. Yoga reshapes our physical and mental energies so they can work together in an optimal way. Then rajas or dynamic energy can be given full play when it's appropriate, such as when we're playing soccer or rushing to an appointment. Tamas or static energy can be called up when that's appropriate, such as when we're sleeping. And sattva or harmonized energy can be brought to bear when we're relaxing with friends, meditating, or doing our Hatha Yoga exercises.

People sometimes fall prey to depression, sloth or greed (tamas), or to anxiety or active aggression (rajas). For yogis though, the material world is a playground for spirit, where they move with calmness, courage, and self-awareness, all gifts of sattva which lead them closer to their Higher Self.

YOGA AND RELIGION

Some communities have reacted to yoga with hostility, feeling it threatens their religious traditions. It is true that yoga developed within the cultural matrix of Hinduism. However, its techniques quickly spread to Buddhist, Jain, Sikh, and Chinese Taoist practitioners for one important reason: Its methods work. Everyone wants to be healthy. And most people see the value in getting more deeply in touch with themselves.

From the monk to the atheist, from the devotee to the scientist, any person can practice yoga and see the benefits. Yoga is one form of physical and spiritual culture that is truly nondenominational.

In the next few chapters you'll learn how you can begin working with your body and breath in a way that enhances your health and happiness, as well as your state of yoga—that is, your link with your Higher Self.

 FYI Although yoga is practiced by adherents of every religion today, it originally developed in the cultural matrix of Hinduism. To learn more about the wisdom of the Hindu tradition, and why many Hindu teachers are so generous in sharing their insights and techniques with others without requiring anyone to convert to their faith, check out my book, *The Complete Idiot's Guide to Hinduism.*

HOUR'S UP!

You might enjoy taking the following quiz to see if you remember the important points made in this chapter. You'll find the answers in Appendix E. Answer true or false to the following statements:

1. One goal of yoga is to "yoke" the different parts of the personality into one harmonious whole.

2. Hatha Yoga was developed by accomplished masters called siddhas, most of whom lived in India.

3. The first Indian yogi to teach yoga in the West was Apollonius of Tyana.

4. It's not possible to integrate yoga with a more aggressive, aerobic-style workout.

5. Traditional yogis believe you not only have a physical body, but four increasingly subtle levels of your personality as well.

6. Prana or life energy keeps the physical body functioning.

7. Yogis say energy can manifest in only two states, active (rajas) and passive (tamas).

8. In emergency situations, people sometimes experience the inner guidance arising from their Higher Self.

9. Yogis believe the world we see around us is really a vast ocean of energy.

10. The highest goal of yoga is to "yoke" you to the center of consciousness within yourself.

Hour 2
Stretch and Release

Chapter Summary

LESSON PLAN:

In this hour you will learn ...

- Although yoga is generally safe and fun, a few medical conditions need special attention before beginning your routine.

- How you dress, when you eat, and the way you breathe affect the quality of your yoga practice.

- Loosening your body's joints before starting the postures helps keep you supple and flexible.

- Stretches energize the spine while toning and relaxing muscle groups.

- Yoga is a noncompetitive form of exercise that emphasizes self-awareness.

In the East, most people think of yoga as meditation practice. In the West, however, the word *yoga* conjures up the picture of a man standing on his head or a woman with her legs twisted like a pretzel. These exercise positions are called Hatha Yoga in India. Their original purpose was to make the body as healthy and long-lived as possible so it could be a fitting vehicle for the soul. Yogis would train their bodies so that they could sit effortlessly in meditation for hours on end without moving a muscle.

Today in the West the health benefits of Hatha Yoga are universally acknowledged. It's common for movie stars and models—professionals who need to look toned and youthful—to practice yoga. But according to the yogis of India, Hatha Yoga's beauty-enhancing abilities are the least of its powers. More importantly, it flushes and reinvigorates the body's major organs, as well as energizing and balancing the nervous system.

You'll notice that many yoga postures involve stretching, bending, or twisting the spine. It's a common belief among traditional yogis that "You're only as old as your spine." If your backbone remains healthy and flexible, the motor and sensory nerves connecting your brain to the rest of your body are able to continue functioning optimally. In India you'll meet yogis in their 80s and 90s who seem as youthful and vigorous as many 20-year-olds in the West. One of the secrets to their excellent health is their supple spines!

PLAY IT SAFE

Before beginning a program of Hatha Yoga postures, there are six safety tips every new student should be aware of. Although Hatha Yoga is one of the safest forms of exercise commonly practiced today, you may inadvertently hurt yourself if you don't bear these points in mind.

CHECK WITH YOUR DOCTOR

If you have any serious health problems, you must check with your physician before beginning a Hatha Yoga routine. He or she can advise you whether there are particular yoga postures you should avoid. In rare instances, a yoga posture may actually aggravate a medical problem. Some of the conditions you need to consult your doctor about include the following:

- Back injury
- Hernia
- High or low blood pressure
- Recent surgery

Always use common sense when beginning a new exercise program. You will need to modify postures that rest part of your weight on your hands and wrists if you have carpal tunnel syndrome, for example. Do not attempt the Head Stand if you have reason to suspect the vertebrae in your neck are somewhat weak. Take it easy and listen to your body. If you have any questions about a particular posture, talk to a certified Hatha Yoga teacher or your physician before proceeding.

TIME SAVER

Want to find the yoga class nearest you? Log on to www.yogafinder.com for worldwide access to teachers, classes, and events related to yoga.

SPECIAL RULES FOR WOMEN

There are two special concerns women yoga students need to be particularly careful about:

- While they are having their menstrual periods, women should avoid postures that put a lot of pressure on the abdomen. On rare occasions, menstruating women have begun hemorrhaging after doing yoga exercises such as the Stomach Lift, which deeply compresses the abdominal cavity. The Stomach Lift is a great technique for preventing constipation, but can cause problems for women during that time of the month. Inverted (upside-down) postures should also be avoided while the menstrual flow is heavy.

- Any woman who is pregnant, or thinks she may be pregnant, should consult a doctor before beginning a yoga routine. Many of the postures are fine for women carrying a child; in fact, some doctors recommend Hatha Yoga as an excellent way to keep relaxed and in shape during pregnancy. However, your doctor will let you know which exercises are safe for each trimester, and which postures to avoid till several weeks after your baby is born.

DRESS FOR MOVEMENT

Tight-fitting clothes will not do for Hatha Yoga. Either they will restrict your movement or you'll rip them apart by the seams as you move into a stretch. Traditionally in the East yogis either wore very little (such as a loin cloth) during a hatha session, or put on very loose-fitting cotton costumes that look similar to pajamas.

Today, leotard-like outfits made of cotton blends are popular for yoga practice. Hatha teachers popularized these close-fitting but nonbinding outfits because they make it easy for your teacher to see exactly how your body is positioned, something the pajama-type clothes tend to cover up. However, a tank top and comfortable, nonbinding shorts or pants will do just as well. Remember, you are looking for clothes that allow a free range of motion and fabric that allows your skin to "breathe" and perspire freely.

PROCEED WITH CAUTION

Your feet should be bare during hatha practice. Doing postures in your stocking feet is particularly hazardous; your feet can slip out from under you as your balance shifts. Shoes obstruct the movement of your feet and ankles in some postures. Remaining barefoot will allow your toes to grip the floor and helps you keep your balance.

EAT LATER

Your stomach should be empty when you begin your hatha practice. This means no heavy meal for four hours before you do the postures, and no snack or light meal for two hours before your hatha session.

It's important to keep yourself hydrated throughout the day, but your stomach should not be full of fluids during hatha practice. You may take a few sips of water during your yoga session if you feel thirsty, but you should not drink a full glass of fluid for at least a half-hour before you begin doing yoga.

Veteran yoga practitioners often do their postures in the morning before breakfast, or in the evening right before supper. Since many of the hatha postures directly affect your abdominal area, doing postures shortly after eating can be very uncomfortable.

BREATHE THROUGH YOUR NOSE

GO TO ▶
Westerners often underestimate the value of coordinating the breath with yoga postures. Yet the yoga masters of India have always insisted breath awareness is one of the most important components of yoga. You'll learn why in Hour 4.

Each person carries a portable air conditioner with them throughout their life. In the yoga tradition, the role of the nose in purifying the air we breathe, as well as moderating its temperature, is never taken for granted. If you find yourself breathing through your mouth while performing a classical yoga routine, you need to slow down and mentally take stock. Bring your attention to your nasal septum (the bridge of cartilage between your nostrils) and consciously breathe through your nose. Your breath should be slow and smooth, deep and even, without jerkiness or long pauses.

Remember not to hold your breath during any postures, unless you are explicitly instructed to do so. Stopping your breath causes toxins to build up in your muscles, leading to a sense of strain and fatigue. For a more pleasant, more productive hatha session, keep breathing!

AVOID FORCE

"No pain, no gain" was the mantra of many avid aerobics exercisers during the late twentieth century. The yogis' attitude is the exact opposite: "No pain means no strain." If you feel pain during a hatha posture, your body is signaling that you've gone too far into the pose and need to back off immediately. Avoid forcing yourself into positions your body isn't ready for yet, and you'll avoid the injuries that could prevent you from advancing much more rapidly in your yoga practice.

While competition may be healthy in certain arenas, such as sports, a competitive spirit is inappropriate in yoga. It's not useful to compare your progress with that of other yoga students since each individual is unique. Your yoga practice will mature at a rate specifically appropriate for you. This laid-back approach helps stave off injuries, sprains, and strains that a more aggressive attitude invites.

LOOSEN UP

Start your Hatha Yoga workout with a series of rolls designed to keep your joints fluid. These simple exercises are safe for virtually everyone. Don't assume that because they're so simple, they may not be worth your time. On the contrary! Arthritis, a painful condition that stiffens the joints, is one of the most common complaints humans experience as they age. These simple exercises help keep the joints flexible, as well as loosening up your body to help prevent injuries as you move into more challenging postures.

These rolls take only moments to do, yet performed on a regular basis they can provide a lifetime of health benefits. In Hour 1, you kept your eyes closed during the concentration and visualization exercises. Keep your eyes open, however, for Hatha Yoga postures, stretches, and rolls. This will help you keep your balance.

HEAD ROLL

First, you'll work with your *cervical vertebrae*, the bones that support your head and neck. When these bones are not well aligned, you might experience headaches, dizziness, fatigue, or upper back pain.

STRICTLY DEFINED

The **cervical vertebrae** are the seven topmost vertebrae of the human spine. These develop a curve in the months after birth as a baby, lying on its belly, struggles to lift its head and see what's happening around it.

1. Stand with your head, neck, and trunk in a straight line.

2. As you exhale, allow your head to drop forward so that your chin falls toward your upper chest. Consciously relax your neck, allowing it to drop a little farther downward.

3. Inhaling, roll your neck clockwise till your right ear rests over your right shoulder. (Don't unconsciously raise your shoulder!) Keep rolling your neck till your head reaches the farthest point backward.

4. Exhaling, continue rolling your neck till your left ear rests over your left shoulder. Keep rolling your neck till your chin once again rests over your upper chest.

5. Roll your neck in a clockwise circle two more times.

6. Now repeat the exercise in the opposite direction, rolling your neck counterclockwise three times.

7. Lift your head, returning to the beginning position. Pay attention to the sensation in your neck.

Don't rush through this exercise; instead perform it with awareness. Especially in the beginning, you might feel points along the roll where your neck muscles seem to catch or snap. Relax through these points. You are releasing years' worth of kinks that have gradually built up in your body.

SHOULDER ROLL

Now shift your awareness from your head and neck to your shoulders and arms.

1. Stand up straight, with your arms dangling, relaxed, at your side. Lift your shoulders upward.

2. Exhaling, roll your shoulders forward and down in as broad a circle as they can comfortably form.

3. Inhaling, continue rolling your shoulders back and upward, completing the circle.

4. Move your shoulders in this circular motion two more times.

5. Now repeat the exercise in the opposite direction three times.

6. Relax your shoulders. Be aware of the subtle feeling of energization this shoulder roll has produced.

JUST A MINUTE

Try this variation of the shoulder roll: Raise your arms straight out to the side. Now roll your entire arm, making small circles at first, then larger circles till you feel your chest opening and closing as your arms swing around in wide arcs. Roll your arms forward first several times, then backward.

In many yoga exercises, even simple ones like this, you will be coordinating your breathing cycle with your motion. At first this might seem awkward, but as you become more sensitive to your body's energy state, you'll soon sense how naturally the breath and body motion work together. The movement of your lungs and intake and outflow of oxygen are actively supporting the movement of your bones and muscles, the different parts of your body working together as one unified whole.

WRIST ROLL

Next, you will work with the delicate muscles and bones in your wrists, hands, and fingers.

1. Stand up straight. Lift your arms directly out in front of you in a straight line.

2. Palms open, lift your hands so that your fingers point straight up.

3. Using your wrists as a pivot point, rotate your hands in a clockwise direction three times. Then rotate them counterclockwise three times. Keep breathing naturally.

4. Now tense your fingers, curling them so they look like curved claws.

5. Rotate your hands clockwise three times, then counterclockwise three times.

6. Bring your arms back down to your side, relaxing your hands and wrists. Be conscious of the sensation there.

HIP ROLL

This exercise pivots around the hips, from which the upper body and legs gently move in a "stirring" motion.

1. Stand up straight with your feet about one foot apart.

2. Place the palms of your hands along the sides of your lower back (the *lumbar spine*), fingers pointing downward. You will keep them there during this exercise. This helps to brace your back, which you will want to keep straight throughout the hip roll.

STRICTLY DEFINED

The **lumbar spine** consists of the five vertebrae of the lower back, just above the sacrum. Like the cervical spine, these vertebrae have a convex curvature, meaning they bulge toward the front of the body. This curve develops as children learn to crawl and stand.

3. Exhaling, gently fall forward from your hips. Extend downward only as far as is comfortable.

4. Swivel your hips clockwise three times, shifting your torso as if it is a spoon stirring your body. Watch your balance. Exhale as your torso moves around backward. Inhale as your torso moves around forward.

5. Repeat three times in a counterclockwise circle.

6. Return to a standing position and release your hands and arms to your side. Pay attention to your internal energy state.

Let your breath be your guide. If you are moving consciously and smoothly, your movement will effortlessly align with your inhalation and exhalation. You won't breathe, or move, too fast or too slow because the natural rhythm of your relaxed breath is setting the pace.

KNEE ROLL

The next two exercises demand a keen sense of balance. If you tend to lose your balance easily, start by placing one hand lightly on the back of a chair to keep you from falling over.

1. Stand up straight. Inhaling, raise your right knee so that your upper right thigh extends out perpendicular from your body. Your lower leg should hang from your knee, not be held upward.

2. Holding the right knee still, move your right foot in a wide clockwise circle three times. Then move it through a counterclockwise circle three times. Keep breathing naturally.

3. Return your right foot to the floor and repeat the exercise three times, using your left knee this time.

4. Return to a two-footed standing position. Be aware of the sense of energization in your knees.

ANKLE ROLL

GO TO ▶
Physical and mental balance are both strongly emphasized in yoga practice. In Hour 3, you'll learn yoga postures specifically designed to help you develop the concentration you need to maintain your sense of balance, even in positions where you normally might start to totter.

Shift your attention to your ankles. During this exercise, be cautious of your balance, or rest one hand on the back of a chair so you don't stumble.

1. Stand up straight. Inhaling, raise your right knee so that your upper right thigh extends out perpendicular from your body.

2. Move your toes in a broad clockwise circle three times, turning from your ankle. Then circle your toes three times counterclockwise.

3. Return your right foot to the floor and repeat the exercise three times, using your left leg and foot this time.

4. Return to a two-footed standing position. Be aware of the sense of energy in your ankles, feet, and toes.

If you have serious problems keeping your balance, you can perform the
ankle roll while sitting in a chair. Sit up straight but sit forward on the chair,
closer to the edge, and lift your leg directly out in front of you. Roll the foot
around the ankle in one direction, then the other.

Mastering the Stretching Poses

Now you're ready for the second portion of your warm-up, the basic yoga
stretches. These involve tensing and relaxing large muscle groups in your
body, gently preparing them for the more challenging postures to come.
They also help to align and adjust your spine, the central axis of your body.

Standing Stretch

This centering exercise gently enlivens the entire body. Don't let your mind
wander but keep it focused, in a relaxed but attentive manner, on the sensations in your body.

1. Stand up straight with your arms hanging down at your side. Your feet
   should be six to eight inches apart.
2. Inhaling, lift both your arms directly out to the side. Keep your elbows
   locked and your fingers extended, palms facing downward.
3. When your arms are pointed straight out, perpendicular to your body,
   flip your hands so that your palms now face upward. As you continue
   inhaling, raise your straight arms so they point directly upward from
   your shoulders.
4. Breathe naturally. Reach up even farther with your hands and arms.
   Hold the position for about 10 seconds.
5. Exhaling, lower your arms, palms facing upward, till they extend
   directly out to your side. Flip your palms downward, and lower your
   arms all the way down to your side.
6. Stand still for a moment, being attentive to your breath and the sensation of aliveness in your body.

Reclining Stretch

Don't be misled by the simplicity of these stretches. If you perform them
carefully, you will notice that your mind feels clearer and more alert. This is
because of the subtle effect on the brain when you release the knots of tension along your spine.

JUST A MINUTE

Some yoga postures are performed in a supine position. You should lie on your back on a thick carpet, a yoga mat, or a blanket rather than on a hard floor, so that your back is straight but comfortable.

1. Lie down on your back on the floor. Your feet should rest no more than six inches apart. Your arms should lie straight up above your head.

2. Reach upward along the floor as far as you can with your right hand, extending up through your fingers. Feel the stretch from your armpits through your arms to your fingertips.

3. At the same time, extend downward along the floor through your right leg. Push your right heel away from your body so that your entire leg is stretched as far as it will go.

4. Remember to keep breathing as you stretch! Keep the left side of your body relaxed.

5. After about five seconds, relax your right arm and leg.

6. Repeat this exercise with your left arm and leg.

7. Alternate two more times, stretching first the right, then the left arms and legs.

8. Now stretch both arms upward and both legs downward simultaneously. Feel the stretch through your entire body. Hold for about five seconds, then relax. Repeat this two more times.

9. Bring your arms down along your side and rest for a moment. Pay attention to the way your body feels.

CAT STRETCH

The Cat Stretch is a superb exercise for maintaining the health and flexibility of the spine. It also helps tone those troublesome muscles of the abdomen and lower pelvis.

You'll notice that many yoga postures, like the Cat Stretch, were named after animals and imitate their movements. Yogis taught their students poses like the Dog, Dolphin, Butterfly, Camel, Cobra, Locust, Fish, Peacock, and even the Crocodile.

FYI *Joints and Glands Exercises* by Rudolph Ballentine, M.D., is one of the finest introductions to very simple stretching and limbering exercises, with a special focus on keeping your joints in excellent working order. These exercises are so easy they're appropriate even for very stiff and elderly students, yet they're impressively effective.

1. Come onto your hands and knees on the floor. Your arms should be straight with your hands positioned beneath your shoulders. Your knees should be slightly apart, positioned beneath your hips.

2. Exhaling, arch your back upward like a cat, as far as it will go comfortably. Tuck your chin in toward your chest and tighten your buttocks.

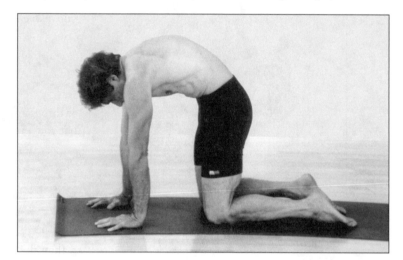

The Cat Stretch, position 1.

(Photo credit: Johnathan Brown)

3. Inhaling, lift your head as far backward as you can comfortably. Simultaneously lift your pelvis. Your stomach and chest move toward the floor.

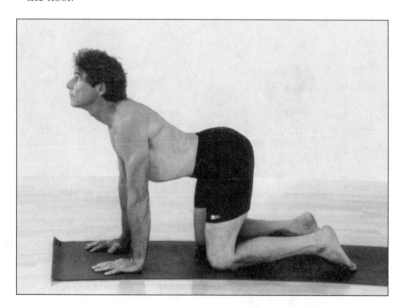

The Cat Stretch, position 2.

(Photo credit: Johnathan Brown)

4. Repeat these two movements, first arching your back upward, then downward, as you exhale and inhale five more times.

5. Now as you exhale and arch upward, bring your left knee up toward your tucked chin.

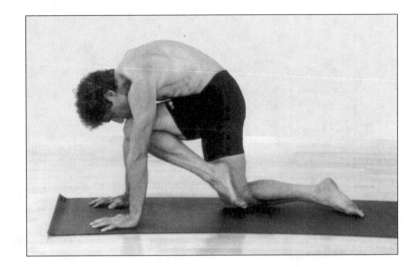

6. As you exhale, stretch your left leg out behind you and lift it upward, away from the floor.

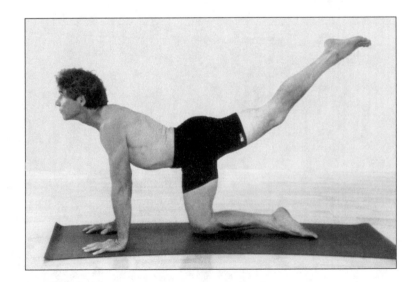

7. Repeat these two movements, first arching your back upward and bringing your left knee toward your chin, then arching downward, lifting your leg up behind you, as you exhale and inhale five more times.

8. Repeat steps 5 to 7, using your right leg this time.

9. Return to your starting position and relax. Be aware of the sensations in your body.

GO TO ▶

In Hours 2 through 12, you'll learn the basic components of a Hatha Yoga routine. In Hour 13, however, you'll learn how to put them together into a program that's appropriate for your fitness and flexibility level.

LUNGE STRETCH

The Lunge is another excellent stretch that helps tone the thigh muscles, as well as aligning the pelvis.

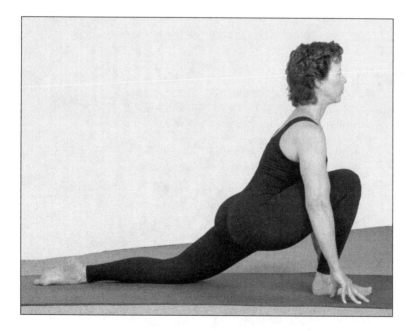

The Lunge Stretch.

(Photo credit: Alex Fernandez & Evolution Visual Services)

1. Come onto your hands and knees on the floor. Your arms should be straight, with your hands positioned beneath your shoulders. Your knees should be slightly apart, positioned beneath your hips. This is the same starting position as the Cat Stretch.

2. Bring your right foot forward so that it rests between your hands.

3. Extend your left leg out behind you, resting your left knee on the floor.

4. Lower your pelvis slightly toward the floor so that your thighs are pushing in opposite directions. Take it easy—move yourself into the pose only as far as feels comfortable.

5. Keep breathing! Hold the pose for about five seconds.

6. Return to the starting position and relax. Be aware of your breath, your heartbeat, and the sensation in your legs.

7. Repeat the posture, bringing the left foot forward this time and extending your right leg out behind you.

8. Return to the starting position and relax.

You have now learned some of the most basic elements of Hatha Yoga. If you find a few minutes each day to do just these few rolls and stretches, you will soon begin to notice a difference in the way your body feels. In the next two hours, you'll learn a few more basics, such as relaxation postures, balance poses, breathing exercises, and body awareness. Once you have these under your belt, you'll have all the elements you need to begin practicing the formal Hatha Yoga postures you'll start learning in Hour 5.

Hour's Up!

Here's a quiz to see if you remember the main points from Hour 2. Answer true or false to the following statements:

1. If you've had surgery recently, you should check with your doctor before beginning a Hatha Yoga program.

2. If you're a woman, it's fine to do all the usual Hatha Yoga postures during your menstrual period.

3. It's best to do yoga poses in your stocking feet, so that your feet stay warm during the routine.

4. You shouldn't have a heavy meal for at least four hours before doing yoga.

5. Breathing through your nose, not your mouth, is recommended during most yoga postures.

6. The best way to check whether you're advancing in yoga is to compare your progress with other students.

7. The cervical vertebrae are the seven bones in the top part of the spine.

8. Stretching postures not only tone the muscles, they may also help align the spinal column.

9. The original purpose of Hatha Yoga was to make the physical body a fitting vehicle for the soul.

10. Claims that yoga helps the body stay youthful are just a myth.

QUIZ

Hour 3

Relax and Focus

LESSON PLAN:

In this hour you will learn ...

- A relaxed, comfortable, and alert state is the foundation of yoga practice.
- Consciously touring your body deepens your self-awareness and state of relaxation.
- Balancing the body contributes to mental and emotional balance.
- Mental discipline is an integral part of physical exercise.

Today, anyone can sign up for a Hatha Yoga class, but in ancient times, students were carefully screened before being allowed to learn the powerful secret practices of yoga. Gurus (a Sanskrit word meaning "mentor" or "instructor"; it often specifically refers to a spiritual teacher) would check whether a potential student was relaxed and receptive or nervous and hostile, self-aware or largely unconscious, mentally balanced or emotionally out of kilter. Gurus were looking for disciples who showed a natural aptitude for self-development. It made their job a lot easier.

These days, yoga instructors can help you master the prerequisites that make success in yoga possible. These include the ability to relax deeply without falling asleep, an intimate acquaintance with the muscle groups and organs of one's own body, and the power to remain balanced and at ease in any physical posture.

In this hour, you'll learn the three foundation stones of yoga: attentive relaxation, a living sense of connectedness with each part of your body, and physical and mental equipoise.

Mastering Relaxation Poses

It's impossible to underestimate the importance of relaxation in yoga. Ironically, Westerners often find relaxation postures the most difficult of all to do properly. People who grow up in the West are trained to constantly be doing something, even if it's something as passive as watching television. The thought of doing nothing sounds boring to some, and perhaps even immoral to others who may have been raised with a strong work ethic.

There are two major reasons why relaxation postures are so important during a Hatha Yoga routine:

- Many yoga postures deliberately compress your muscles and internal organs. When you relax, these tissues resume their natural shape and normal blood flow resumes. If you rush through your yoga routine, ignoring the relaxation phase, then the proper delivery of oxygen throughout your body, as well as the removal of toxins that build up while you hold a posture, are prevented. You will quickly begin to feel strained and fatigued, while the cleansing and revitalizing effects of the yoga postures are partially blocked.

- Deeply relaxing, even if just for a moment, has an effect on the brain similar to pushing the reset button on your computer. "Programs" you no longer need to run are shut off and your mental "desktop" is cleared. You experience this as the quieting of random thoughts, and the releasing of mental energy constellated on the last posture you performed. Your awareness shifts into the present moment, and your energy state is "cleared" so that it can move into the next pose freshly and cleanly.

Relaxation is not something you do, but something you allow to happen. Just as you cannot make yourself go to sleep, but must surrender to the process of falling asleep, so the harder you try to make yourself relax, the more tense you'll become. In the reclining relaxation poses you do not fight with your body or force it do anything. Instead you release your body as if you were dropping a piece of clothing on the floor.

 FYI *Relax and Renew: Restful Yoga for Stressful Times* by Judith Lasater can help you understand the importance of relaxation, as well as demonstrating a variety of techniques to help you release stress.

From this point forward, you'll be learning the Sanskrit names for each formal yoga posture you practice. Don't worry about memorizing these; the Sanskrit names will not be included in the quizzes at the end of each chapter. However, it's useful to be generally familiar with these terms because you'll run across them in any yoga classes you may attend and in yoga books and magazines. You'll notice that the names of most yoga poses end with the Sanskrit word *asana*, which means "posture" or "pose" and is pronounced *AH-sun-uh*.

MOUNTAIN POSTURE

Tadasana is the root posture from which almost all standing yoga poses begin. *Tada* is Sanskrit for "mountain"; an asana means a yoga posture. In this pose you are standing as firm as a mountain, rooted in the earth, and unmoving.

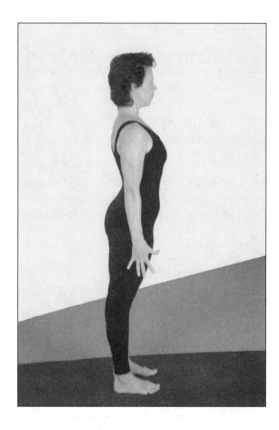

The Mountain Pose.

(Photo credit: Alex Fernandez & Evolution Visual Services)

1. Stand up straight with your feet flat on the floor, about six inches apart. Your feet should be parallel to each other, with your toes pointed forward, not inward or out to the side.

2. Pull your shoulders up and back. Then let them relax so that your arms hang naturally at your side.

3. Your back should be straight upright, but not tense as if you were standing at military alert.

4. Your weight should be balanced over the arches of your feet, not shifted forward toward your toes or back onto your heels.

5. Your eyes should remain open, but your mental focus should be inward.

To make sure you're standing straight, imagine there's a hook attached to the top of your skull. A cable is gently pulling the hook upward. Feel your body straightening and your mental attention shifting upward.

When you are holding this pose correctly, you will not feel the tendency to rock either forward or backward. Instead, you are centered squarely over your feet. There is a deep sense of being grounded and still.

Physicists describe two states of energy: potential and kinetic. Kinetic energy is in motion, producing an effect. Potential energy is motionless. It appears inert but in reality it contains enormous power simply waiting to be activated, like a battering ram that looks like a useless log but can knock down a wall if you swing it properly. In the Mountain Posture, the body's energies remain in a potential state. The mind remains quiet but alert, like the body.

In the Mountain Posture, no random thoughts move across in your mind. You're not mentally picturing the next posture you plan to do. Instead your awareness remains centered in your body, solid, silent, and strong. From the starting point of this stable pose, the kinetic energy of your body and mind will be harmoniously released in the more active postures.

CHILD'S POSTURE

Balasana is the counterpose to many backward bending postures you will perform while lying on your stomach on the floor, such as the Cobra and the Boat. It is especially helpful in releasing tension that may have built up in your back. *Bala* means "child." This posture imitates the fetal position into which young children sometimes fold themselves.

1. Sit back on your heels. Your feet should be together.
2. As you exhale, lean forward till your forehead touches the floor. Close your eyes. Your lower pelvis remains resting on your heels.
3. Lay your arms down along the side of your legs, palms facing upward.
4. Breathe naturally, allowing your body to relax deeply.
5. If you're uncomfortable, rock gently from side to side to help relieve tension.

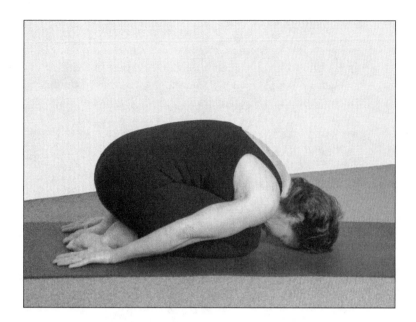

The Child's Posture.

(Photo credit: Alex Fernandez & Evolution Visual Services)

This simple-looking posture has deep effects, stretching and relaxing the spine, especially the lumbar area. It also eases tension in your hamstrings and the adducting muscles in the thighs. (The adductors are the thigh muscles that pull your legs together.)

Because this is such a powerful relaxation pose, it's worth taking the time to adjust to it comfortably. If you're not flexible, a couple small pillows can help during the first few weeks, while your body is learning to accommodate the pose. If your head doesn't want to reach the floor, place a pillow under your forehead. If you back hurts, trying slipping a pillow between your thighs and torso. If your knees ache, a pillow between your thighs and legs will minimize the discomfort.

PROCEED WITH CAUTION

 Even simple-looking yoga postures can be uncomfortable for people whose bodies are very stiff. Practice the stretches and rolls outlined in Hour 2 to loosen your muscles. Use pillows to support body parts that need a little lift so you can fully relax into a posture.

KNEES-TO-CHEST POSTURE

Apanasana is the counterpose to many backward bending postures you will perform while lying on your back on the floor, such as the Plow and the Arch. *Apana* refers to the downward moving energies in the body, which are said to be activated when the legs are pressed into the chest.

The Knees-to-Chest Posture.

(Photo credit: Alex Fernandez & Evolution Visual Services)

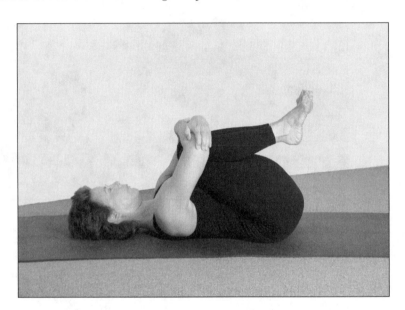

1. Lie on your back on the floor.
2. Raise your knees to your chest. Your head and your hips remain on the floor. Your legs are bent at the knee.
3. Wrapping your arms around your legs, draw them closer to your chest. Keep breathing!
4. If you're uncomfortable, rock gently from side to side.

This is an excellent posture for relieving strain in the lower back.

CROCODILE POSTURE

Yoga instructors often ask students to lie in *Makarasana* because this posture virtually forces people to breathe diaphragmatically, as the yoga masters do, rather than using their chest muscles to breathe. *Makara* means "crocodile." In this pose you lie on your stomach without moving (except to breathe), like a crocodile underwater.

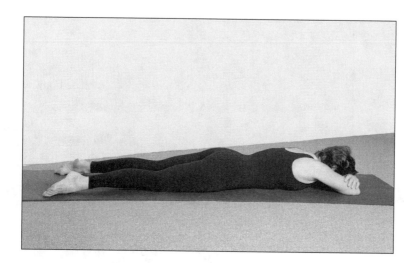

The Crocodile Posture.

(Photo credit: Alex Fernandez & Evolution Visual Services)

1. Lie on your stomach on the floor. Your legs should be stretched out straight with your feet about eight to twelve inches apart. Turn your toes away from each other.

2. Fold your arms in front of you. Gently grasp your right upper arm with your left hand and your left upper arm with your right hand.

3. Rest your forehead on your crossed lower arms. The bottom of your face is tipped slightly upward so your nose is not pressed into your arms or the floor. Close your eyes.

4. Breathe naturally. Allow yourself to relax deeply.

When you are holding this pose correctly, your chest is raised slightly up off the floor.

FYI *The Muscle Book* by osteopath Paul Blakey will help you understand the major muscle groups in your body, and how they're affected by exercise, stretches, and massage.

GO TO ▶
When you are at rest or exerting yourself minimally, you should use your diaphragm, not your chest muscles, to drive your breathing cycle. In Hour 4, you'll learn why diaphragmatic breathing is so important, and how to check if you're doing it properly.

CORPSE POSTURE

Shavasana is the king of relaxation postures, although it has a rather unsavory name. *Shava* is Sanskrit for "corpse." When yoga adepts perform this posture they relax so completely and breathe so subtly that, except for the healthy color of their skin, they look as if they could be dead. They have attained a level of physical and mental stillness that most ordinary people don't experience even in deep sleep.

The Corpse Posture.

(Photo credit: Alex Fernandez & Evolution Visual Services)

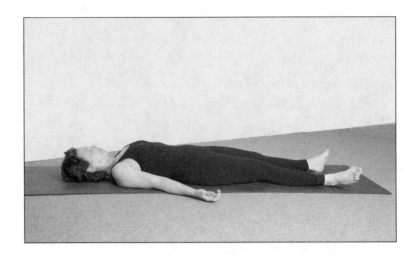

1. Lie on your back on the floor. Place your feet a comfortable distance apart.

2. Rest your arms alongside your body. Your hands should lie six to ten inches from your body, with your palms turned upward.

3. Close your eyes. Pay attention to the sensation of the breath passing in and out of your nostrils. Relax deeply for two to five minutes.

Most yoga sessions end with the Corpse Posture. It's not unusual to hear at least one student in a typical class begin to snore while lying in this pose. However, the point is to relax, not to fall asleep! To help students relax more deeply yet stay awake, instructors will often lead them through a systematic tension and relaxation exercise while they lie in the Corpse Posture. Try this one.

1. Rest on your back in the Corpse Posture, with your eyes closed.

2. Bring your full awareness to your forehead. Wrinkle your forehead tightly, then allow the muscles in your forehead to relax like butter melting in the sun.

3. Widen your mouth in a grimace, tensing your cheek muscles. Then allow the muscles in your face to relax.

4. Tense, then relax, your shoulders.

5. Tense, then relax, your arms.

6. Tense, then relax, your hands.

7. Lift, then relax, your upper torso.

8. Lift, then relax, your lower torso.

9. Tense, then relax, your thighs.

10. Tense, then relax, your legs.

11. Tense, then relax, your feet.

12. Tense, then relax, your legs.

13. Tense, then relax, your thighs.

14. Lift, then relax, your lower torso.

15. Lift, then relax, your upper torso.

16. Tense, then relax, your shoulders.

17. Tense, then relax, your arms.

18. Tense, then relax, your hands.

19. Tense, then relax, your shoulders.

20. Tense, then relax, your arms.

21. Tense, then relax, your face.

22. Tense, then relax, your forehead.

23. Bring your full awareness to your breath. Watch your body breathe for a minute or so.

24. Gently move your fingers and toes. Place your cupped hands over your eyes. Open your eyes, put your hands down, and sit up. Notice how calm and refreshed you feel.

JUST A MINUTE

You should be comfortable in the Corpse Posture, but not so cozy that you fall asleep. Throw a light blanket over yourself if you are cold, and place a small pillow under your head if your neck feels strained. But do the pose on the floor rather than in bed to prevent yourself from nodding off.

TRAVEL THE BODY

From ancient times to the present, pious Hindus have traveled around the Indian subcontinent, visiting some of the innumerable pilgrimage sites throughout the country. This was a difficult and sometimes dangerous undertaking. The yogis, however, claimed that there was no site more sacred than one's own Higher Self, and no country more worthy of touring than one's own body.

For India's traditional yogis, physical exercises were more than health-promoting techniques. They were also the means to enhance self-awareness. Postures that particularly flexed and strengthened the spinal column, as well as many of the breathing exercises, were specifically designed to optimize the functioning of the nervous system. Mental clarity, emotional tranquility, and the unimpeded expression of enlightened will have always been valued highly in the yoga tradition.

The yogis developed the 61 Points exercise, a concentration technique in which you "make a pilgrimage" to 61 sacred sites in your body, in order to increase your body awareness and your ability to remain intensely focused while deeply relaxed in the Corpse Posture. This double ability to remain physically tranquil yet intently mentally concentrated is believed to open the doors to higher states of consciousness. Yogis believe this state helps you tap into the full depths of your creative power, intellectual genius, intuitive insight, and spiritual illumination.

GO TO ▶
In Hour 14, you'll learn more about the mental and spiritual benefits of more advanced yoga techniques such as meditation.

VISIT THE 31 POINTS

The Corpse Posture, which you've just learned, is the basis for one of yoga's most famous concentration techniques, the 61 Points exercise. In this exercise you shift your mind through 61 distinct points in your body, mentally speaking the appropriate number between 1 and 61 as you pause at each point.

This technique is by no means as easy as it sounds. Most students find themselves continually distracted by random thoughts and reverie, or abruptly drift off to sleep. Yoga instructors usually have students begin with the first 31 points. Only after you can remember all 31 points in order and move through each one without losing count or getting distracted should you attempt the more challenging 61 Points exercise.

Lie in the Corpse Posture. Bring your full awareness to each of the following points in turn, speaking the corresponding number in your mind as you feel that spot in your body.

*The 31 and 61
Points.*

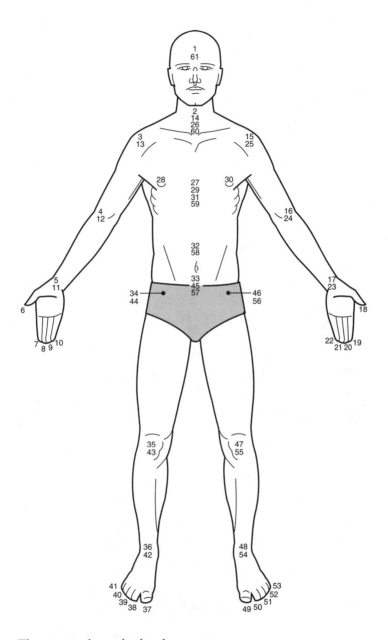

1. The center of your forehead.
2. The center of your throat.
3. Your right shoulder.

4. Your right elbow.

5. Your right wrist.

6. Your right thumb.

7. Your right index finger.

8. Your right middle finger.

9. Your right ring finger.

10. Your right little finger.

11. Your right wrist.

12. Your right elbow.

13. Your right shoulder.

14. The center of your throat.

15. Your left shoulder.

16. Your left elbow.

17. Your left wrist.

18. Your left thumb.

19. Your left index finger.

20. Your left middle finger.

21. Your left ring finger.

22. Your left little finger.

23. Your left wrist.

24. Your left elbow.

25. Your left shoulder.

26. The center of your throat.

27. The point between your breasts.

28. Your right nipple.

29. The point between your breasts.

30. Your left nipple.

31. The point between your breasts.

You'll notice that you visit a number of spots, such as the point between your breasts, repeatedly. Your consciousness is following the natural contours of your body just as if you were retracing your steps through the countryside, returning to certain central locations. You'll find yourself visiting higher priority spots in the upper and central parts of your body more often.

TIME SAVER

If you have trouble remembering all the points in the 61 Points exercise, an inexpensive cassette is available that will lead you through the technique. Call the Himalayan Institute Press at 1-800-822-4547 and ask for the tape called *31 and 61 Points: A Technique for Health and Relaxation.*

VISIT THE 61 POINTS

When you are able to move through all 31 points with full attention, you're ready to move on to the rest of the exercise.

Lie in the Corpse Posture. Bring your full awareness to each of the spots detailed in the 31 Points exercise, mentally saying the corresponding number at each place. Now continue moving your awareness through your body to the following points.

32. Your navel.

33. The point between your two hipbones.

34. Your right hip.

35. Your right knee.

36. Your right ankle.

37. Your right big toe.

38. Your right second toe.

39. Your right middle toe.

40. Your right fourth toe.

41. Your right little toe.

42. Your right ankle.

43. Your right knee.

44. Your right hip.

45. The point between your two hipbones.

46. Your left hip.

47. Your left knee.

48. Your left ankle.

49. Your left big toe.

50. Your left second toe.

51. Your left middle toe.

52. Your left fourth toe.

53. Your left little toe.

54. Your left ankle.

55. Your left knee.

56. Your left hip.

57. The point between your two hipbones.

58. Your navel.

59. The point between your breasts.

60. The center of your throat.

61. The center of your forehead.

You can learn a great deal about yourself from the 31 Points and 61 Points exercises. Though there were some points in your body you could sense effortlessly, there may have been other spots that were harder for you to mentally locate. Which parts of your body do you feel less connected with? The Hatha Yoga postures you learn in Hours 5 through 12 will help you develop greater awareness of parts of your body you may have "tuned out" for years.

You probably also learned how easily distracted you are. How many points could you feel before your mind began to wander? In the yoga tradition, the ability to concentrate is directly correlated to the ability to achieve one's goals in life. Learning to focus, staying on track till you reach the sixty-first point, is an excellent exercise in mental self-discipline.

Mastering Your Balance

Another important preliminary to a Hatha Yoga program is developing a sense of balance. In some yoga postures you will be standing on one leg, or shifting your weight while you are bending or twisting, so being able to keep your balance is important.

There can be no physical balance without mental balance. You'll be amazed at how quickly you start teetering out of a hatha posture the moment your mind begins to wander. An unwavering mind is a prerequisite for an unwavering body.

You are about to learn two balancing exercises—one fairly easy, the other a little harder. Keep your eyes open; most people will begin to fall over if their eyes are closed for any length of time in these poses. Find a reference point in the room around you, and keep your eyes trained on that one point while you hold the posture.

JUST A MINUTE

Your sense of equilibrium is controlled by the vestibular system in your inner ear. However, the vestibular nerve receptors are closely tied in with vision and body positioning. If you experiment with shutting your eyes during the Tip Toe Stretch or Tree Posture, you'll discover it's much harder to maintain your balance!

TIP TOE STRETCH

The Tip Toe Stretch is the easiest balancing posture. However, even in this pose beginners often notice that when their mind starts to wander, they instantly lose their sense of stability and come out of the pose. In yoga, mind and body are perfectly integrated. Balancing postures give you immediate feedback when your mind-body coordination is broken. You suddenly find it difficult to remain in the pose.

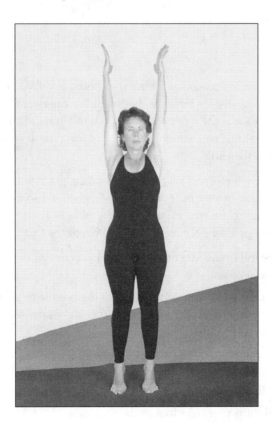

The Tip Toe Stretch.

(Photo credit: Alex Fernandez & Evolution Visual Services)

1. Stand in the Mountain Posture. Fix your eyes on a stationary object directly in front of you.

2. Inhaling, raise your arms straight out to your sides, then straight up above your head.

3. As your raise your arms, simultaneously lift yourself up on your tip toes.

4. Balance on your toes for 15 to 30 seconds. Be fully attentive to your breath and energy state while holding the pose.

5. As you exhale, simultaneously lower your arms and lower your feet back onto the floor.

6. Repeat the Tip Toe Stretch two more times.

7. Now repeat the exercise three more times. This time raise your arms directly in front of you, then over your head, rather than lifting them out to the side.

TREE POSTURE

Vrikshasana is a more demanding yoga posture. *Vriksha* is Sanskrit for "tree." In this pose, one leg serves as the "trunk" of the tree, while your other leg and arms act as the tree's limbs. Just as a tree stands firmly without trembling or falling over, you should stand in this pose as sturdily as if you were rooted to the earth.

If you have a problem keeping your balance, practice the Tree Posture while standing next to a table or the back of a chair. As soon as you feel yourself beginning to lose your balance, use the table or chair to steady yourself. Hold the pose for no more than five seconds the first few times you try it.

1. Stand in the Mountain Posture. Fix your eyes on a stationary object in front of you.

2. Standing on your left foot, place the bottom of your right foot against the inner side of your left calf. Your right knee should point directly out to your right side.

3. Place your palms together in front of your chest, fingers pointed upward.

4. Hold this posture for 5 to 15 seconds, if you can comfortably.

5. Return your right foot to the floor and relax for a moment. Be aware of the sensations in your body.

6. Repeat the Tree Posture, this time standing on your right foot and placing the bottom of your left foot against the inner side of your right calf.

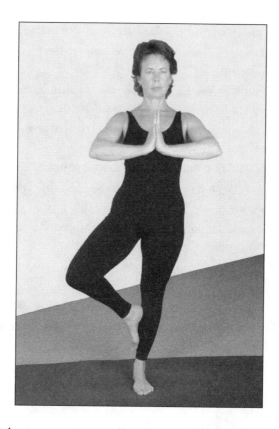

The Tree Posture.

(Photo credit: Alex Fernandez & Evolution Visual Services)

As your flexibility improves, you will gradually be able to place the sole of your foot against your knee, then against the top of the inner thigh of your other leg. As your balance improves, you will be able to stretch your arms above your head, still pressing your palms against each other.

Physical, emotional, and mental balance are important goals of yoga. Yogis believe that when the Lower Self (the body, breath, and mind) is in harmony, the light of the Higher Self (the divine spirit) can shine through unimpeded, and life becomes illumined.

QUIZ

Hour's Up!

Here's a quiz that reviews the main points from Hour 3. Answer true or false to the following statements:

1. In yoga you learn to relax deeply without falling asleep.
2. Relaxing between yoga postures helps replenish oxygen to your internal organs.
3. Hatha Yoga emphasizes awareness of the Inner Self, and discourages you from focusing on your physical body.
4. The Mountain Posture teaches you to vent your emotions, like a volcano spewing lava.
5. The Child's Posture mimics the fetal position.
6. You should hold your breath in the Crocodile Posture, like a crocodile underwater.
7. You should hold your breath in the Corpse Posture, as if you were actually dead.
8. The 61 Points exercise involves mentally traveling throughout your body.
9. It's easier to keep your balance when your eyes are open.
10. Physical, emotional, and mental balance are major goals of yoga practice.

HOUR 4

Ride Your Breath

CHAPTER SUMMARY

LESSON PLAN:
In this hour you will learn ...

- Prana or vital energy is the connecting link between body and mind.
- Biological processes that people can't normally control can be partially regulated through breath control.
- Diaphragmatic breathing is the foundation of physical and mental health.
- Alternate nostril breathing helps balance the nervous system.
- Vigorous breathing techniques oxygenate the brain and invigorate the mind.

According to the yoga masters, breath is the basis of life. Our experience in this plane of reality began at the moment of our first inhalation and ends with our last exhalation. The yogis point out that you can lose any of your senses, your sight or hearing for example, or even lose your mind, and still go on living. But when the breath departs from the body, all other physical functions cease.

While some Westerners believe each person is allotted a certain number of years to live, yogis believe every soul is assigned a certain number of breaths. So if you breathe slowly, you'll live longer! That sounds silly, until you pause to consider that animals that breathe the fastest, like hummingbirds, have very short lives. However, animals that breathe comparatively slowly, such as some turtles and whales, have exceptionally long lives. The breath drives the metabolism. Creatures that breathe rapidly simply "burn out" much more quickly because they're literally aging faster.

THE LINK BETWEEN BODY AND MIND

For thousands of years, yogis have recognized breath as the flywheel of life, an important connecting link between different functions of the body. Some bodily activities are under your conscious control, such as walking or talking. Others are unconscious; you're not consciously aware of making your heart beat or of your liver extracting toxins from your bloodstream because these essential functions are governed by your "involuntary" nervous system. Your breath is one activity that is both involuntary (it goes on whether you're aware of it or not) and voluntary (you can control it to a certain degree when you want to).

Because of this double function, your breath gives your conscious mind a key it can use to open the controls of the involuntary nervous system. In the early 1970s, Swami Rama demonstrated under strict laboratory conditions that while lying unmoving he could manipulate the beating of his heart, the operation of his brain waves, his body temperature, and other functions that Western scientists had previously believed were beyond our ability to consciously control.

Even more important from the perspective of yoga, your breath is the connecting link between your body and mind. You'll notice that if you're upset, you breathe in an agitated way. If you're sitting calmly but force yourself to breathe quickly and erratically, after only a moment your body and emotions will start to feel unsettled. Long ago, the yoga masters noted that no matter how dangerous or disturbing the circumstances they found themselves in, if they made themselves continue breathing calmly, their minds would stay centered. This technique for maintaining inner tranquility has also been used by martial arts masters and saints. This open secret lies at the very heart of yoga practice.

 FYI Why bother with breath? How does breathing affect your energy level? How do yogis use breathing exercises to induce higher states of consciousness? *Science of Breath: A Practical Guide* by Swami Rama, Rudolph Ballentine, M.D., and Alan Hymes, M.D., answers these and other important questions about the yoga of breath.

MASTERING THE BASICS OF BREATH

The way we breathe has an enormous impact on how we feel physically and emotionally. Apnea, a condition where a person periodically stops breathing, has been associated with heart damage and other serious medical problems. Chronic rapid breathing, on the other hand, is associated with hyperthyroidism (a condition where the thyroid gland is overstimulating the body), anxiety or panic disorder, and other maladies.

Because the link between breath and mind was so obvious, yogis devoted centuries to studying the effects of breathing, and developed a sophisticated science of breath called *Svarodaya*. It was a preeminently practical science designed not only to cultivate health and vitality, but ultimately to propel the mind into deeper states of self-understanding.

Here are the basic breathing exercises every yoga student should know. Don't underestimate the power of these practices because they appear simple. Each produces dramatic effects on the nervous system when performed for several minutes with full awareness.

DIAPHRAGMATIC BREATHING

The diaphragm is the large, flat, horizontal muscle lying toward the bottom of your rib cage that separates your chest from your upper abdomen. When you exhale the diaphragm pushes upward into a dome shape, forcing much of the air out of your lungs. As your diaphragm relaxes back downward, fresh air rushes into your lungs.

Pranayama means "breath control" or "control of the vital force" and refers to the many breathing exercises developed by yogis to energize the body and focus the mind. Of the dozens of these techniques, diaphragmatic breathing (shown in the following illustration) is the most important. You'll be asked to breathe diaphragmatically during most yoga postures and during meditation.

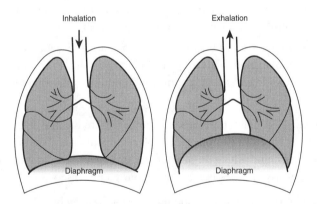

Diaphragmatic breathing.

The first two exercises that follow will help you understand how it feels to breathe diaphragmatically. The third will help you get in the habit of breathing this way on a regular basis.

1. Lie on your stomach in the Crocodile Posture, which you learned in Hour 2. Breathe through your nostrils. Your mouth should be closed.

2. Feel your abdomen pressing into the floor as you inhale, and moving back up from the floor as you exhale.

3. Be attentive to the sensations in your lungs and abdomen. This posture is forcing you to breathe diaphragmatically.

Most people breathe shallowly, preventing the body from being properly oxygenated. When you breathe diaphragmatically, your lungs get the amount of fresh air nature intended. Carbon dioxide, a natural waste product of your respiration, is properly expelled from your lungs. The diaphragmatic movement is massaging not only your lungs but your abdominal organs, ensuring that they're getting enough richly oxygenated blood and eliminating toxins.

When you breathe shallowly, you are relying more on the muscles between your ribs to breathe, and less on your diaphragm. This type of chest breathing is associated with stress. If you watch friends or co-workers when they're obviously stressed, you'll almost always see they're breathing fairly rapidly from their upper chest, rather than smoothly and evenly from their upper abdomen.

Now try the following exercise to ensure you can still feel the diaphragmatic movement in other positions.

1. Lie on your back in the Corpse Posture you learned in Hour 3. Breathe through your nostrils.

2. Rest your left hand on your chest near your heart and your right hand on your abdomen just below your rib cage.

3. If you are still breathing diaphragmatically, your left hand will not move at all. Instead, your right hand will slowly and gently move up and down as your diaphragm compresses and then releases your abdominal organs.

GO TO ▶
In Hour 14, you'll learn the basic sitting postures yogis use for doing breathing exercises and meditation. In yogic breathing, a comfortable, upright posture and mental attentiveness are important prerequisites.

Notice how comfortable and natural it feels to breathe diaphragmatically. This style of breathing automatically places you at ease. This is in part because you're using the least amount of energy to get the most amount of fresh oxygen, nearly effortlessly rebuilding your energy reserves.

Beginning yoga students should do the following breathing exercise for three to five minutes several times daily. This will help you get into the habit of breathing diaphragmatically throughout the day.

1. Sit upright in a comfortable position with your head, neck, and trunk straight.

2. Bring your awareness to your breath. Feel it flowing naturally in and out through your nostrils for a half-minute or so. Your breathing will slow down and deepen as you begin to relax.

3. Feel your upper abdomen moving slightly forward and backward as you breathe. Your chest should be motionless.

4. Your breath should be smooth and even, without jerks or pauses. Inhalation and exhalation are approximately equal in length. Don't stop breathing between the inflow and outflow of your breath. Your breath should keep flowing in a soft, smooth, continuous cycle.

5. Breathe diaphragmatically for three to five minutes. Notice how calm and centered you feel. Repeat this exercise three times each day for the first month of your yoga practice, until diaphragmatic breathing becomes the normal way you breathe, if it isn't already.

JUST A MINUTE

Yoga teachers sometimes use sandbags or "breath pillows" to help beginning students learn diaphragmatic breathing. Placed below the ribs while you're lying on your back in the Corpse Posture, a five-pound sandbag can help you develop greater breath awareness. It also strengthens the diaphragm. Sandbags are available from most shops that sell yoga gear (see Appendix C for more information).

When you are breathing diaphragmatically, you'll sense the movement of your upper abdomen. Note that there should be no dramatic movement in your lower abdomen. If this occurs, you are practicing "belly breathing," not diaphragmatic breathing.

Diaphragmatic breathing is baseline breathing for the yogi. It's the way nature intended you to breathe under most circumstances. However, it's not appropriate for certain types of activities, such as aerobic exercise, when you'll need more oxygen than diaphragmatic breathing can provide, or during deep states of meditation, when you'll need less oxygen to maintain your inner focus.

COMPLETE BREATH

The Complete Breath is an exercise yogis use when they need more oxygen because they're about to perform some activity that's very energy intensive, like climbing a Himalayan foothill to their cave! For beginners, this is also an excellent way to get in touch with the different compartments of your respiratory system.

1. Sit upright in a comfortable position with your head, neck, and trunk straight. Remember to breathe through your nose, not your mouth.

2. Exhale as much air out of your lungs as you can comfortably.

3. Inhale deeply, feeling the fresh air filling the bottom lobes of your lungs.

4. Continue inhaling until the middle portion of your lungs is filled with air. You should feel your rib cage expanding to accommodate this much air.

5. Continue inhaling as if you are "topping off" your lungs. As the top lobe of your lungs fills with air, your clavicles (shoulder bones) will lift a little.

6. Begin exhaling, emptying the top lobes of your lungs. Your shoulders will settle back downward. There should be no momentary pause in your breathing cycle between the inhalation and exhalation (or between the exhalation and inhalation).

7. Empty the middle portion of your lungs. Your rib cage will contract.

8. Empty the bottom of your lungs. Your upper abdomen will move backward slightly toward your spine.

9. Continue these slow, deep breaths for one or two minutes.

By the time you have completed a series of Complete Breaths, you will feel remarkably energized. If you should start to feel lightheaded, you have exceeded your comfortable capacity. Next time take fewer breaths. Increase your capacity to take in air gradually over the next few weeks.

PROCEED WITH CAUTION

Sometimes young children deliberately hyperventilate in order to experience the sense of giddiness it produces. Mental clarity and energization are the goal of vigorous breathing exercises, not lightheadedness. If you start feeling dizzy during the breathing exercises described here, stop immediately and allow your body to breathe normally.

Alternate Nostril Breathing

One of the most highly praised yogic practices is called *Nadi Shodhana*, which is Sanskrit for "Channel Purification." It sounds almost outrageously simplistic, yet students who've worked conscientiously with this technique often report its impact on their level of awareness is truly astonishing. It's a real "consciousness-raiser."

Nadi can refer to any type of channel from a river to a nerve fiber. In Nadi Shodhana it refers to conduits of energies in the subtle body. Western science has not yet recognized the existence of these structures, but Hindu, Buddhist, and Chinese medical traditions all make extensive use of them. There are said to be 72,000 nadis in the subtle body. Because these are the conduits along which the energy of consciousness travels from the mind into the body, keeping them viable and unobstructed is a major goal in yoga practice. When the nadis flow smoothly, awareness remains clear and the body is enlivened.

There are two phases to Channel Purification. As soon as you begin practicing them, you'll see why the technique is commonly called Alternate Nostril Breathing.

1. Sit with your head, neck, and trunk straight.

2. Mentally settle into your breathing process. Watch your breath; allow yourself to breathe diaphragmatically. Remember to breathe only through your nose during this exercise; never breathe through your mouth.

3. Use the thumb of your right hand to gently block your right nostril. Exhale slowly and smoothly, in a relaxed manner, through your left nostril.

4. Use the fingers of your right hand to block off your left nostril. Inhale slowly and smoothly through your right nostril.

5. Repeat steps 3 and 4 two more times.

6. You are about to begin your fourth exhalation. Leave your right fingers on your left nostril and exhale through your right nostril.

7. Block your right nostril with your right thumb and inhale through your left nostril.

8. Repeat steps 6 and 7 two more times.

9. Put your right hand down. Exhale and inhale through both nostrils three times.

Now move on to the second phase. You will repeat the same procedure, but will start with the other side.

1. Use the fingers of your right hand to gently block your left nostril. Exhale slowly and smoothly, without jerks or pauses, through your right nostril.

2. Use the thumb of your right hand to block off your right nostril. Inhale slowly and smoothly through your left nostril.

3. Repeat steps 1 and 2 two more times.

4. You are about to begin your fourth exhalation. Leave your right thumb on your right nostril and exhale through your left nostril.

5. Block your left nostril with your right fingers and inhale through your right nostril.

6. Repeat steps 4 and 5 two more times.

7. Put your right hand down. Exhale and inhale through both nostrils three times.

GO TO ▶

Having trouble breathing through your nose? In Hour 20, you'll learn the Nasal Wash. This easy but amazingly effective technique has been used by yogis for centuries to clear the nasal passages, as well as to stave off colds, asthma, allergies, and other problems associated with the upper respiratory tract.

The following table clarifies the steps of this important technique. One session of Nadi Shodhana involves three full repetitions of steps 1 through 18. Your breath should be slow, smooth, and even, with no jerks or pauses.

Breath No.	Exhale	Inhale
1.	Left	Right
2.	Left	Right
3.	Left	Right
4.	Right	Left
5.	Right	Left
6.	Right	Left
7.	Both	Both
8.	Both	Both
9.	Both	Both
10.	Right	Left
11.	Right	Left
12.	Right	Left
13.	Left	Right
14.	Left	Right
15.	Left	Right
16.	Both	Both
17.	Both	Both
18.	Both	Both

If your nose whistles or wheezes as you breathe, there is a minor obstruction in your nasal passageway. Blow your nose and try to breathe more quietly. Practicing the Nasal Wash (see Hour 20) will also help alleviate this problem.

Long-time yoga students often use a particular *mudra* or hand position when practicing Alternate Nostril Breathing. These hand positions are said to produce specific energetic effects in the subtle body. The index finger and middle finger of the right hand are folded down. The student uses the right thumb to gently close the right nostril, and the right ring finger to gentle press closed the left nostril.

FYI *The Breathing Book* by Donna Farhi is a fine introduction to the rationale and techniques of yogic breathing. It explains what prana (vital energy) is in Western terms, and clarifies the effects of breathing exercises on the body and brain.

In the past few decades, Western science has identified personality characteristics generally associated with the two sides of the brain. One side is related to rationality and logic while the other relates more to intuition and artistic expression. Curiously, these two behavioral patterns were identified by yoga masters centuries ago and associated with the two nadis or nerve currents flowing out of the brain and down the spine. The right nadi, called *pingala*, is associated with logical, purposeful thinking and assertive action, while the left nadi, called *ida*, is connected with imagination, reverie, and more passive behaviors. One of the goals of Alternate Nostril Breathing is to balance these two currents so that life force flows not through one or the other but through the central canal between them, called the *sushumna*. When the sushumna is activated, a deep state of calmness and balance is experienced. In Western terms, the two hemispheres of the brain are now integrated and function in tandem.

STRICTLY DEFINED

The **pingala** is the primary right energy channel of the subtle body, associated with logical thinking and assertiveness. The **ida** is the primary left energy channel of the subtle body, associated with reverie and passiveness. The **sushumna** is the primary central energy channel of the subtle body, associated with heightened states of consciousness.

You'll learn more about how yoga students work with the state of sushumna awareness in Hour 15. But you can already have actual experience of what the yogis are talking about by practicing Alternate Nostril Breathing. Ordinarily you breathe primarily through one nostril for about two hours, then in the span of several minutes the active nostril spontaneously closes up and the formerly passive nostril opens (most people don't even notice this happening). You then breathe primarily through the other nostril for about another two hours.

When you practice Alternate Nostril Breathing with full attention, you'll notice that by the end of the session both your nostrils are flowing equally freely. This stimulates nerves located at the top of your nasal passage that lead directly into the brain and harmonize its two hemispheres. You'll experience this as a relaxed, alert, expansive state of consciousness. It's a natural high which, when deepened through meditative practice, leads to greatly expanded states of awareness.

Advanced yogis monitor their breathing cycle throughout the day. Merely by mentally focusing on one nostril they can shift the flow of their breath into that nasal passageway from the other. By focusing on the septum between their nostrils, they can make both nostrils open within a few seconds. When both nostrils are flowing equally freely it's the optimal time to sit for meditation as the brain has now been switched into a balanced state through the mechanism of the breath. If you practice Alternate Nostril Breathing attentively for several weeks, you'll quickly develop this ability also, and you'll be able to see for yourself how the way you breathe influences your state of mind.

ENERGIZE YOUR AWARENESS

Yoga includes several breathing techniques that are simple but quite vigorous. These forcefully clean your respiratory passages and stimulate your heart, lungs, and abdominal organs. The whole body is energized and mental alertness is intensified. You will feel invigorated when you do these exercises properly. However, you should *not* hyperventilate to the point that you feel dizzy, faint, or spacey. The point is to oxygenate your body and brain, not to knock yourself out.

GLOWING FACE BREATHING

Kapalabhati literally means "shining skull." This exercise brings color to your cheeks and fresh oxygen to your cells, and activates your digestive organs through the sharp movement of your abdominal muscles.

1. Sit comfortably with your head, neck, and trunk straight. Breathe only through your nose during this exercise. Do not use your mouth to breathe.

2. Bring your full awareness to the muscles in your abdomen. Use those muscles together with your diaphragm to quickly and forcefully exhale.

3. Release your mental grip on your abdominal muscles. Allow fresh air to spontaneously refill your lungs. Do not actively inhale but simply allow air to rush back into your body through your nostrils.

4. Exhale forcefully and inhale passively seven times.

As you work with this exercise over the course of several weeks, work up to repeating the Glowing Face Breath 21 times.

PROCEED WITH CAUTION

 The psychiatric institute in Bangalore has a special wing for "kundalini cases." Here Indian doctors treat overzealous yoga students who have damaged their nervous systems by doing advanced breathing exercises without proper supervision. Sophisticated breathing techniques explained in some yoga manuals should never be practiced without the guidance of a competent teacher.

BELLOWS BREATHING

Bhastrika means "bellows." The Bellows Breath is an intensified form of the Glowing Face exercise in which you rapidly force air both in and out of your lungs as if they were a blacksmith's bellows. The effect is tremendously energizing.

1. Sit comfortably with your head, neck, and trunk straight. Breathe through your nose, not your mouth.

2. Use the muscles in your abdomen as well as your diaphragm to quickly and forcefully exhale.

3. Now quickly and forcefully inhale, without pausing between breaths.

4. Exhale and inhale forcefully seven times.

Gradually work up to repeating the Bellows Breath 21 times. Stop immediately if you feel yourself becoming lightheaded.

HUMMING BREATH

Ujjayi means "victory through expansion." Unlike the last two techniques, which are quite forceful and produce dramatic physiological effects, Ujjayi is a slower, more relaxed technique that produces a more subtle but pleasant sensation. Like the other techniques, it ventilates the lungs and helps clear out phlegm, but this exercise also soothes the nerves while gently vitalizing the body.

Ujjayi can be a little tricky for beginners to learn because it involves controlling the glottis, the cleft in your vocal cords through which air passes when you speak, in a way most people have never learned to do consciously. However, once you get the knack of it, you'll never forget how to do it, like riding a bike or typing.

1. Sit comfortably with your head, neck, and trunk straight. Use your nose, not your mouth, to breathe during this exercise.

2. As you slowly and smoothly exhale, make a continuous humming sound. The sound should come from the front of your upper throat, not so much from your mouth.

3. Now, as you slowly and smoothly inhale, keep humming. The pitch of your hum will spontaneously rise.

4. Continue humming as you exhale and inhale for a half-minute to a minute.

The trick to performing the Humming Breath is to keep humming as you breathe in. Most people are used to making sounds only as they exhale, so it may take a few tries before you learn to keep humming even as you inhale. You will find yourself making a sound that vaguely resembles the buzzing of a bee. To check that you're doing the Humming Breath properly, place your fingers lightly over your throat just above your Adam's apple. You should feel this area vibrating intensely as you hum.

A FEW WORDS OF CAUTION

The breathing exercises you've just learned are simple but powerful. Provided you don't overdo the more vigorous techniques so much that you hyperventilate, you will discover that each exercise has substantial physical and mental benefits.

However, you should be cautious about performing yogic breathing exercises more advanced than those described in this book, particularly ones that involve holding your breath. Breath retention is for advanced students only, and even then only when practiced under the close supervision of an experienced teacher. You should not be holding your breath during any of the breathing exercises taught in this book. Breath retention is an important technique used by advanced yogis, but without proper preparation and a teacher's guidance, regularly stopping your breath can lead to serious problems like apnea or even brain damage.

It's true that yogic adepts can virtually stop their breath for extended periods of time, not unlike hibernating mammals. (Advanced yogis can place their bodies in a state much like suspended animation while they focus exclusively on their inner world.) However, they have done years of preparatory exercises before attempting these potentially dangerous techniques.

FYI *Breath, Mind, and Consciousness* by Harish Johari offers an advanced yogi's perspective on yogic breathing exercises. It's a fascinating introduction to an ancient science that Western researchers are only beginning to discover.

RECOGNIZING LIFE FORCE

As you learned in Hour 1, life force, or vital energy, is called prana in Sanskrit. It manifests in three forms. First there is the cosmic prana or universal life-giving energy. According to the yoga tradition, the source of life energy for our world system is our Sun, a veritable fountain of prana. Its heat, light, and the other forms of energy it emanates make life possible on our planet.

The second form of prana is the energy we assimilate from the air. Humans take in life force primarily through respiration. Food and water are also essential for survival, although we can live for a few days without water, and much longer without food. Without air, however, we'd be dead in a matter of minutes. Oxygen is the most basic form of prana, but vital energy is more than just oxygen. It's the intelligence inherent in living energy that transforms a mixture of biochemicals into an eating, growing, reproducing cell.

Third, yogis break prana down into five separate vectors active in the physical body:

- *Udana* operates in the head and controls the senses based there: sight, hearing, taste, smell.

- *Prana* operates in the throat and upper chest, controlling speech and respiration.

- *Samana* operates in the area between the heart and navel, and governs digestion.

- *Apana* operates in the abdomen below the navel and regulates the expulsion of waste materials.

- *Vyana* pervades the body, and governs movement.

Note that one of the five forms of prana is also called prana. This is because it relates specifically to the breath, just as the planetary prana relates to the atmospheric energy, and cosmic prana represents the universal life force.

Yoga works with all five forms of prana. In this hour, you learned several ways to work with the second form of life force. In future hours, you'll learn Hatha Yoga exercises such as the Stomach Lift that work directly with apana and concentration exercises that control udana.

In classical yoga texts, breath or the life force is often compared to a horse. The soul "rides" this horse throughout its travels through the physical world. A yogi aspires to be like a skilled rider who controls her mount masterfully. Then the tremendous power of the cosmic life energy helps "carry" the soul to optimal health and well-being.

Hour's Up!

Test your knowledge of yoga breathing techniques with the following quiz. Answer true or false to the following statements:

1. Animals that breathe more rapidly live longer.
2. Respiration goes on automatically, whether you're aware of it or not, but you can also consciously control your breathing.
3. In yoga, the breath is considered the connecting link between the body and mind.
4. Nature intended you to breathe shallowly, from the upper part of your lungs, throughout the day.
5. People breathe primarily through one nostril for about two hours and then shift to breathing primarily through the other nostril in a continuous cycle.
6. The diaphragm is a form of life force that governs digestion.
7. Vigorous yogic breathing exercises help oxygenate the body.
8. Holding your breath for several minutes at a time is an excellent beginning-level yoga exercise.
9. The Humming Breath requires you to hum continuously, even while you're inhaling.
10. Prana or life force transforms chemicals into living matter, according to the yogis.

PART II
Basic Hatha Yoga Postures

Hour 5 Beginning Hatha Yoga

Hour 6 More Basic Postures

Hour 7 Beginning Bends

Hour 8 Basic Twisting Poses

Hour 9 Strengthen Your Abdomen

HOUR 5

Beginning Hatha Yoga

CHAPTER SUMMARY

LESSON PLAN:

In this hour you will learn ...

- The Cobra, Locust, Boat, and Bow Postures strengthen and tone the back muscles.
- The Arch and Bridge Postures flex and align the spinal column.
- The Child's Posture is the appropriate counterposture for prone backward bending poses.
- The Fish Posture opens the chest, helping ventilate the upper lobes of the lungs.
- Diaphragmatic breathing should be maintained through all backward-bending exercises.

You have already learned a few stretching exercises to help warm up your musculoskeletal system for your Hatha Yoga session. You've also mastered some limb rolls to help keep your joints in good working order. In addition, you've learned some important relaxation postures, two of which you'll practice again during this hour. And you've studied the fundamental breathing practices all yoga students should know, including Diaphragmatic Breathing, which you'll be using continuously as you learn the seven new postures detailed here.

Now it's time to move on to some of the most popular Hatha Yoga postures of all time. You'll learn the basic poses, as well as some variations, and you'll also discover a few of the health benefits associated with these classic exercises.

MASTERING THE BASIC POSTURES

You will begin this series of yoga postures with the four basic backward bending poses performed while prone (lying on your stomach), then progress to the three backward-bending poses you'll do while supine (lying on your back).

It's a good idea to use a yoga mat or do the postures in a room with carpeting. Performing the poses on a hard wood or linoleum floor is rather uncomfortable for all but the hardiest yoga students.

In Hour 4, you learned to breathe diaphragmatically. In every posture taught in this book, remember to breathe with your diaphragm. This will help keep you relaxed and focused throughout your yoga routine. If you find yourself breathing shallowly, or needing to breathe through your mouth, you are probably pushing yourself too hard, and straining, not strengthening, your muscles.

COBRA POSTURE

The Cobra Posture is one of the best known and most distinctive yoga postures. It's called *Bhujangasana* in Sanskrit, after the snake whose characteristic striking posture it imitates. This is a superb exercise with a host of benefits, including increasing the flexibility and proper alignment of your upper back. It's great for the circulation in the disks in your spine, and even enhances the elasticity of your lungs, helping you breathe better.

One of the most important benefits of the Cobra is that it strengthens the muscles in your back, shoulders, and neck, helping to improve your posture generally. This pose, when done regularly and correctly, is great for preventing and relieving many types of backache. This is good news for employers because severe backaches are one of the most common reasons workers call in sick.

The Cobra Posture.

(Photo credit: Alex Fernandez & Evolution Visual Services)

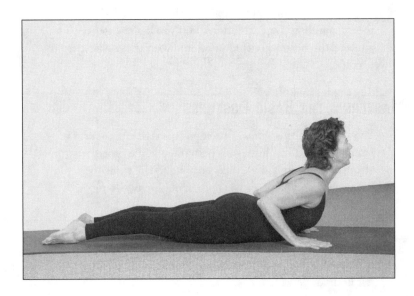

1. Lie on your stomach on the floor. Your legs should lie next to each other, straight but relaxed. Your forehead should rest on the floor. Breathe diaphragmatically.

2. Place your palms on the floor at your side. Your fingers should line up with your breasts.

3. As you inhale, slowly lift your face forehead first, then your nose, then your chin.

4. Continue lifting till your shoulders and upper chest come up off the floor. Do not use your hands or arms to push yourself up from the floor! Instead use the muscles in your neck and back to raise yourself.

5. When you have lifted your head and upper chest as far off the floor as you can comfortably without using your hands, hold the position for about five seconds. Keep breathing!

6. As you exhale, slowly lower yourself back down to the floor, upper chest first, then shoulders, then chin, nose, and forehead.

7. Turn your face to the side and rest your cheek on the floor. Allow your body to relax for a moment. Pay close attention to how your body feels, especially your spinal column. Then repeat the Cobra Posture two more times.

8. When you have completed three repetitions of the Cobra Posture, fold back into the Child's Posture.

JUST A MINUTE

You learned the Child's Posture in Hour 3. This important yoga exercise is the counter-posture to the backward-bending poses you perform while lying on your stomach. It will release any tension that may have accumulated in your back and shoulders.

Slowly work up to holding the Cobra for 10 to 30 seconds during each repetition. Remember to breathe diaphragmatically throughout the practice. This will help you hold the posture more comfortably.

Try turning your eyes upward to look at the ceiling as you hold the pose. This has a psychological effect that helps some people extend their necks further back into the pose.

The most common mistake beginning students make when they learn the Cobra Posture is they push themselves up off the floor using their arms. This seems natural to do, but it sabotages the fundamental purpose of the pose. Your goal is to strengthen the muscles in your back, not in your arms! Bear in mind that cobras don't have arms to lift themselves up with. Don't confuse the Cobra with the push-up exercises you perform in calisthenics classes, where the focus is on building muscle mass in your upper limbs.

In more advanced yoga classes, you might be asked to momentarily push up farther with your arms after you have assumed the classical pose. This is to help develop increased flexibility in your spine. Beginners should not strain their backs, however, but work slowly and carefully to increase how far you can raise yourself in the Cobra using your neck and back muscles alone.

PROCEED WITH CAUTION

 Performing reclining yoga postures directly on a hard floor can strain the vertebrae in the spine. It's always best to have at least a little padding when doing your postures. Carpeting should be cleaned before yoga practice. Remember, you'll be placing your face on the carpet during poses like the Cobra.

LOCUST POSTURE

The next yoga posture you'll learn is called *Shalabhasana*, after the grasshopper or locust. These small creatures move their tail ends up and down in a distinctive manner the yogis duplicate in this posture.

This pose gives the muscles of your lower back a great workout, and in fact is often recommended by physical therapists for patients with lower-back problems. It also helps tone the muscles at the back of your thighs.

The Locust Posture.

(Photo credit: Alex Fernandez & Evolution Visual Services)

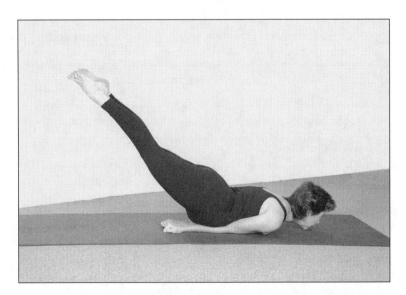

1. Lie on your stomach on the floor. Your legs should lie right next to each other, straight out along the floor. Your chin should rest on the floor. Breathe diaphragmatically.

2. Your arms should lie extended along your sides. Now make fists with both your hands and slip your fists underneath your body so that your pelvic bones rest on them.

3. As you inhale, slowly lift both of your legs upward, without bending your knees. Raise your legs as far as you can comfortably, and then hold the position for about five seconds. Don't hold your breath! Focus your awareness on the sensations in your body.

4. As you exhale, slowly lower your legs and place your arms back out along your sides.

5. Turn your face to one side and relax for a moment. Then repeat the Locust Pose two more times.

6. When you're done, fold back into the Child's Posture and relax.

Gradually work up to holding the posture for 10 to 20 seconds with each repetition.

FYI For a superb and comprehensive introduction to yoga, pick up a copy of *The Yoga Tradition: Its History, Literature, Philosophy and Practice* by Georg Feuerstein, Ph.D. Dr. Feuerstein is director of the Yoga Research Center in California and is one of the foremost authorities on yoga in the English-speaking world.

Beginners with very weak lower back musculature may find this posture difficult. Also, some sensitive individuals find that resting part of their weight on their fists is too uncomfortable. If either problem is the case for you, try the following easier variation of the Locust Posture.

1. Lie on your stomach on the floor. Turn your head back slightly so the only part of your head touching the floor is your chin.

2. Your arms should lie extended along your sides. Turn them so that your palms face your body and make fists with your hands, but do *not* place your hands underneath your body.

3. As you inhale, slowly lift your right leg upward, bending your right knee only slightly, if necessary. Focus on your thigh muscles to ensure that you are holding your right knee aloft using the muscles in your right thigh and the rear of your pelvis only. You should not be leaning toward the left, using the left side of your body to prop you up. Hold the position for about five seconds. Keep breathing.

4. As you exhale, slowly lower your right leg and relax for a moment. Then repeat this Half-Locust Pose two more times.

5. Now repeat the same exercise three times, lifting your left leg this time. Focus intently on each movement, sensing your energy state as you hold the posture and making sure you don't push yourself too hard.

6. When you're done, fold back into the Child's Posture and relax.

BOAT POSTURE

The next exercise is called *Naukasana*, which literally means "boat pose." This posture combines the effort you made in both the Cobra and the Locust. Yet surprisingly, many students actually find this posture easier than holding the Locust Posture alone because in this exercise the upper and lower parts of the body feel more balanced.

The Boat is another posture with powerful conditioning effects. It's excellent for strengthening the back. But also, because of the pressure it places on the abdominal organs, it dramatically helps improve circulation in the midsection of your body. This might be why, although the pose is mildly strenuous, you feel invigorated afterward.

The Boat Posture.

(Photo credit:
Alex Fernandez &
Evolution Visual
Services)

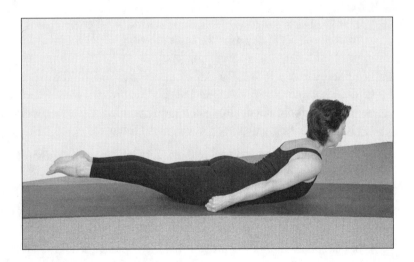

1. Lie on your stomach on the floor, facing down into the floor. Your legs should be straight, with your feet about eight inches apart.

2. Your arms should lie extended along your sides. Turn them so that your palms face your body. Fold your hands into fists.

3. As you inhale, raise your head, neck and upper trunk up off the floor without using your arms to lift or support yourself.

4. At the same time that you lift your upper body, also lift your legs straight upward. Your legs may spontaneously move farther apart from each other as you assume this pose.

5. Keep breathing. Hold the pose for five seconds. Notice that your breath feels like it's supporting your body.

6. Exhaling, lower your upper and lower body back to the floor.

7. Relax for a moment, then repeat the exercise two more times.

8. Fold back into the Child's Posture, to release any tension that may have built up in your back, thigh, and neck muscles.

As you begin feeling more comfortable in the pose, try holding it for 10 to 20 seconds. Don't overextend yourself if holding it this long feels strenuous in the beginning! If you practice the Boat regularly, you'll be amazed at how soon you'll be able to hold it much longer without any discomfort.

Here are two of the many variations of the Boat Posture. The first is for students who find the Boat Posture easy and would like to make it a little more challenging.

1. Lie on your stomach on the floor. Extend your arms directly above your head, along the floor.

2. Lift yourself into the Boat Posture as described above, but this time lift your arms, too. Your arms stay in line with your raised head.

The second variation is just for fun. This pose is called *Vimanasana* in Sanskrit. Ancient Hindu texts claim that thousands of years ago, Indian scientists had developed flying vehicles called *vimana,* which great kings and sages used to quickly shuttle back and forth across the Indian subcontinent. In this pose you hold your body as if you were flying like a bird.

1. Lie on your stomach on the floor. Extend your arms directly outward, perpendicular from your body, along the floor. Move your legs about two feet apart.

2. Lift yourself into the Boat Posture as you inhale. Simultaneously raise your arms out to the sides.

It's important to keep breathing in the Boat Posture. Beginners usually want to hold their breath, but this quickly increases the sense of strain in the pose, as carbon dioxide builds up in the body. You'll find that if you continue breathing diaphragmatically, you can hold the pose longer with less effort.

 Yoga International magazine offers an excellent series of inexpensive pamphlets introducing various practical facets of yoga such as "Yoga Therapy for Knees and Shoulders" and "Yoga and Pregnancy." To learn more, log on to www. himalayaninstitute.org.

Bow Posture

Dhanurasana means "Bow Pose" in Sanskrit. In this posture, you shape your body as if it is a tautly strung bow. This pose enhances the suppleness of the entire back as well as your shoulders.

The Bow Posture.

(Photo credit: Alex Fernandez & Evolution Visual Services)

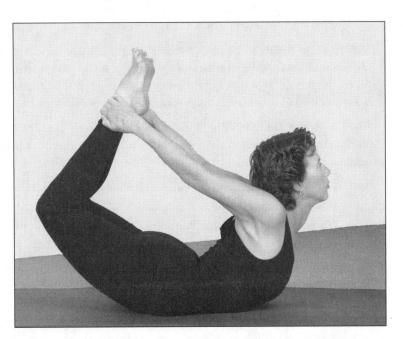

1. Lie on your stomach, resting your chin on the floor. Your arms should lie along your sides.
2. Bending your knees, lift your lower legs upward behind you. Inhale during this motion.

3. At the same time, lift your head and chest up off the floor. Reach backward with your hands and grasp your ankles.

4. Keep breathing. Hold the pose for about 10 seconds, or as long as you can comfortably. Repeat the posture two more times.

5. Fold back into the Child's Posture to relieve any tension in your spine.

For most people this is the most challenging of the backward-bending exercises you've learned so far. If this posture is difficult for you, try reaching back and grasping only one ankle, while balancing yourself by extending your other forearm along the floor in front of you and the other leg along the floor behind you. Then relax and repeat, grasping the other ankle with the other hand. You will gradually develop more flexibility and be able to hold both ankles at once.

FYI Are you interested in learning more about the specific anatomical effects of each yoga posture? Want to know exactly which muscles, bones, and organs are being worked? *Anatomy of Hatha Yoga: A Manual for Students, Teachers and Practitioners* by H. David Coulter, Ph.D., is an excellent technical reference book that will satisfy your desire for detailed information about yoga and biology.

HALF FISH POSTURE

Now it's time to roll over onto your back for the classic supine backward bending yoga exercises.

Ardha Matsyasana means "Half Fish Posture" in Sanskrit. Fish breathe oxygen like humans do, but they are able to extract it from water. In the fish pose your chest expands, allowing you to take in more air and breathe more fully. Your upper and middle back is also extended and flexed, promoting the health and suppleness of your spine.

1. Sit on the floor with your legs together, extended in front of you. Breathe diaphragmatically.

2. Lower yourself backward onto your elbows, placing your elbows and lower arms on the floor alongside your body.

3. Arch your back, and bend your neck backward till the top of your head touches the floor. Support your upwardly extended chest with your elbows and head.

4. Resist the temptation to open your mouth while holding this posture. Keep breathing through your nose. Remain in the pose for 10 to 20 seconds, depending on your capacity. Mentally focus on the sensations in your body and on your energy state.

GO TO ▶
The version of the Fish Posture described here is technically called the Half Fish. The fully formed posture is somewhat more difficult. In the full Fish, you would begin by sitting in the Lotus Posture, described in Hour 14. As you lean back onto your elbows and hold the pose, your legs remain folded together on the floor.

5. Carefully lower yourself onto your back and relax for a moment. Repeat the Fish Posture twice more.

6. When you're done, relax deeply in the Knees-to-Chest Posture, which you learned in Hour 3. This will help relieve any remaining tension in your lower back.

The Half Fish Posture.

(Photo credit: Alex Fernandez & Evolution Visual Services)

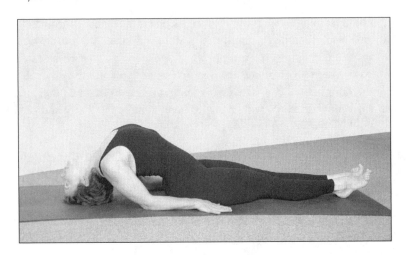

ARCH POSTURE

Dvipada Pitham is called the Arch Posture in English, or sometimes the Desk Pose or Half Wheel. The deep back muscles are stretched and energized, as are the muscles that link the pelvis and thighs.

The Arch Posture.

(Photo credit: Alex Fernandez & Evolution Visual Services)

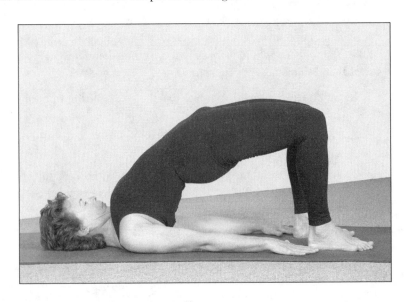

1. Lie on your back on the floor with your arms lying along your side. Turn your palms downward.

2. Bend your knees, bringing your heels as close to your lower pelvis as you can comfortably. Your feet remain flat on the floor, your knees raised. Your feet should be eight to ten inches apart.

3. Inhaling, lift your lower back, middle back, then upper back up off the floor, in that order, as high as you can without straining. Raise yourself slowly, paying attention to the lifting movement. The vertebrae in your spine will rise from the floor one by one as the lifting motion moves from your lower pelvis to your shoulders.

4. Your breastbone will lift toward your chin. However, keep your head and neck on the floor and keep breathing. Your arms and hands remain motionless on the floor.

5. Hold the pose for 10 to 20 seconds, depending on your capacity.

6. Now as you exhale, lower yourself back down to the floor in reverse order. Your breastbone moves down first, then your upper back, and finally your lower torso, vertebra by vertebra.

7. Pause for a moment, allowing your knees to rest against each other. Then repeat the Arch Posture two more times.

8. When you're finished, relax deeply in the Knees-to-Chest Posture.

If you are flexible enough and have long arms, you can grasp your ankles with your hands while holding the Arch Posture. This makes holding a more rounded arch easier.

This pose puts a lot of pressure on the knees and should not be practiced by anyone with serious knee problems.

The Arch and the Fish, which you've just learned, are counterpostures to poses you'll learn in Hour 6 such as the Shoulder Stand and Plow.

BRIDGE POSTURE

Setu (pronounced *say-two*) *Bandhasana* means "bridge" in Sanskrit and is the name of a posture that looks similar to the Arch but works quite differently anatomically. You'll notice you feel less pressure on your knees and on the muscles in your lower pelvis and back upper thighs. This is because your hands and upper arms are relieving much of the strain by bracing your weight against your elbows. The Bridge also allows you to flex your spinal column more dramatically than the Arch.

The Bridge provides a good stretch for your lower back and abdominal muscles. It also strengthens and tones the thigh muscles.

The Bridge Posture.

(Photo credit: Alex Fernandez & Evolution Visual Services)

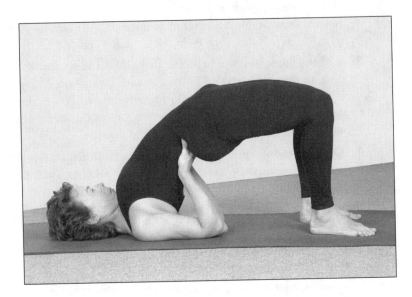

1. Lie on your back on the floor with your arms alongside you and your feet about ten inches apart.

2. Bend your knees and slide your feet close to your buttocks. Your feet should be flat on the floor, and your knees are raised.

3. As you inhale, lift your pelvis as far off the ground as you can comfortably. Your breastbone will move upward, perpendicular to your chin. Resist the temptation to stop breathing.

4. Press your hands into your mid-back to help support your back. Your elbows remain on the floor. You may find that you can now lift your pelvis a little farther, thanks to the extra support from your upper arms.

5. Hold the pose for 10 to 20 seconds.

6. Lay your arms down alongside you and lower your body. Relax for a moment, then repeat the Bridge Posture two more times.

7. When you're done, fold up into the Knees-to-Chest Posture to release any accumulated tension in your spine.

An easy variation of the Bridge Posture is to leave your arms lying on the floor and not lift your pelvis very high. With each repetition of the posture, lift your body up a little bit higher.

If you have yoga-savvy friends who've been doing these postures for some time, you'll probably find they come into the Bridge Posture in a different way. Experienced students use the Bridge as a sort of "half-way posture" when they're coming out of the Shoulder Stand (which you'll learn in Hour 6). They'll lower themselves into the Bridge to help release tension in their back before coming all the way down into the Corpse Posture. However, this is suitable only for students who're already fairly experienced with hatha postures and have a good sense of balance.

PROCEED WITH CAUTION

The backward-bending postures are excellent beginning-level yoga postures. However, if you suffer from heart disease or high blood pressure, or if you've suffered serious knee injuries or other knee joint problems, check with your doctor first. Skip these postures if you're pregnant or having your menstrual period.

KNOW YOUR LIMITS

Everyone wants to excel. Of course you want to do your best, whether you're in a Hatha Yoga class with 30 other students, or you're alone in your living room at home. But your Hatha Yoga session is not the place to push your limits, especially in the beginning. The price for overextending yourself in a hatha posture today may be stiff and sore muscles that prevent you from doing any hatha at all tomorrow. Take it easy! Let your body adjust to these new postures gradually.

It's important to remember that a lot of what makes Hatha Yoga so rejuvenating has to do with the way it affects your blood circulation. By tensing and straining yourself, you block the very circulation the posture is meant to enhance. So relax! Have a good time with the poses and don't feel you have to compete with anyone else, and especially not with yourself. If you take it easy each day, forming the postures only to your comfortable capacity, you'll be amazed at how much progress you make in just a few weeks.

QUIZ

HOUR'S UP!

Try taking this quiz to see if you remember the important points from Hour 5. Answer true or false to the following statements:

1. Breathing deeply and rapidly increases the effectiveness of Hatha Yoga postures by filling your lungs with oxygen.

2. Doing yoga postures on a hard floor without any cushion provides optimal support for the vertebrae of your spine.

3. The Cobra Pose is often effective in relieving many types of backache.

4. To get maximum benefit from the Cobra Pose, push yourself up as far as you can using your arms.

5. The Locust Pose requires you to lift the lower part of your body upward while lying on your stomach.

6. The Boat Posture places the entire weight of your body on the abdomen.

7. The Fish Posture is the one yoga pose performed while breathing through your mouth.

8. No one who has suffered a knee injury should practice the Arch Pose.

9. In the Bridge Posture, you support your arched back with your hands.

10. Pushing yourself strenuously to excel will help you progress much faster in your yoga practice.

Hour 6

More Basic Postures

In Hour 5, you learned seven of the most important Hatha Yoga postures, all performed while you're lying on the floor. Before you get up, there are five more excellent exercises you'll want to incorporate into your Hatha routine. Two standing poses will help round out the session and aid you in making the transition into the standing bends and twists you'll practice in Hours 7 and 8.

Mastering More Floor Postures

At the end of a vigorous calisthenics program, you'll feel the breath rushing in and out of your lungs and blood surging through your body as the aerobic effects of the exercises work your cardiovascular system. You will probably also feel fatigued and perhaps stiff and sore.

Yoga postures have a dramatically different effect. If you're doing the poses correctly and carefully pacing yourself, you won't feel sore afterward because you have never exceeded your comfortable capacity. Rather than feeling exhausted from your yoga workout, you'll feel relaxed, centered, and alert, ready to meet the challenges of the day.

Here is a series of five more postures that you perform while you're down on the floor.

Staff Posture

The Staff Posture is an excellent pose particularly for Western yoga students who're not used to sitting on the floor. It looks deceptively simple, but students raised in

Chapter Summary

LESSON PLAN:

In this hour you will learn …

- The Staff Pose will help loosen your hamstrings and lower back muscles so you can sit comfortably on the floor.
- The Pigeon improves circulation in your visceral organs.
- The Plow and Shoulder Stand are excellent for strengthening the musculature in your back and improving your posture.
- The Warrior, Horse Riding, and Down Facing Dog poses are superb stretching and toning exercises.
- While aerobic exercises work the cardiovascular system, Hatha Yoga works on your muscles, internal organs, and glands.

Western countries generally find it surprisingly challenging the first time they try it. Most of them have grown up sitting in chairs and sofas, often generously padded ones at that, rather than on the ground. The result is that their lower back and hamstring muscles are usually tight. This pose will help loosen those muscles and can do wonders for your posture.

This pose is called *Dandasana* in Sanskrit after the *danda* or staff that many yogis carry with them. Your goal is to sit up as straight as a staff.

The Staff Posture.

(Photo credit: Johnathan Brown)

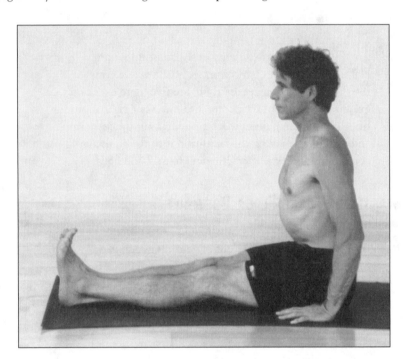

1. Sit on the floor with your legs together, extended straight out in front of you. Place your palms on the floor beside you, next to your hips.

2. Sit up straight. Inhaling, draw your spine up as if someone is gently pulling upward on your head.

3. Keep your knees straight. Press your heels away from your body to further lengthen your legs.

4. Hold the position for 10 to 20 seconds. Breathe diaphragmatically. Your back and neck muscles are working to keep you upright but the rest of your body should be relaxed. Mentally scan your body to make sure none of your other muscles are tense.

5. Come out of the pose, bend your knees, and relax for a moment.

The Staff Posture is an important pose that will help loosen and strengthen the muscles in your lower back. However, if the posture is painful in the beginning, sit on a cushion such as a pillow, folded blanket, or meditation seat while you hold the pose. It's important that you keep your back and knees straight, but lifting your hips slightly off the floor is fine in the beginning. The first few times you do the Staff Posture you may want to push upward with your hands, which rest on the floor beside you. This will help you straighten your spine.

When you attend a yoga class, you'll find quite a number of hatha poses begin from the Staff Posture or one of its variants. You'll learn a few of these in Hours 7 and 8. It will be helpful for you to spend some time mastering this pose, because it's excellent for improving your posture. You'll discover more about why yogis consider an upright posture so important in Hour 8.

 One of the finest introductions to Hatha Yoga postures to come out in recent years is *Yoga: Mastering the Basics* by Sandra Anderson and Rolf Sovik, Psy.D. This beautifully illustrated book is accompanied by two videotapes, *Flexibility, Strength and Balance* and *Deepening and Strengthening*, which guide you through a beginning-level yoga routine.

SHOULDER STAND

The Shoulder Stand is called *Sarvangasana* or "All Limbs Posture" because it has a powerful affect on virtually every part of your body. It is often called the queen of Hatha Yoga postures because of the high esteem in which yogis hold it. (The king is the Headstand.)

The Shoulder Stand turns you upside down, which enhances circulation and prevents blood from pooling in the lower portions of your body. The pose is especially valued for its ability to nourish and balance the thyroid and parathyroid glands, which help control your metabolism, temperature, body weight, and heart rate.

1. Lie on your back with your arms along your sides, palms down. Your legs should be together.

2. As you inhale, lift your legs straight up in the air, perpendicular to your body.

3. Swing your legs down over your head. This provides a counterweight, which makes it easy for you to now lift your pelvis and torso up off the floor. Bracing your elbows into the floor, use your hands to help push your back upward and to steady it when your spine has reached a position at a right angle to the floor.

4. Lift your legs straight up in the air. Do not bend your knees. Your head, neck, shoulders, and upper arms remain on the floor. Every other part of your body is now upside down in the air.

5. Keep breathing. Hold the posture for 30 seconds if you can comfortably, or up to a minute if you can do so without strain. Use the time to enjoy the sense of balance you are experiencing.

The Shoulder Stand.

(Photo credit: Alex Fernandez & Evolution Visual Services)

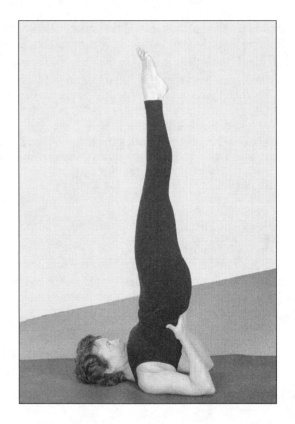

To come out of the posture, allow your straight legs to dip halfway toward your head, place your arms back down at your side, and slowly roll your back down onto the floor as you exhale. Lower your legs and relax in the Corpse Pose.

The Shoulder Stand is another posture that feels quite pleasurable once you've mastered your balance in the posture. More advanced yoga students hold this pose up to five minutes while moving through several variations. While holding the posture, for example, they spread their legs apart in a wide angle forming a V shape. Others spread their thighs apart but press the soles of their feet together, forming a diamond shape with their legs.

If you're particularly inflexible or are completely new to upside-down postures, you may want to exercise extra care in trying this pose for the first time. Fold a couple of blankets into squares of about two feet by two feet and lay them on the end of your yoga mat. This should form about four inches of padding. Lie down on the blankets so your head extends over the end of the blankets but your shoulders are supported. Lifting yourself into the Shoulder Stand with padding under your shoulders will prevent excess strain on the vertebrae in your neck.

You need to be careful not to fall or injure yourself in this posture. If you have serious problems balancing upside down in the pose, don't try it again without seeking help from an experienced yoga teacher. If you're just mildly shaky in the posture, have a friend hold your legs steady for a few moments till you get a feel for staying balanced in the posture.

The numerous benefits of the Shoulder Stand go beyond obvious ones like strengthening the back, arms, and shoulders. It also gives the cervical vertebrae (the bones at the top of your spine) some traction, helping alleviate problems in this area. It dramatically increases blood flow to the important endocrine glands in the throat. Because it helps move stagnant blood out of the lower limbs, the Shoulder Stand can help improve conditions like varicose veins.

This posture is said to improve digestion and to energize the liver, pancreas, gall bladder, and spleen. As its Sanskrit name claims, this posture is an "all around" winner.

GO TO ▶
In India, many yogis will immediately move into the Fish Posture after holding the Shoulder Stand and the Plow. This helps relieve any tension that might have built up in the back and balances the flexing motion of the spine. Refer to Hour 5 to review the Half Fish Pose.

PLOW POSTURE

The Plow Posture, called *Halasana* in Sanskrit, is one of the best possible postures for toning your abdominal muscles. *Hala* actually means a "plow." If your belly needs some shaping up, you should be practicing this pose.

The Plow has some features in common with the Shoulder Stand. Many yogis go into the Shoulder Stand immediately before or after the Plow without pausing to rest in between. Both poses begin by lying on the floor and lifting your straightened legs vertically in the air, then down over your head. In the Plow, you keep going until your toes touch the floor. In the Shoulder Stand, however, once your torso is upright in an inverted position, you lift your legs straight up in the air.

The Plow Posture.

(Photo credit: Alex Fernandez & Evolution Visual Services)

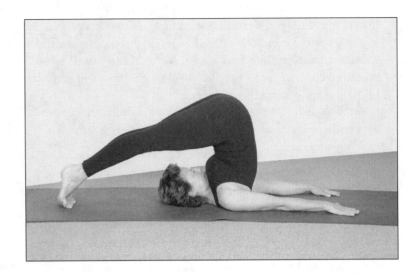

1. Lie on your back on the floor with your arms lying along your sides, palms facing down. Your legs should be straight and lying close together.

2. As you inhale, lift your legs straight up in the air, perpendicular to your body.

3. Raise your pelvis so your lower torso comes up off the floor. Use your back and abdominal muscles, the momentum from raising your legs in step 2, and the bracing action of your arms, which remain on the floor, to accomplish this.

4. Keep swinging your straight legs until they come over your head, parallel to the floor. Your toes are now pointed toward the floor. Focus on your breath. Make sure you are breathing diaphragmatically.

5. Relax in this position for 10 to 15 seconds.

6. If you feel comfortable and your back is flexible enough, continue rolling backward till your toes touch the floor.

7. If your back feels slightly uncomfortable, brace your elbows against the floor and press your hands into the middle of your back to support it. Keep your mental focus on your body. Enjoy the yoga posture.

8. To come out of the posture, swing your legs back up till they are vertical, then slowly roll your back down onto the floor and lower your legs.

9. Relax for a moment in the Corpse Pose, then repeat the Plow Posture one more time.

If your back feels a bit tense after completing the Plow, assume the Arch Posture or the Half Fish, which you learned in Hour 5, to help relax your back muscles.

Like the Shoulder Stand, the Plow has a glowing reputation in the yoga tradition. According to the yogis, it's one of the most rejuvenating of all postures. This may be in part because of its beneficial action on the thyroid gland. However, it also revitalizes your spleen, liver, small intestines, and colon. It's said to prevent constipation when practiced regularly.

PIGEON POSTURE

Now you'll move on to two poses that begin from a crawling position.

Kapotasana means Pigeon Pose in Sanskrit. (A *kapota* is a pigeon.) This posture is not only beautiful to look at, it offers a host of health benefits. It stimulates your lungs, kidneys, and back muscles as well as the glands of your *endocrine system*.

STRICTLY DEFINED

The **endocrine system** is made up of glands whose secretions are released directly into your blood. This includes, for example, your thyroid and pituitary glands.

For people who're already somewhat flexible, the Pigeon is an enjoyable pose to hold. If you find the position too intense in the beginning, place a cushion under the lower pelvis of your folded leg, or under the thigh and groin of your straight leg. This will relieve some of the pressure and help you feel more at ease.

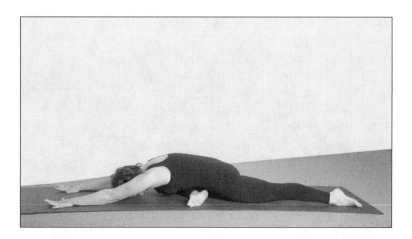

Preparation for the Pigeon Posture.

(Photo credit: Alex Fernandez & Evolution Visual Services)

1. Begin on your hands and knees on the floor.

2. Pull your right knee up as close to your hands as it will come comfortably. Now shift your right foot to the left, so that it's lying beneath you, perpendicular to your torso.

3. Extend your left leg straight out behind you. The leg stays on the floor. Point your left toes away from your body.

4. Lower your upper torso so that you are lying down on top of your right leg. Rest your forehead on the floor. Slide your arms along the floor till they extend out straight above your head.

5. Hold this position for five to ten seconds, feeling the stretch. Remember to breathe smoothly and quietly through your nostrils.

6. Slide your hands back toward your body and lift your head and torso upward as far as you can comfortably. Use your arms and hands to support yourself.

7. Hold this position for another 10 seconds. Don't strain. Keep breathing!

8. Roll slightly to your right and release your right leg. Relax in the Crocodile Pose, which you learned in Hour 3. Mentally scan your body to check how each part feels.

9. Repeat the Pigeon Posture, folding the left leg under your body this time.

The Pigeon Posture.

(Photo credit: Alex Fernandez & Evolution Visual Services)

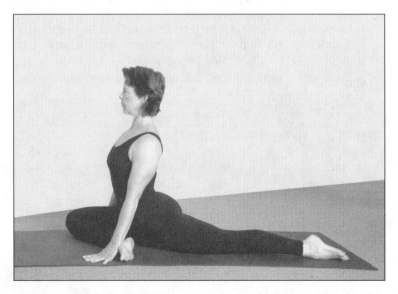

If you're not particularly flexible, you may not be able to raise your head and torso very far in step 6. That's fine. Don't push your body any farther than feels comfortable. Advanced students can hold their trunk up in a vertical line from the floor or even bend backward in this pose.

FYI If you're ready for a book that guides you through a wide variety of yoga postures with a wealth of anatomical explanations, try *Yoga Mind, Body and Spirit: A Return to Wholeness* by Donna Farhi. Farhi is one of the most respected yoga teachers of the twenty-first century.

DOWN FACING DOG POSTURE

There are a variety of yoga poses called the Dog Posture. This version is specifically called *Adho Mukha Svanasana* in Sanskrit, which means the downward *(adho)* face *(mukha)* dog *(svana)* pose *(asana)*.

This pose will strengthen your arms and wrists, as well as stretching the hamstrings and Achilles tendons in your legs. It also sends rejuvenating blood to your lungs, head, and neck.

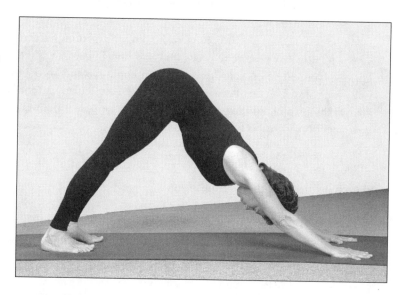

The Down Facing Dog Posture.

(Photo credit: Alex Fernandez & Evolution Visual Services)

1. Begin on your hands and knees. Your toes should be on the floor but your heels are raised.

2. Lower your pelvis onto your heels.

3. Slide your arms out in front of you along the floor. Keep them straight and don't sit up off your heels. Don't lower your head all the way to the floor.

4. Now raise your pelvis into the air. Drop your heels to the ground as you do so. Your hands and the soles of your feet are now the only parts of your body on the floor, while your pelvis is lifted as high as possible.

5. Hold your feet and arms straight. Keep your head in line with your arms. Your body looks like an upside-down V.

6. Hold the pose for about 10 to 15 seconds, if you can do so comfortably. Breathe diaphragmatically. Be attentive to your body and adjust any parts that may feel strained.

7. Drop down to your knees, sit back on your heels, and relax for a moment. Then repeat the Down Facing Dog two more times.

PROCEED WITH CAUTION

If your hamstrings or ankle muscles feel too strained in the Down Facing Dog posture, allow yourself to bend your knees slightly, or brace your heels against a wall so the wall bears part of your weight. Remember, you should never feel pain in a yoga posture. If you do, adjust the posture so that you're comfortable.

Don't be intimidated by the complex-sounding instructions for this pose. This is a fairly easy posture to do if you know how to get into it properly. Basically you just sit on your heels, run your hands forward on the floor, and hoist your hips. The first few times you try it, be particularly attentive to your wrists as you hold the posture. Drop out of the pose if the weight of your upper body creates too much strain for them.

The Down Facing Dog is particularly valuable because it combines some of the benefits of an inverted posture like the Shoulder Stand with a good leg stretch, while strengthening the arms.

PROCEED WITH CAUTION

Carpal tunnel syndrome is an increasingly common problem in the West today, where so many people spend time at a keyboard. If you have this condition, be very careful with postures like the Down Facing Dog, which shift much of your weight onto your wrists. Trying forming your hands into a fist while holding the pose, or check with your doctor whether you should use a wrist brace or avoid this type of yoga pose altogether.

MASTERING MORE STANDING POSTURES

Now it's time to get up off the floor and start working with a few of the easier yoga postures that begin from a standing position. The next two poses are excellent stretches and are quite energizing.

WARRIOR POSTURE

If you browse through different yoga manuals, you'll find there are several different exercises called the Warrior Posture *(Virabhadrasana)*. A virabhadra is a hero or warrior; *vira* means "virile man" and *bhadra* means "fierce." The version you're about to learn is a distant relative of the Lunge Stretch, which you practiced during Hour 2. It's as if you're doing the Lunge Stretch in a standing position. Both postures strengthen and firm the muscles of your legs.

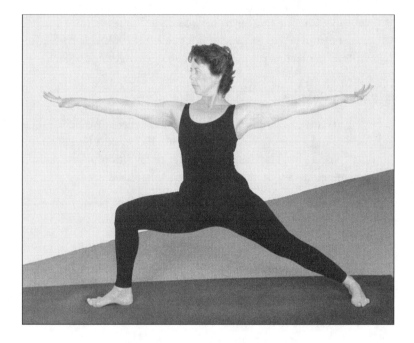

The Warrior Posture.

(Photo credit: Alex Fernandez & Evolution Visual Services)

1. Stand up straight in the Mountain Pose, which you learned in Hour 3.

2. Step your right foot forward two and a half to three feet (depending on how tall you are).

3. Step a bit farther back with your left foot. Your right knee should now be bent at about a 90-degree angle, while your left leg remains straight. Turn your left foot outward slightly so you have a good grip on the floor.

4. Swivel your torso 90 degrees to the left so that you are facing away from the line formed by your two legs.

5. Raise your arms directly out to your sides. Your right arm now extends over your right leg while your left arm extends over your left leg. Stretch out through your fingertips.

6. Turn your head to the right so you're looking directly over your right shoulder.

7. Hold the Warrior Pose for 15 to 30 seconds. Breathe diaphragmatically. Pay attention to the way your body feels.

8. Return to the Mountain Pose and relax for a moment. Then repeat the Warrior Posture, placing your left leg forward and your right leg back this time.

You'll feel the stretch in your thigh muscles particularly. Don't overdo this posture, especially the first few times you do it. However, once you're comfortable in the posture you'll discover why it's called the Warrior Pose. It seems to automatically generate a psychological state of strength and vigor.

HORSE RIDING POSTURE

In *Utkatasana* you sit down on a chair, except there isn't a chair there. Perhaps this should be called the "air chair" pose! Utkatasana literally means "horse rider" posture because the pose imitates the position of a rider except that your legs are held together rather than straddling a saddle.

The Horse Riding Posture works the muscles of the pelvic floor and inner thighs.

1. Stand in the Mountain Posture with your feet together.

2. Inhaling, stretch out your arms, lifting them straight out to the side, then up directly over your head till your palms touch. Don't bend your elbows. Stretch up all the way through your fingertips.

3. Now bend your knees and lower your pelvis as if you were going to sit down. Move downward as far as you can comfortably without losing your balance or overstraining your leg muscles.

4. Hold the pose for 15 to 30 seconds. Keep breathing. Be attentive to your physical state.

5. Inhaling, rise back up into a standing position. Exhaling, lower your arms to your sides.

6. Repeat the Horse Riding Posture two more times.

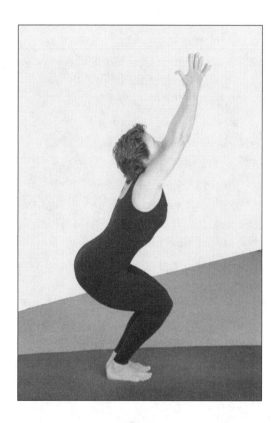

The Horse Riding Posture.

(Photo credit: Alex Fernandez & Evolution Visual Services)

Here's an important key to performing this stretch with a minimum of strain. Start the pose with your feet right next to each other. As you lower yourself toward the nonexistent chair, press your knees together. Your knees are now braced against each other rather than bearing the full brunt of your weight as you settle down onto them.

With practice you'll be able to "sit" more deeply into the posture. Take it easy especially the first few times you do the pose. Resist the temptation to overstrain your thigh muscles or you'll feel sore later.

In the next hour you'll move on to some of the most important bending exercises in the yoga repertoire.

JUST A MINUTE

Most people do just fine during their first attempt at yoga postures. Remember, you don't have to be perfect the first time! However, if you are not limber at all, some of the postures can be a challenge when you first start out. Go back to the stretching and limbering exercises you learned in Hour 2 and practice those for a few weeks. Soon you'll be in better shape to progress to the classic yoga poses.

QUIZ

HOUR'S UP!

You've just learned seven new Hatha Yoga postures. Can you remember a few basic points about each of them? Take this quiz and find out. Answer true or false to the following statements:

1. The Staff Posture trains you to sit comfortably on the floor.

2. The Shoulder Stand is especially valued for its effect on the thyroid and parathyroid glands.

3. The Plow Pose is excellent for toning the abdominal muscles.

4. The Pigeon Pose requires you to hold yourself upside down.

5. The Down Facing Dog Posture offers both the benefits of an inverted posture and strength training.

6. The Warrior Pose is similar to the Lunge Stretch but is performed lying on the floor.

7. In the Horse Riding Posture you stand with your legs separated, as if you were straddling a saddle.

8. Aerobic exercises focus on stimulating the endocrine system, while Hatha Yoga postures emphasize cardiovascular fitness.

9. It's helpful to assume a backward bending pose like the Half Fish after the Shoulder Stand and Plow.

10. People with carpal tunnel syndrome need to be cautious performing Hatha Yoga poses that shift their weight onto their wrists.

Hour 7

Beginning Bends

Chapter Summary

LESSON PLAN:
In this hour you will learn …

- Hatha Yoga bending exercises stretch and tone the major muscle groups of your body.
- Many of the bending postures also promote the action of your abdominal organs.
- Forward-bending exercises tend to calm the nervous system.
- The Churn and the Butterfly require you to keep moving rather than remain still in a yoga posture.
- Several of these postures have advanced versions appropriate for more limber students.

Backward-bending yoga postures, like the Cobra and the Arch, which you learned in Hour 5, have an invigorating effect physically and psychologically. This is in part because of the way they activate your sympathetic nervous system, the part of your nervous system that gears you up for emergencies, preparing you for action. Forward-bending exercises, on the other hand, generally have a calming effect on your body and mind.

The bending exercises you'll learn in this hour not only help you become more supple, they also provide a massage for your abdominal organs, including your stomach, liver, small intestine, and colon. In this way, they promote digestion and the prompt elimination of waste from your body. You should not be surprised to find some improvement in these areas if you practice these postures regularly.

Mastering the Bending Poses

In this hour, you will learn a series of simple but effective bending exercises that begin in both standing and sitting positions. You'll also learn some "active" yoga exercises—postures in which you keep moving rather than hold still.

Remember to take it easy, especially the first few times you're holding the poses while you're still learning your limits. Never force yourself past your capacity or push through pain in any yoga exercise. Yoga is meant to be safe and enjoyable. It will stay that way if you respect your body's present limitations.

PROCEED WITH CAUTION

There is an important contraindication for the bending postures you need to be aware of. If you have serious back pain, check with your doctor before attempting these poses. Hatha Yoga actually helps with many types of back problems, but can aggravate serious pre-existing conditions.

STANDING SIDE BEND

The Standing Side Bend is basic, yet learning to do this posture well will help you enormously when you move on to the somewhat more challenging postures in Hour 8. Focus on cultivating flexibility and maintaining your balance.

The Standing Side Bend.

(Photo credit: Alex Fernandez & Evolution Visual Services)

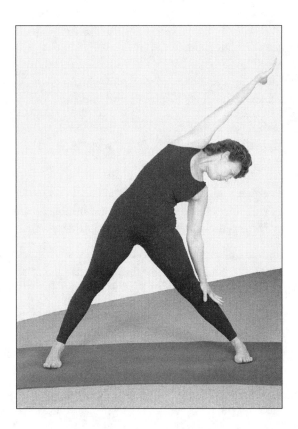

1. Stand up straight with your legs two and a half to three feet apart. Your toes point forward.

2. Inhaling, raise your right arm directly out to your side. Keep your right arm straight. Your palm should face downward.

3. When your right arm is positioned horizontally, flip your palm so that it faces upward. As you continue inhaling, lift your right arm straight up above your head. Stretch upward through your fingertips.

4. Exhaling, bend to the left, allowing your left hand to slide down your left thigh. Bend only as far as you feel comfortable. Don't tilt forward or backward as you bend, but lower your upper body directly to the side. Glance down toward your left foot if you need to check your alignment. Then face directly forward, which will help you keep your balance.

5. Hold the posture for five to ten seconds, or to your comfortable capacity. Breathe diaphragmatically. Mentally scan your body to make sure you're holding the position correctly and no part of your body feels strained.

6. Inhaling, straighten back up, sliding your left hand back up your left thigh.

7. Exhaling, lower your right arm until it points directly outward to the side from your body. Flip your palm so it faces downward. As you continue exhaling, lower your arm all the way back down to your side.

8. Repeat the Standing Side Bend, raising your left arm this time and bending to the right.

GO TO ▶

In Hour 8, you will learn more side bends that will add a twisting motion to the posture. This increases the stimulating effect of the pose on your abdominal organs, including your liver and intestines.

STANDING BACKWARD BEND

You've already learned a number of backward bending yoga exercises, particularly in Hour 5. The Standing Backward Bend is especially valuable because it serves as a counterposture to the forward bending poses you're about to learn. If your back starts feeling cramped or uncomfortable in any of the following postures, stand up straight and ease back into the Standing Backward Bend. It will release the tension. It also opens your chest and improves the elasticity of your lungs.

1. Stand in the Mountain Pose, which you learned in Hour 3.

2. Place the palms of your hands on either side of your spine as far up your back as you can comfortably. Your fingers should point downward.

3. Inhaling, bend your neck backward. Then bend your back backward, helping support the bend with your hands. Bend only as far as you can without straining or losing your balance.

4. Hold the posture for 10 to 20 seconds. Breathe diaphragmatically. Remain relaxed but balanced in the posture.

5. Exhaling, stand back up straight and release your arms.

6. Repeat the Standing Backward Bend two more times.

The Standing Backward Bend.

(Photo credit: Alex Fernandez & Evolution Visual Services)

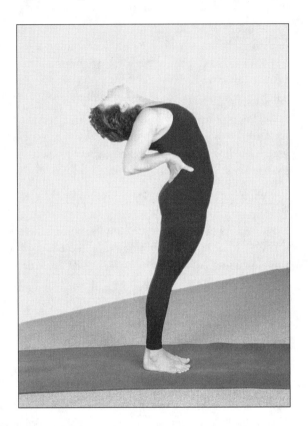

Here is a more advanced version of the Standing Backward Bend that allows you to bend back farther and has the additional benefit of gently stretching the inner thigh muscles.

1. Stand up straight with your legs about three feet apart, toes pointing forward.

2. Place your palms on the backs of the tops of your thighs, fingers pointing downward.

3. Inhaling, bend your neck backward and arch back with your spine. Then bend backward from your hips, running your hands down the back of your thighs.

4. Hold the posture for 10 to 20 seconds. Breathe diaphragmatically. As you relax in the posture you may find you can bend backward a little bit more.

5. Exhaling, stand back up straight, release your arms, and bring your legs together in the Mountain Pose.

6. Repeat this Standing Backward Bend two more times. Notice how it makes you feel.

Students often feel a sense of heightened alertness and clarity following this posture. Don't rush through your yoga postures, but watch to see how your body and mind respond during and after the pose.

 Yoga Mind and Body by Sivananda Yoga Vedanta Center is a charming and beautifully illustrated introduction to some of the fundamental yoga postures. Sivananda was a highly respected yogi from northern India. A number of the most influential yoga teachers working in the West were his students.

STANDING FORWARD BEND

The Standing Forward Bend is called *Padahastasana* in Sanskrit. *Pada* means "foot." (Related English words include "podiatrist," a foot doctor.) *Hasta* means "hand," and *asana*, of course, means "yoga posture." So the Padahastasana literally means the hand-to-foot posture.

This posture helps mobilize your intestines to action. It also stimulates many of your abdominal organs including the liver, kidneys, stomach, pancreas, and spleen. In addition, it increases the suppleness of the hip and hamstring muscles.

1. Stand in the Mountain Pose. Keep your feet together.

2. Inhaling, stretch your arms straight out in front of you, palms facing down. Without pausing, keep lifting them till they extend straight over your head.

3. Exhaling, bend forward from your hips. Keep your back, arms, and legs as straight as you can comfortably.

4. Touch your shins, ankles, feet, or the floor with your hands, depending on how far down you can reach without straining yourself.

5. As you hold the pose, be attentive to your breathing. Make sure you're breathing diaphragmatically in a smooth and relaxed manner.

6. As you relax into the posture, you may find that you can bend forward a little bit more. Feel the muscles around your hips relaxing, allowing you to deepen the bend. Hold the pose for 10 to 20 seconds.

7. Inhaling, return to a standing position with your arms straight above your head.

8. Exhaling, lower your arms directly out in front of you, then down to your sides.

9. Repeat the Standing Forward Bend two more times. Then stand in the Mountain Pose for a moment and relax.

The Standing Forward Bend.

(Photo credit: Alex Fernandez & Evolution Visual Services)

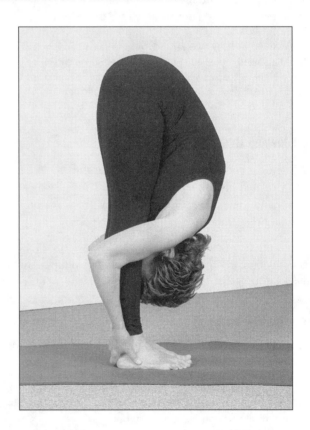

You will feel the blood rushing to your head in this posture. Never hold the pose so long that you become dizzy or lightheaded.

As you become more limber, you can deepen the Standing Forward Bend by grasping your shins and gently pulling your chest closer to your legs. Remember, deepen the posture by relaxing into it, not by forcing or straining yourself.

SITTING FORWARD BEND

The Sitting Forward Bend is known as *Paschimottanasana* in India. Paschi-mottana refers to the Western direction, so Paschimottanasana is the yoga posture that stretches the back side of the body, which some yogis call "the west end." This posture gives many of the same benefits as the Standing Forward Bend. In addition, it's said to improve circulation between your spinal disks, stimulate digestion, and prevent constipation.

In Indian folklore, this pose is said to be particularly helpful for diabetics, and to help trim the waist and hips.

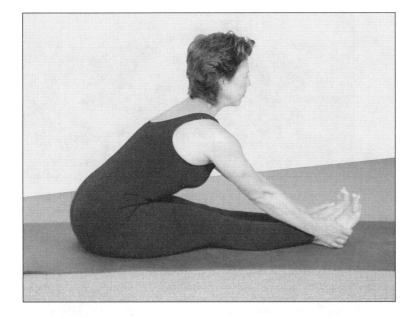

The Sitting Forward Bend, version 1.

(Photo credit: Alex Fernandez & Evolution Visual Services)

1. Begin sitting on the floor in the Staff Pose, which you learned in Hour 6.

2. Inhaling, raise your arms straight out in front of you and stretch through your fingertips. Raise your arms till they're straight up above your head.

3. Exhaling, bend forward from your hips. Keep your back straight and your head in line with your arms. Bend down as far as you can without strain.

4. Now rest your hands on your feet or along your lower legs, however far down you can reach comfortably. Keep your knees straight.

5. Breathe diaphragmatically. Hold the posture for 5 to 15 seconds. Scan your body for pockets of tightness and stress. Allow those areas to relax, or back up out of the posture slightly so you feel less stress.

6. Inhaling, sit back up with your arms above your head.

7. Exhaling, lower your arms straight out in front of you, then down to the floor.

8. Relax. Then repeat the Sitting Forward Bend two more times.

The Sitting Forward Bend, version 2.

(Photo credit: Alex Fernandez & Evolution Visual Services)

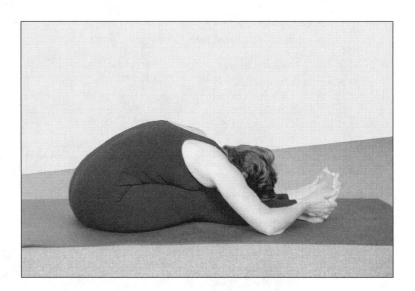

If you're fairly flexible and have long arms, you might be able to reach beyond your feet. In this case rest your elbows on the floor and grasp your big toes with your fingers.

There is a second version of the Sitting Forward Bend that you'll often see students doing in yoga classes. Some people find this variation a bit easier.

1. Sit in the Staff Pose. Draw your right foot up toward your groin and place the bottom of the foot against your left inner thigh.

2. Inhaling, lift your arms straight forward from your body, then straight upward above your head.

3. Exhaling, bend forward from your hips till your face rests on your left leg, or as far downward as you can comfortably. Grasp your left foot with your hands.

4. Hold the pose for 5 to 15 seconds. Breathe diaphragmatically. Ease back out of the posture slightly if you feel any discomfort. If your left thigh aches, bend your left knee a little bit.

5. Inhaling, sit back up, raising your arms above your head. Exhaling, lower your arms and relax for a moment.

6. Repeat the exercise with your left foot pressed into your right inner thigh and your right leg extended directly forward this time.

JUST A MINUTE

In both versions of the Sitting Forward Bend explained here, it's important that you bend from your hips, not from your waist. Your whole back should come down toward your legs, not just your upper back. You will feel the stretch in your lower back.

CHURN

Chalan, or the Churn, is one of the comparatively few classical Hatha Yoga postures in which you remain in motion throughout the exercise, rather than firmly holding a pose.

The Churn is superb for improving flexibility in the hips, thighs, and lower back.

1. Sit on the floor in the Staff Pose, which you learned in Hour 6.

2. Shift your legs as far apart as you can without feeling any sense of strain in your inner thighs. Keep your legs straight, with your toes pointing up.

3. Turn your torso to the right. Exhaling, bend from your hips and reach toward your right toes with your left hand. Try to keep your back as straight as possible.

4. Inhaling, sit back up straight and turn forward.

5. Turn your torso to the left. Exhaling, bend from your hips and reach toward your left toes with your right hand.

6. Inhaling, sit back up straight and turn back to center.

7. Repeat the Churning motion 10 to 20 more times. Remember to coordinate your movements with your breath.

If you're not very flexible and find this exercise difficult, try keeping your legs extended directly in front of you rather than out to the sides. Allow your knees to come up slightly and your back to bend a bit as you churn.

If the Churn seems easy for you, instead of reaching for your foot, run your extended hand along the floor to the outside of your opposite foot, deepening the bend.

Churning.

(Photo credit: Alex Fernandez & Evolution Visual Services)

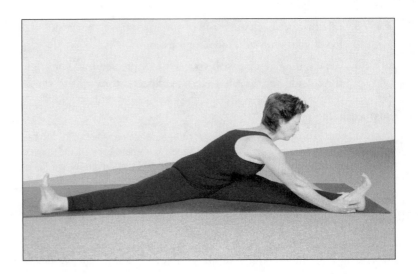

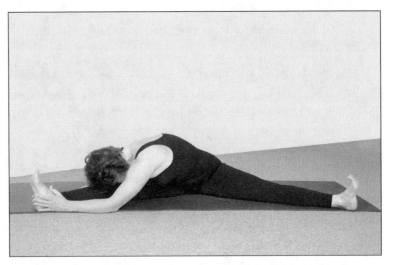

SYMBOL OF YOGA

Yoga Mudra means the "gesture" or "symbol" of yoga. It is valued not only for the stretch it provides, but for the gentle pressure it applies to the abdomen. This stimulates peristalsis, the rhythmic contraction of the intestines that propels waste matter through your bowel. The proper and regular elimination of waste is considered essential to good health in the yoga system.

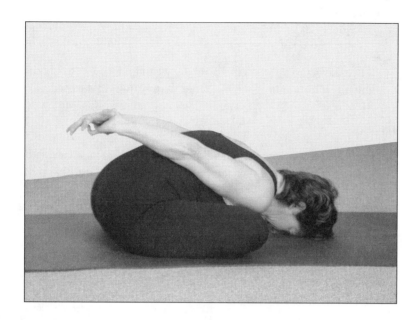

The Symbol of Yoga.

(Photo credit: Alex Fernandez & Evolution Visual Services)

1. Sit cross-legged on the floor with your back straight.

2. Reach behind your back and catch hold of your left wrist with your right hand.

3. Exhaling, bend forward from your hips. Keep your back straight as long as you can.

4. Bend forward until you can rest your forehead on the floor in front of you. Try not to roll forward from your seat. Keep your lower pelvis on the floor.

5. Get comfortable in the posture. This may mean adjusting the pose so that you're not bent as far forward. Breathe diaphragmatically. Stay in the pose for 20 to 30 seconds if you are at ease doing so.

6. Sit back up, release your hands and legs, and relax. Pay attention to the sensations in your body and energy field.

If you are too stiff to relax in this posture, there is an easier version that can also be quite beneficial.

1. Kneel on the floor. Then sit down on your heels.

2. Place your fists against your lower abdomen, just above your legs, between your hipbones.

3. Bend forward until your forehead rests on the floor.

GO TO ▶

In Hour 9, you'll learn the Stomach Lift and Stomach Roll, two of the most effective yoga exercises for stimulating the bowels and helping keep the elimination of waste regular and complete. Yogis believe that your awareness becomes clearer and your health more vibrant when wastes and toxins are promptly expelled from the body.

4. Breathe diaphragmatically. Hold the pose for 10 seconds, then sit back up and relax.

When advanced yogis do this pose, they bend forward in the Lotus Posture, which you'll learn in Hour 14, rather than sitting cross-legged.

BUTTERFLY

The final yoga exercise you'll learn in this hour does not involve bending your back, but folding your knees. This is one of the best yoga poses for stretching and firming your thigh muscles. Like the Churn, it's one of the few Hatha Yoga poses that involves continuous movement, rather than requiring you to hold still in one position.

The Butterfly is called *Baddha Konasana* in Sanskrit, which literally means "folded angle."

PROCEED WITH CAUTION

 Don't force your knees down farther than they'll move comfortably in the Butterfly exercise. If they're still a few inches off the floor when you've bounced them down as far as you can comfortably, that's fine. You'll find that if you repeat this exercise regularly for a few weeks, your knees will move lower without any sense of strain or pain.

---

1. Sit on the floor in the Staff Posture.

2. Bending your knees, bring your feet together as near your groin as they'll come comfortably. Press the soles of your feet against each other. Cup your fingers around your toes if you can do so without having to lean forward. Keep your knees down.

3. Maintaining this position, gently bounce your knees up and down on the floor. With every few bounces, raise them a little higher and let them bounce a little lower.

4. Continue fluttering your knees up and down as if your legs were butterfly wings for a half minute or so. Don't use force! Don't go too fast. Stay relaxed, remain attentive to the sensations in your legs and lower back, and keep breathing slowly and smoothly.

5. Stretch your legs out in front of you and relax for a moment.

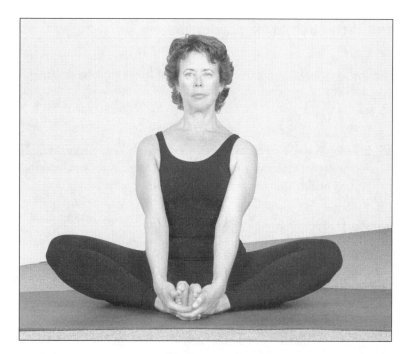

The Butterfly.

(Photo credit: Alex Fernandez & Evolution Visual Services)

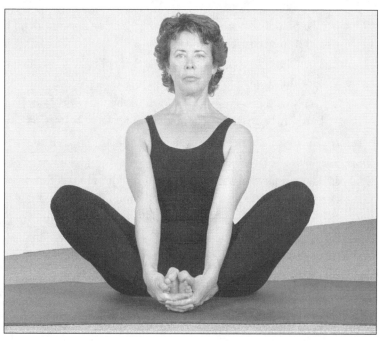

BEND WITHOUT BREAKING

You'll notice that in each posture, you are always encouraged to be aware of how your body feels. It's important that you continually scan your body for areas of pain, tension, or discomfort so you can ease up in the pose until that part of your body relaxes or becomes more flexible. Yoga is not mindless exercise. It demands continuous awareness.

In Hour 8, you'll go on to add twists to your bends, working more deeply with a part of your body the yogis consider absolutely fundamental in maintaining health and youthfulness: your spinal column.

HOUR'S UP!

QUIZ

Take this quiz to see if you've absorbed this hour's main points. Answer true or false to the following statements:

1. Backward-bending exercises tend to make you feel more alert.

2. Forward-bending exercises tend to make you feel more relaxed.

3. Many bending exercises improve your digestion by massaging your abdominal organs.

4. The Standing Forward Bend and the Sitting Forward Bend have completely different biological effects.

5. The Churn, the Butterfly, and the Symbol of Yoga require you to be in continuous movement.

6. You should press your knees down to the floor with your hands in the Butterfly to ensure you're holding the posture correctly.

7. The Yoga Mudra helps stimulate peristalsis, which is the rhythmic beating of your heart.

8. The primary function of the Sympathetic Nervous System is to make you feel sympathy for other living beings.

9. Holding yoga postures requires full, continuous mental attention.

10. In India, Hatha Yoga is considered both a system of physical exercises and a form of mental discipline.

HOUR 8

Basic Twisting Poses

CHAPTER SUMMARY

LESSON PLAN:

In this hour you will learn ...

- Twisting motions affect your body in a more complex manner than bending postures.

- The spinal column is the second most important part of your nervous system, after your brain.

- Yoga exercises like the Torso Twist, Half Spinal Twist, and Reclining Twist stretch and energize the entire spine.

- The angle and twisting poses taught in this hour also massage the abdominal organs.

- The Rocking Chair Roll allows you to gently massage your own back.

In Hour 7, you learned more of the basic yoga bending exercises. Now it's time to learn some twists. Twists add another dimension to a posture. They involve swiveling around an axis in a way that's not symmetrical, as bends usually are. They require more complex movements that, like wringing a wet cloth, compress or extend different parts of your body in opposite directions at the same time.

Twists squeeze your inner organs, forcing blood from one area of your body into another. This is how they mobilize your circulatory system and is part of the reason why you feel so good after you've done a couple of them.

MASTERING THE TWISTING POSTURES

You are about to learn some of the best known of the yoga twisting postures. However, there are two preparatory poses you need to learn first: The Angle and Triangle will get you ready for the Revolving Triangle. After this you'll master the relatively easy Torso Twist, a posture that also helps you work on your balance. Remember that physical balance requires mental poise, so the Torso Twist is also an exercise in balanced awareness.

Next you'll learn the Half Spinal Twist, which begins in a sitting position. You'll learn both the easy and the more challenging versions. You can choose which you prefer depending on your level of flexibility. After this comes the Reclining Twist, a powerful twist you'll do lying on your back.

Finally you'll learn the Rocking Chair. This is one of the moving poses yogis use to release tension in their back following a series of spine twisting postures.

Angle Pose

The Angle Pose is called *Parshvottanasana*, which literally means "side bend posture." Sometimes it's also called *Konasana*, which means simply "angle posture." This position helps improve the strength and flexibility of the leg and pelvic muscles.

The Angle Pose.

(Photo credit: Alex Fernandez & Evolution Visual Services)

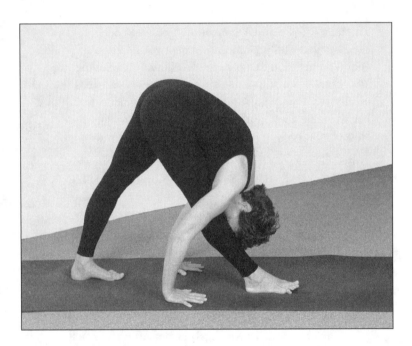

1. Begin in a standing position with your arms at your sides.

2. Step your right foot forward so that it is about three feet ahead of your left foot. Keep your legs straight. Turn your left toes out from your body about 45 degrees (one eighth of a circle) to help you keep your balance.

3. Inhaling, raise your arms straight above your head and lean as far backward as you can comfortably. Roll your head back and look up at the ceiling.

4. Exhaling, pivot forward from your hips. Bend as far forward as you can without discomfort. If you are limber, your face may reach your right leg. Place your hands on the floor to steady yourself.

5. Hold the pose for 15 to 20 seconds. Breathe diaphragmatically. Be aware of the feeling of living energy coursing through your body.

6. Inhaling, lift yourself into an upright position. As you continue to inhale, raise your arms straight in the air, lean backward, and look up at the ceiling.

7. Exhaling, return to an upright position and lower your arms. Note how your body feels.

8. Repeat the Angle Pose, this time placing your left foot about three feet forward. Remember not to bend your knees.

If you have trouble balancing in the full pose, place your left hand on your right leg (the leg that's extended forward) to steady yourself. Put your right hand on your back above your right hip. This will help support your weight.

 FYI Want to know which yoga postures India's yogis recommend for particular ailments? Or how using props can help you progress in your yoga practice? Try *Yoga: The Path to Holistic Health* by B.K.S. Iyengar. Iyengar is widely considered one of the greatest Hatha Yoga masters of the twentieth century.

TRIANGLE POSE

Trikonasana, or the Triangle Pose, is a deep side bend. It's a very popular pose in the yoga tradition because it provides a superb stretch for all the muscles on the outer sides of the body. The posture also stretches and compresses your abdominal organs, aiding in digestion and elimination.

Note that while in the Angle Pose, you placed one foot a giant step in front of the other, but in the Triangle Posture your feet are placed out to the side from each other.

1. Stand up straight with your legs two and a half to three feet apart. Your left toes point straight forward, your right toes should point out away from your body at about a 45-degree angle to help you keep your balance.

2. Inhaling, raise your arms directly out to your sides. Keep your arms straight. Your palms should face downward.

3. Exhaling, bend directly to the right until your right hand reaches your right leg or foot. Don't tilt forward or backward, but keep your entire body in one plane.

4. Lift your left arm so that it points straight upward. Stretch out through your fingertips. Turn your head to the left so that you are looking up at the ceiling.

5. Hold the pose for 5 to 20 seconds, if you can do so comfortably. Be aware of your breath. If you feel any tremors in your body, ease up on the posture a little bit.

6. Inhaling, raise your body back up to a vertical position, with your arms pointing straight out to your sides.

7. Exhaling, bend to the left till your left hand reaches your left leg or foot. Point your right arm straight upward and turn your head to the right.

8. Hold the pose for 5 to 20 seconds. Don't strain. Breathe diaphragmatically.

9. Inhaling, lift your upper body back up to a vertical position.

10. Exhaling, lower your arms and move your legs back, together into the Mountain Pose. Relax for a moment, sensing the energy in your arms, legs, and side muscles.

The Triangle Pose.

(Photo credit: Alex Fernandez & Evolution Visual Services)

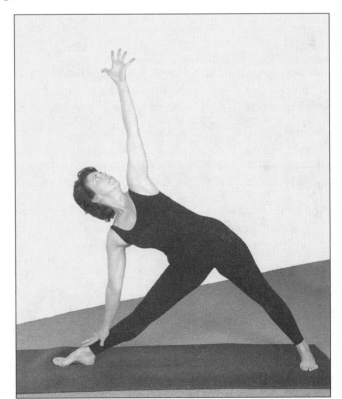

This pose helps adjust the vertebrae in your lower back, including your *sacrum*, as well as stretching the muscles in the back of your legs. It also gently flexes your hip joints.

STRICTLY DEFINED

The **sacrum** is the bony bottom portion of your spine. It's a composite of five vertebrae at the bottom of your spinal column that are fused together into one unit.

One of the most notable benefits of the Triangle Pose is the powerful stretch it provides for each side of your body. To deepen this stretch, try the posture again. This time, after holding your free arm directly upward in the pose, turn your head forward and swing the arm down till it's positioned next to your ear. Stretch the arm through your fingertips, feeling the stretch through that whole side of your body. (Your other hand is still holding on to your leg or foot.) Hold the pose for a few moments, and see how this feels different from the first version of the Triangle Pose. Then return to a standing position and relax.

Now you're ready to progress to the twisting postures.

REVOLVING TRIANGLE

The Revolving Triangle is a popular yoga pose that has several variants. Here you'll learn a version called *Parivritta Trikonasana*, which literally means "twisting triangle pose."

JUST A MINUTE

In the Revolving Triangle, resist the temptation to twist and bend from the middle of your torso. If you do this, it's unlikely you'll be able to reach your leg with your opposite hand. The twist should come from your hip area. This will allow you to both twist and bend down much farther.

1. Begin standing in the Mountain Pose. Then step your feet three feet apart (or farther, if you're tall). Your toes should point forward.

2. Inhaling, raise your arms directly out to your sides. Stretch out through your fingertips. In this pose, your palms face forward.

3. Exhaling, bend at your hip and twist downward so that your right hand touches your left foot (or your left leg, if that's more comfortable). Keep your arms and legs straight.

4. Extend your left arm straight upward. Turn your head to face up toward your left hand.

5. Hold the pose from 5 to 15 seconds, depending on your comfortable capacity. Breathe diaphragmatically. Scan your body and relax any tense muscle that's not directly involved in maintaining the posture.

6. Inhaling, lift your torso back into an upright position.

7. Exhaling, lower your arms to your sides and bring your legs together.

8. Repeat the Revolving Triangle, twisting down to the right this time.

The Revolving Triangle.

(Photo credit: Alex Fernandez & Evolution Visual Services)

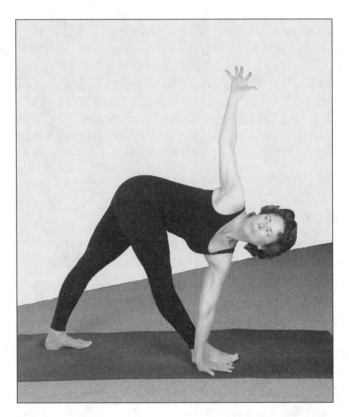

Beginners often cannot reach their leg with their other hand when they hold this posture correctly. That's okay. Move into the pose only as far as you can comfortably. Over the course of the next few weeks, you'll be impressed at how much deeper into the posture you'll be able to go.

FYI *Structural Yoga Therapy: Adapting to the Individual* by Mukunda Stiles will help you understand anatomy and kinesiology in relation to Hatha Yoga. It lays out a program of 24 yoga postures for use in maintaining health and achieving healing.

TORSO TWIST

Tadasana Parshvabhangi or the Torso Twist is perhaps the easiest of all yoga twisting exercises. Yet to hold it correctly you must enter and remain in the posture consciously. When the Torso Twist is held properly, it gives a complete twist to the entire spinal column, helping to enliven your nervous system.

1. Stand in the Mountain Pose. Extend your arms out to your sides, stretching through your fingertips. Your palms should face downward.

2. Exhaling, twist from your hips as far as you can to the right. Your arms continue pointing straight out to your side. Your knees should still be pointing forward. The twist starts at your pelvis, not your legs.

3. Turn your neck as far to the right as you can comfortably.

4. Hold the pose for 10 to 30 seconds, depending on your capacity. Breathe diaphragmatically.

5. Inhaling, swivel back to face forward again.

6. Exhaling, lower your arms. Notice the rush of energy through your body caused by the posture's stimulation of your nervous system.

7. Repeat the Torso Twist, twisting left this time.

Don't rush through the Torso Twist, but move into the posture with awareness. Feel the twisting motion from the root of your spine to the top of your neck. The lower vertebrae of your spinal column will participate more fully in the pose if you twist from the bottom of your pelvis rather than from your legs, as you may unconsciously be tempted to do. Keep your knees facing forward to prevent this from happening.

JUST A MINUTE

Many bending and twisting yoga postures require you to do the pose twice, the first time holding the position to the right, the second time to the left. Try to maintain the posture for about the same amount of time in both directions. This tones both sides of the body equally.

Try this more advanced version of the Torso Twist to make the pose more challenging. When you start the posture in the Mountain Pose, stand on your toes. Stay on your tiptoes throughout the exercise. This is not as easy as you might suppose and will demand extra concentration.

The Torso Twist is a remarkably energizing posture. Be sure to take the time to twist in both directions, so the stretch to your spine is balanced.

The Torso Twist.

(Photo credit: Alex Fernandez & Evolution Visual Services)

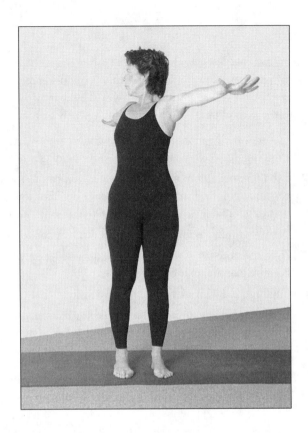

HALF SPINAL TWIST

GO TO ▷
Kundalini is the energy of consciousness that galvanizes the brain to higher states of awareness. You'll learn more about this form of energy and the way yogis work with it in Hour 18.

The Half Spinal Twist or *Ardha Matsyendrasana* (*ardha* means "half") is usually the most complex posture new students learn in a beginning-level Hatha Yoga class. You'll learn two versions in this hour. The first is for students who're not very flexible. The second is a more advanced variation, and it should be practiced only by more supple students.

This pose is named after the great Indian sage Matsyendra, who used the Full Spinal Twist, together with advanced breathing techniques, to help raise the kundalini or spiritual energy in his spine.

1. Sit cross-legged on the floor. Rest your left palm on your right knee. Place your right hand (or your right fingertips, if your arms are short) on the floor immediately behind the center of your back.

2. Inhaling, gently push up with your right hand to help you straighten your back as much as possible.

3. Exhaling, twist your back around to the right as far as you can comfortably. Turn your head farther to the right. This motion should come from your back muscles themselves, not from your arms.

4. Hold the posture from 10 to 20 seconds, as long as you feel comfortable.

5. Inhaling, twist back to face the front.

6. Place your hands in your lap and breathe slowly and smoothly. How does your back feel? How about your abdomen? Are your arms and legs relaxed?

7. Repeat the posture with your right hand on your left knee and your left hand directly behind your back, twisting to the left this time.

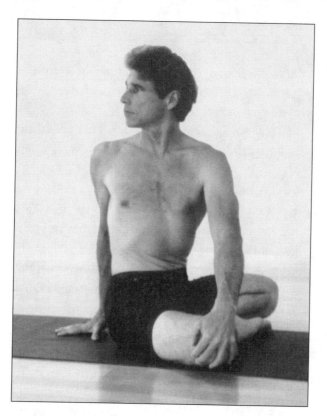

The Half Spinal Twist, version 1.

(Photo credit: Johnathan Brown)

There are numerous versions of the Half Spinal Twist. See if you are comfortable in the following one.

The Half Spinal Twist, version 2.

(Photo credit: Alex Fernandez & Evolution Visual Services)

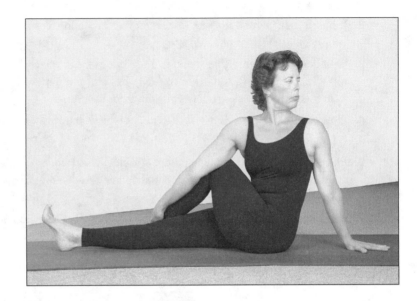

1. Sit on the floor in the Staff Pose, which you learned in Hour 6.

2. Lift your left foot over your right leg and position it against the outside of your right upper thigh.

3. Inhaling, twist your torso to the left. Twist from the pelvis.

4. Rest your left hand on the floor about six inches behind your left hip.

5. Lift your right arm over your left knee and take hold of your left foot with your right hand.

6. Turn your head as far as possible to the left, looking over your left shoulder. Keep your back as straight as you can without a sense of strain.

7. Keep breathing! Hold the posture for 5 to 10 seconds.

8. Exhaling, release the twist and return to the Staff Pose.

9. Repeat the Half Spinal Twist, but exchange leg and arm positions, and twist to the right this time.

GO TO ▶
The Full Spinal Twist is an advanced posture. You'll learn how it's done in Hour 11. Long-limbed, limber students may already be capable of the full version of this pose, but others should work with the Half Spinal Twist for some months before attempting the full version.

The Half Spinal Twist may be particularly challenging for students with petite-length arms and legs, for the obese, and for individuals who are quite stiff. Work with the first version of the posture, which is accessible to just about everyone if the second one is too difficult.

The Half Spinal Twist is excellent for improving the health and elasticity of the spinal column. Because it provides a powerful twist for the abdominal organs, it promotes digestion and elimination of wastes. Both the kidneys and intestines benefit.

RECLINING TWIST

Now lie back on the floor for the Reclining Twist. You'll learn two versions of this posture. The first is especially for strengthening your abdominal muscles while enhancing the suppleness of your middle and lower spine. The second variation works the entire spine.

The Reclining Twist is called *Jathara Parivartanasana* in Sanskrit. *Jathara* means "stomach," and *parivartana* means "flipped around." This is another of the yoga poses in which you'll be in motion throughout the exercise.

1. Lie on the floor in the Corpse Posture, which you learned in Hour 3.

2. Extend your arms out directly to your sides, keeping your arms straight and your palms down. You will be using your arms to brace your body in this posture.

3. Lift your knees but keep your feet flat on the floor. Keep your legs together throughout this exercise.

4. Keeping your head, arms, shoulders, and upper back in the same place on the floor, lower your knees to your right toward the floor. In one continuous movement, raise your knees back up and lower them to the left toward the floor. Raise them back up.

5. Roll your legs from one side to the other 10 to 20 times. Breathe diaphragmatically. Enjoy the massaging sensation in your middle and lower back.

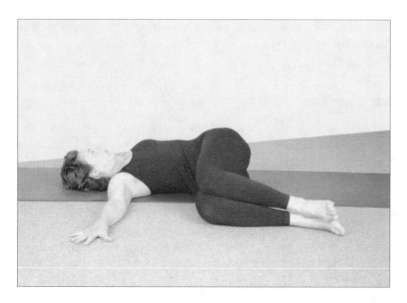

The Reclining Twist.

(Photo credit: Alex Fernandez & Evolution Visual Services)

Now try the more advanced version of the same posture. In this variation, you will hold still in the pose rather than moving back and forth.

1. Lie on the floor with your arms extended straight out to your sides, palms facing downward. Your legs should be straight with your feet together.

2. Place your right foot on your left knee. Keep your left leg straight.

3. Roll to the left so that your right knee moves downward toward the floor to the left of your left knee. Swing from your pelvis. Your shoulders and arms don't move—they stay in the same position on the floor throughout this pose.

4. Turn your head to the right. Keep your shoulders and arms squarely on the floor in their original position.

5. Hold the pose and relax deeply for 15 to 20 seconds. Feel the twist along your entire spine. Breathe diaphragmatically.

6. Return to your starting position. Repeat the pose, stretching in the opposite direction this time.

Relaxing into the Reclining Twist is a great way to get the kinks out of your back. This pose should be comfortable. If any part of your body feels strained, back off a bit till you can lie in the position at ease.

STRAIGHTEN YOUR BACK

After all these back-bending and torso-twisting postures, it's time to learn a yoga exercise that massages the spinal column and relieves tension in the back muscles.

ROCKING CHAIR ROLL

Yogis in India use the Rocking Chair Roll both before and after a series of exercises. By stretching your back muscles and limbering the spinal column, it prepares the body for back-bending and twisting poses. After the session, it helps relieve residual strain in the back.

PROCEED WITH CAUTION

Before attempting the Rocking Chair Roll, make sure there are no objects (furniture, other yoga students, etc.) for at least three feet in front of you and five feet behind you. You don't want to accidentally hit something or someone during the rolling movement.

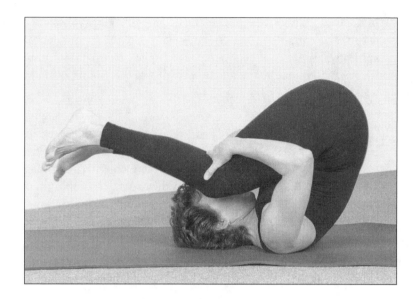

The Rocking Chair Roll.

(Photo credit: Alex Fernandez & Evolution Visual Services)

1. Sit on a cushioned surface, such as a carpet or yoga mat. Don't do the Rocking Chair Roll on a hard, unpadded surface.

2. Sit in the Staff Pose. Lift your knees and grasp the underside of your thighs near the knees. Your feet remain flat on the floor.

3. Round your back and lower your chin.

4. Roll backward toward your shoulders. As your feet come up off the floor, straighten your legs part way. This adds momentum and helps you roll back a little farther. Do not roll all the way back as if you were doing a backward somersault.

5. Without stopping, begin to roll forward again, bending your knees once more as you roll. This adds momentum in the forward direction.

6. Roll back and forth 5 to 10 times.

7. Sit back up in the Staff Pose. Allow your breathing to return to normal.

RESPECT YOUR SPINE

The spinal column is the second most important part of your nervous system. Only your brain itself is more vital. The spine is the nerve channel that connects the master glands and gray matter of the brain to the rest of your body. Most of your sensory nerves, which are responsible for feeling your body and the world around it, as well as most of your motor nerves, which allow you to move and handle objects, "hook up" to your brain through this conduit. Nearly every Hatha Yoga exercise is designed to work with the spine.

GO TO ▶
While yoga postures are ideal for exercising the spinal column, yogis use concentration and meditation techniques to exercise their brains. Hour 15 will introduce you to the yogic world of "exercise without movement" where exercise occurs in the field of consciousness itself.

In the yoga tradition, the health of the spine is a primary concern. So is the posture you typically sit, stand, and walk in. Do you slump when you stand up? Do you tilt to one side when you sit? Yogis note that poor posture affects the field of awareness. You are not as alert when you don't hold your head, neck, and trunk straight.

One major purpose of the many yoga postures, including the angle poses and twists taught in this hour, is to build strength and flexibility into the spinal column so that you can sit, stand, and walk with your head, neck, and trunk in a straight line. That's something no creature on earth other than *homo sapiens* can do. Yogis claim that only in the human can kundalini or the energy of consciousness flow fully. They say this is in part because of our vertical spinal column, which is capable of conducting kundalini more freely than an animal's horizontal spine.

In Hour 9, you'll turn your attention to yoga exercises that firm and tone your abdominal muscles, while exercising your inner abdominal organs.

HOUR'S UP!

QUIZ

Here's a quiz to help you review some of the ideas and practices presented during this hour. Answer true or false to the following statements:

1. Twisting postures have a "wringing" effect on your internal organs.
2. The Angle Pose involves moving one leg forward from the other while the Triangle requires you to move your legs to the side from each other.
3. The Half Spinal Twist requires you to stand on your toes and twist half way around to your side.
4. It's best to do the Rocking Chair Roll directly on a hard surface like a wood or cement floor.
5. The Revolving Triangle is far more effective if you twist from the middle of your torso rather than from your hips.
6. The Torso Twist gives a complete twist to the entire spinal column.
7. The spinal column is the channel linking most of your body with your brain.
8. Yogis aim to sit and stand with their backs straight but relaxed.
9. If you feel tremors while holding a yoga posture, you should continue holding the pose till the tremors stop.
10. Yoga twisting poses massage the abdominal organs.

HOUR 9

Strengthen Your Abdomen

CHAPTER SUMMARY

LESSON PLAN:
In this hour you will learn ...

- Maintaining the health and motility of the abdominal organs is a top priority in Hatha Yoga.
- The Stomach Lift and Stomach Roll provide a deep internal massage to the stomach and intestines.
- The Leg Lift and Balance Pose develop strength and firmness in the abdominal muscles.
- Excellent digestion and proper elimination of waste are imperative for physical vitality and mental clarity.
- Precautions must be taken before undertaking the extremely powerful abdominal exercises of Hatha Yoga.

Modern Western society devotes a lot of attention to the abdominal area. If you want to look good your tummy must be firm. The exercise industry has made hundreds of millions of dollars peddling devices that are supposed to help you tone your abs.

The yoga tradition also focuses on the abdomen, though for different reasons. In yoga, the concern was never so much about how you look as how you feel. When your body is in top shape, your mind is free to focus on the attainment of your life goals. You're much less distracted by disease, injury, and the general aches and pains associated with life in a physical body. Also, your awareness is clearer because your liver and intestines have effectively removed the toxins that cloud your consciousness, and excess energy is not being wasted on digestion. The fact that you look better when your body is healthier was simply a happy by-product of yoga to the ancient adepts. A trim, radiant body was a signal that you were making good progress in your yoga practice.

MAINTAIN YOUR CENTER

Ayurvedic physicians, the native Hindu doctors of India, believe that many disease processes, even some that appear completely unrelated, begin in one of three sites in the body: the stomach, small intestine, or colon.

- An unhealthy stomach can lead to bloating, indigestion, and a sense of physical, mental, and emotional lassitude.

GO TO ▶
The traditional medical system of India is called *Ayurveda,* which literally means "the knowledge that bestows a long life." You'll learn more about Ayurveda in Hour 20.

- An unhealthy small intestine is associated with fever, hyperacidity, anger, and irritability.

- An unhealthy colon is said to produce constipation, gas, fatigue, insomnia, and an anxious, fearful, unsettled mental state.

The abdominal exercises taught in yoga not only tone your abs, they also work the organs responsible for digestion and elimination. When your stomach and gut are in good working order, your energy level improves significantly, your skin begins to clear up, and your mood is lifted.

MASTERING THE ABDOMINAL POSES

When Swami Rama of the Himalayas, one of the best known yogis of the twentieth century, was asked which one yoga posture was the most important for people in Western countries, he responded, "They should all do *Uddiyana Bandha* (the Stomach Lift)." When asked why, he explained, "People in the West eat mostly refined foods. They don't get enough fiber and they don't get enough exercise. So their digestive fire is weak. Because of this they become sick. If they did no other asanas at all, but still did Uddiyana Bandha, they would be much healthier."

The abdominal exercises described in this hour are powerful, deep-acting poses that have a dramatic effect on the body. For most people, they're superb health promoters. But the very fact that they're so powerful also means they must be undertaken with special care. The precautions you need to respect if you're going to do a Hatha Yoga routine were outlined in Hour 2. However, several vitally important points bear repeating especially in the context of these deep-acting postures:

- People who have serious abdominal conditions such as a hernia or colitis should not do these poses.

- People who have blood pressure imbalances should avoid these poses unless they are approved by a doctor.

- People who have a heart condition should avoid these poses unless they are approved by a physician.

- Women: Never do the abdominal poses while you are menstruating. There is a small chance these poses could cause hemorrhaging if you do them during your menstrual period.

- Women: Do not do the abdominal poses if you are pregnant.

- Don't attempt these postures if you've just eaten. Ideally, at least four hours should have passed since your last meal.

If you have any questions about whether your medical condition might be adversely affected by these deep-acting exercises, consult your doctor!

 FYI The postures in this hour are not for women who are pregnant. If you're expecting, "Prenatal Yoga" from Gaian, Inc. (put together by the folks at *Yoga Journal*), is a video you'll want to see. Yoga instructor Shiva Rea advises you how to work with the special needs of your changing body, and teaches yoga exercises that will help you prepare for labor and delivery.

Stomach Lift

The Stomach Lift, or *Uddiyana Bandha* (*Uddiyana* means "moving upward," and *Bandha* means "lock"), is one of the most highly praised of all yoga postures. Indian yogis claim there is no internal organ that doesn't benefit from this powerful exercise.

The first version of the Stomach Lift is one of the extremely few yoga poses in which you will be asked to hold your breath.

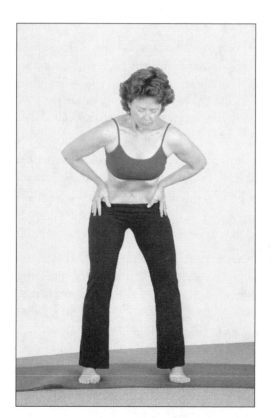

The Stomach Lift.

(Photo credit: Alex Fernandez & Evolution Visual Services)

1. Stand with your feet about two feet apart. While bending your knees slightly, lean forward from your pelvis. Your back should be straight.

2. Put your palms on your thighs just above your knees.

3. Exhale forcefully, pressing as much air out of your lungs as you can.

4. Without inhaling, drop your head forward, pressing your chin into your throat.

5. Vigorously pull your abdominal muscles in and up. This pulls your entire stomach area backward in the direction of your spine.

6. Hold the posture until you need to take a breath. Then release your abdominal muscles and lift your head. Breathe!

7. Repeat the Stomach Lift three more times.

Lowering your chin against the hollow of your throat is called the Chin Lock or *Jalandhara Bandha* in the yoga tradition (*Jala* refers to the nerves in the back of the neck, while *Dhara* means "pulling upward"). Lowering your chin helps prevent you from breathing in or out during exercises in which it's important that you hold your breath. It also pulls the top of the spinal column upward.

Here is a second, more dynamic version of the Stomach Lift. Many yogis practice both versions during the same yoga session for their slightly different effects. This variation gives a more vigorous massage to your internal organs. You will keep breathing during this exercise. Your breath will be forceful, similar to the breathing technique called the Bellows, which you learned in Hour 4.

1. Hunch over your slightly bent legs with your hands resting on your thighs, as directed in the previous version. Do not bend your back!

2. Exhale vigorously, forcefully lifting your abdominal muscles in and up.

3. Inhale quickly, allowing your abdominal muscles to fall back into their normal place.

4. Continue forcefully exhaling and inhaling, as you lift and release your abdominal region. Repeat this 8 to 20 times, depending on your comfortable capacity. If you feel yourself getting dizzy or lightheaded, stop immediately!

5. Stand up in the Mountain Pose and allow your breathing rate to return to normal. Be aware of the movement of energy in your abdominal region.

STOMACH ROLL

Nauli or the Stomach Roll is an advanced version of the Stomach Lift. Some students pick it up quickly, others never quite get the hang of it. It seems to be like that trick of rolling the tongue into a cigar shape that some children learn in grade school and others never master.

Nauli involves a great deal of concentration in the beginning. You need to be able to isolate the muscles on the right side of your abdomen from those on your left side. Most people go through their entire lives without ever needing to do this, so this is a new and for some people difficult skill to pick up. However, it provides a thorough massage for your abdominal organs and works the muscles of your stomach area like no other exercise—yogic, aerobic, or calisthenic—can do.

You will need to hold your breath during this exercise. Never hold it longer than your comfortable capacity.

1. Stand with your feet about two feet apart. Lean forward from your pelvis, keeping your back straight. Your legs should be slightly bent.

2. Put your palms on your thighs just above your knees. This is the same starting position as the Stomach Lift.

3. Exhale completely. You will hold your breath through the rest of this exercise.

4. Lift the abdominal muscles on the right side of your abdomen in and up. Then release them. The muscles on the left side of your abdomen remain relaxed throughout this step.

5. Lift the abdominal muscles on the left side of your abdomen in and up. Then release them. The muscles on the right side of your abdomen remain relaxed throughout this step.

6. Relax your belly, stand up straight, and take a few breaths. Then repeat steps 4 and 5 three more times, pausing when you need to take a breath.

When advanced students do the Stomach Roll, you will see the muscles in their abdomen contracting and releasing in a rolling fashion, as if a wave were moving over their abdominal area.

LEG LIFT

The single Leg Lift is called *Utthita Ekapadasana* in Sanskrit (*eka* means "one"). The double Leg Lift is called *Utthita Dvipadasana* (*dvi* means "two"). *Pada* is Sanskrit for "leg" or "foot," and *utthita* means "upward motion."

The Leg Lift.

(Photo credit: Alex Fernandez & Evolution Visual Services)

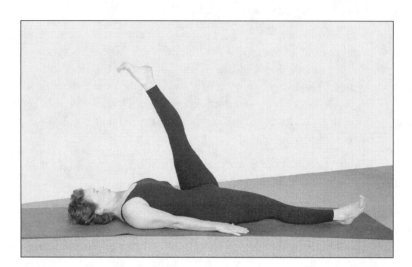

1. Lie on your back on the floor with your hands by your sides, palms down. Your legs should be straight.

2. Inhaling, lift your right leg upward very slowly (for the full length of your inhalation). Keep lifting until it's lifted straight up.

3. The moment you begin exhaling, very slowly lower your right leg back to the floor.

4. Repeat the Leg Lift, raising your left leg this time.

5. Repeat the exercise alternating both legs three more times. Then relax in the Corpse Pose.

JUST A MINUTE

If the Leg Lift is difficult for you, before lifting your right leg, bend your left leg at the knee and rest the sole of your left foot on the floor. This will take some of the strain off the muscles in your lower abdomen. Reverse legs and repeat the exercise lifting your left leg.

Use the muscles in the lower section of your abdomen, as well as those in the thigh muscles of the leg you're raising, to accomplish this posture. Avoid the temptation to roll slightly to the side and brace yourself on the other leg while you hold your leg up.

There are several worthwhile variations to the Leg Lift, though these are more challenging. The first is to lift both legs at the same time. Keep the parts of your body that are not involved in lifting your legs relaxed. Breathe diaphragmatically.

The second variation is to lift one leg at a time as you inhale, but hold it steady four to five inches above the floor rather than raising it farther. Hold the pose for several breaths, then lower the leg on an exhalation. This is superb for conditioning the muscles of the lower abdomen, but is a surprisingly demanding pose to hold if you're not already quite fit.

The third version is for the most limber students. Lift only one leg at a time; make sure the other remains flat on the floor. As you lift your leg, simultaneously raise your head, neck, and shoulder area up off the floor. Grasp your raised shin with your hands and press your head into your raised thigh. Hold for about 15 seconds, being careful not to strain yourself. Then release and relax.

At the beginning level, a little bit of cheating in yoga is okay, provided you know what you're doing and don't inadvertently hurt yourself. If it's too difficult to keep your legs straight during a pose, it's okay to bend them a little—you won't cause any harm. However, you should be aware that this does detract from the overall value of the pose. Try to work toward being able to keep your legs completely straight at some point in the future.

 FYI One of the easiest and clearest introductions to Hatha Yoga is put out by *Yoga Journal* magazine. Check out *Yoga Journal's Yoga Basics* by Mara Carrico for an excellent overview of the fundamental postures taught in the yoga tradition.

BALANCE POSE

Utthita Hastapadasana means "the posture in which the hands and feet are raised" (*Utthita* means "raised," *hasta* means "hand," and *pada* means "foot"). In this pose you balance on your hips, which is why it's generally called the Balance Pose in English.

The moment you first hold this yoga posture you will instantly understand why the yogis say it's so good for strengthening your abdominal muscles. You'll feel them working hard. Because this is a strenuous workout for those muscles, begin by holding the pose for only a few seconds. You are better off holding the pose for just a moment, relaxing, and repeating it again than straining to hold the posture longer and then not having the strength to repeat it a second time.

The Balance Pose.

(Photo credit: Alex Fernandez & Evolution Visual Services)

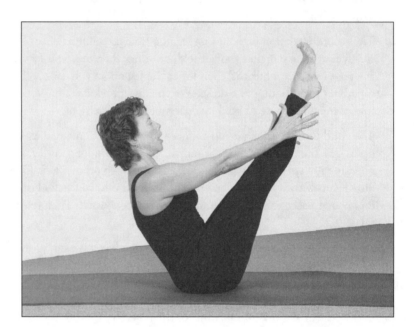

1. Lie on the floor with your legs straight and your arms at your sides.

2. Inhaling, lift your legs upward till they point diagonally in the air. Keep your legs straight.

3. At the same time, lift your torso up off the floor so that only the bottom of your pelvis remains on the ground. Keep your arms straight, positioned horizontally so that they're parallel to the floor. Your palms face downward. Stretch out through your fingertips. Your body should look like a V with your arms extended like a crossbar horizontally through the middle of the V.

4. Hold the pose for 5 to 10 seconds. Do not hold your breath! Be aware of the sensations in your body, and adjust any muscle groups that feel overly strained.

5. Exhaling, lower your body back to the floor.

6. Relax for a moment, breathing evenly. Then repeat the Balance Pose three more times.

If you've been working out in the gym or doing crunches at home, your abdominal muscles may already be in good shape. In that case, try a more challenging version of the Balance Pose.

1. Sit on the floor in the Staff Pose, which you learned in Hour 6. Lean backward, keeping your back straight.

2. At the same time, place your palms on the floor about six inches behind you. They should be positioned, palms down, just to the outside of your hips.

3. Using your arms to support your torso and inhaling slowly, lift your legs into the air till they point in a steep diagonal line. Keep them straight. Don't raise your legs all the way up into a vertical position; if you do, your legs will be braced against your pelvis on the floor and you will lose the toning effect of this posture. Keep your legs together. Stretch out through your toes.

4. Hold the pose for 5 to 10 seconds. Keep breathing!

5. Exhaling, lower your legs. Return to the Staff Pose and relax for a moment. Feel the energy in your stomach area.

6. Repeat this version of the Balance Pose three more times.

Because you are supporting the upper half of your body with your arms, you can lift your legs much higher in this second variation of the Balance Pose. This gives more of a workout to your lower abdominal muscles.

You're now ready to go on to Part 3, in which you'll be introduced to some intermediate and advanced level postures. You'll also learn how to set up a yoga routine that's designed specifically for you.

Hour's Up!

Here is the quiz for Hour 9. How many points from this hour can you remember? Answer true or false to the following statements:

1. You should hold your breath while you're doing the first version of the Stomach Lift.

2. In the more dynamic version of the Stomach Lift, you should breathe forcefully, as you did in the Bellows Breathing exercise.

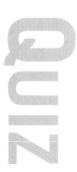

QUIZ

3. The Stomach Roll involves isolating the muscles on both sides of your chest.

4. Women benefit most from abdominal exercises by doing them during their menstrual periods.

5. The Stomach Lift is particularly effective in helping to treat hernias.

6. If you lift your legs all the way into a vertical position in the Balance Pose, you will lose much of the toning effect on your abdominal region.

7. In the Leg Lift, you should raise your leg to a vertical position and hold it there for one or two minutes.

8. The Chin Lock helps you take deeper, more even breaths.

9. Ayurvedic doctors believe many disease processes begin in the stomach, small intestine, and colon.

10. Indian physicians associate an unhealthy colon with constipation, gas, and an unsettled mental state.

PART III

More Challenging Yoga Poses

HOUR 10   Intermediate Hatha Yoga

HOUR 11   Advanced Hatha Yoga

HOUR 12   Flowing Postures

HOUR 13   Your Hatha Routine

HOUR 10

Intermediate Hatha Yoga

CHAPTER SUMMARY

LESSON PLAN:
In this hour you will learn ...

- Intermediate level yoga postures build on the poses you already learned in the beginning level hours.

- The Eagle and the King Dancer Postures promote the development of concentration and poise.

- The Back Bending Monkey Posture is an advanced variation of the Lunge Stretch.

- The Camel is the intermediate posture between the simple Backward Bend and the advanced Wheel Pose.

- Use common sense in testing your ability to move into more difficult poses.

Now it's time to begin building on the fundamental postures you've already learned. The Standing Backward Bend, which you learned in Hour 7, as well as the Fish, Arch, and Bridge Postures from Hour 5, have prepared you for the Camel and the Inclined Plane. The Tree Posture from Hour 3 was the foundation for the Eagle. The Lunge Stretch, which you practiced in Hour 2, will help you assume the Back Bending Monkey Pose.

The Sitting Forward Bend from Hour 7 helped you develop the flexibility you need to correctly assume the Archer Posture. And when you begin practicing the King Dancer Pose, you may experience a mental attitude similar to the one you cultivated in the Warrior Pose during Hour 6.

EXPAND YOUR LIMITS

In this book and most other yoga manuals you see, as well as in most yoga classes you may take, you will continually be asked to remain mentally present as you hold the postures. You need to be aware of what's happening with your body, what's going on with your breath, and what's transpiring in your mind. Remaining in an attentive state has three purposes:

- By constantly monitoring your muscles and other internal tissues and organs, you can prevent injuries while gently guiding yourself further into a posture day by day or week by week.

- Maintaining an inward focus teaches you to become sensitive to your energy state, a level of their being most people ignore.
- Focusing your awareness inward introduces you to yourself and prepares you for more advanced concentration and meditation techniques.

In yoga as it's classically taught, it's important to be gentle with yourself. That does not mean, however, that you should be complacent. In India, hatha yogis achieve dramatic levels of physiologic control. They can virtually stop their heartbeat for minutes at a time and slow their respiration to one or two breaths a minute for hours on end. They achieve these extraordinary accomplishments one step at a time, mastering one stage completely before moving on to the next. But they don't stop until they have achieved their goal of complete self-mastery.

Most people in the West are not interested in attaining the same level of proficiency as the yoga masters of India. Good health and a firm, toned body is a more common goal for Westerners. The postures you've already learned are enough to contribute significantly to your health and well-being. If you're interested in learning more, developing a finer level of attunement to your body as well as greater strength and suppleness, then either now or at some more appropriate time in the future you will want to move on to Intermediate and Advanced level yoga postures.

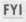 **FYI** The late Swami Vishnu-Devananda is author of two yoga classics: *The Sivananda Companion to Yoga,* which has sold more than 700,000 copies; and *The Complete Illustrated Book of Yoga.* Vishnu-Devananda was a famous hatha yogi and peace activist who was a disciple of the great Indian saint Swami Sivananda.

MASTERING THE INTERMEDIATE POSTURES

In this hour, you will learn six new postures and their variants. Use common sense in testing whether you are ready for these new poses. If you feel discomfort, or if your body simply won't stretch that far, or you just can't balance on one foot that long, continue working with the beginning level postures. Remember, beginning poses are not less effective than more advanced ones. They're just easier to do!

INCLINED PLANE POSTURE

Purvottanasana is the Inclined Plane Posture. *Purva* means "first" or "front of the body," and *uttana* means "stretch." The Inclined Plane Posture gives an excellent workout to your back muscles and helps to tone the muscles in your arms, abdomen, pelvis, and thighs. It also opens your shoulders and chest, facilitating respiration.

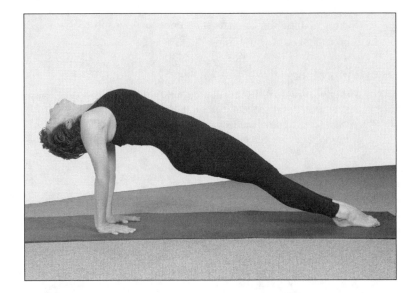

The Inclined Plane Posture.

(Photo credit: Alex Fernandez & Evolution Visual Services)

1. Sit on the floor in the Staff Pose, which you learned in Hour 6.

2. Lean backward. Put your hands on the floor about ten inches behind your hips.

3. Inhaling, lift your body until it forms a straight line pointed diagonally upward from your toes to your head. Only your hands and the soles of your feet remain on the floor. Your arms are straight. Let your head fall backward.

4. Hold the pose for 5 to 10 seconds. Breathe diaphragmatically. Pay attention to your body. Where do you feel surges of energy? Where do you feel strained? Try to stay as relaxed as you can while still maintaining the pose.

5. Exhaling, lower your hips to the floor and return to the Staff Pose.

When you become comfortable in this pose, try this variation. Holding the full posture, arch your back as far as you can without straining, and drop your head way back. This gives a superb stretch to your entire body.

CAMEL POSTURE

Ustrasana means "Camel Pose" in Sanskrit. This is a backward-bending exercise in which you will need to support yourself with your arms. This pose is terrific for helping increase the suppleness of your spine. It also helps ventilate the top lobes of your lungs.

PROCEED WITH CAUTION

 Some beginning students may never before in their lives have bent backward as far as the Camel Posture requires. If you think you're flexible enough to try it but bending that far still makes you feel uncomfortable, have a friend "spot" you, kneeling nearby to catch you in the unlikely event that you fall backward.

The Camel Posture.

(Photo credit: Alex Fernandez & Evolution Visual Services)

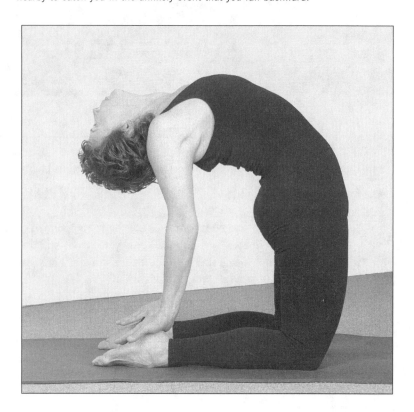

1. Kneel on the floor. Keep your legs together. Stretch upward through your head, neck, and trunk.

2. Inhaling, bend slowly backward from your waist. Reach straight down with your arms and catch hold of your ankles or rest your palms on the underside of your feet. Reach down with your right arm first, then your left. Your spine should be arched back.

3. Drop your head backward. Relax your neck.

4. Hold the pose for 10 to 30 seconds, depending on your capacity. Keep breathing! Be conscious of the way this posture makes your body feel.

5. Exhaling, lift yourself back up into a kneeling position. Take a few resting breaths, then repeat the posture one more time.

Don't rush into the pose! Take your time bending backward so you don't lose your balance or get dizzy. Bend from the top of your pelvis if you can.

In Hour 11, you will learn the ultimate backward-bending yoga exercise, called the Wheel. Don't even think about attempting the Wheel till you can hold the Camel comfortably for at least half a minute.

EAGLE POSTURE

Garudasana means Eagle Posture. (Garuda was the greatest of the eagles in Hindu mythology.) If you have a good sense of balance, this posture will be easy and fun. Don't attempt this pose unless you've already mastered the Tip Toe Stretch and the Tree Posture, which you learned in Hour 3. These preliminary balancing exercises will have prepared you for the Eagle Pose.

Balancing poses are important in yoga because they help you develop poise and concentration. The Eagle Pose in particular also develops strength in your ankles and flexibility in your arms, wrists, and shoulders.

1. Stand in the Mountain Pose, which you learned in Hour 3.

2. Bend your right leg slightly. You will be balancing on this leg, so don't bend too much! Then wrap your left leg around your right leg. Your left knee goes over and above your right knee. Your left foot wraps behind your right leg and rests above the outside of your right ankle.

3. Cross your left arm over your right arm so your arms form an X shape. Wrap them farther until your can place your palms together.

4. Hold the pose as long as you can without losing your balance. Work toward standing in the pose for 30 seconds.

5. Unwrap your arms and legs and return to the Mountain Pose. Relax for several breaths.

6. Repeat the Eagle Posture, standing on your left leg this time.

The Eagle Posture.

(Photo credit: Johnathan Brown)

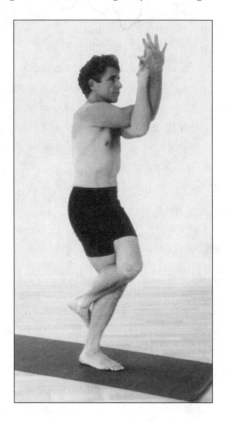

JUST A MINUTE

The Eagle and the King Dancer Postures, both require an excellent sense of balance. Do these postures in your bare feet. Keep your eyes open and fixed on an unmoving object in your line of sight. Don't allow your mind to wander. Remember, it's a balanced mental state that creates physical balance.

KING DANCER POSTURE

In the Indian tradition, the divine spirit is believed to be the greatest dancer of all. The eternal flux of matter and energy is said to be his dance. *Natarajasana* or the King Dancer Pose honors the endless balance of the divine nature as it swirls dynamically through all the cycles of time. *Nata* means "dance." *Raja* is Sanskrit for "king."

The King Dancer is another balancing pose, yet like the Warrior Posture it is a dynamic and assertive stance. Like the Eagle Posture, it helps you gain poise and concentration. It's also extremely good for loosening the pelvic ligaments.

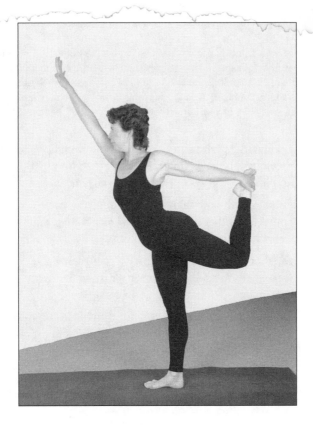

The King Dancer Pose.

(Photo credit: Alex Fernandez & Evolution Visual Services)

1. Stand up straight in the Mountain Pose.
2. Bending your right knee, lift your right foot up behind you toward the back of your pelvis. Keep your right thigh in line with your left leg.
3. Reach down with your right hand and grab your right foot, if you can do so without straining or losing your balance. Try to keep your back straight.
4. Inhaling, raise your left arm straight out in front of you, then upward till it points up straight in the air. Stretch through your left fingertips.
5. Keep your eyes trained on a point in front of you to help you keep your balance. Hold the pose as long as you can, up to 30 seconds. Be aware of your posture as well as your balance. Breathe diaphragmatically.

6. Exhaling, release your right foot and lower your left arm. Relax in the Mountain Pose for a moment.

7. Repeat this pose, lifting the left leg and right arm this time.

When you can hold this preliminary posture comfortably for 15 seconds or more, try extending yourself into the full posture.

FYI Some yoga students decide they'd like to learn a little about Sanskrit when they discover that the names of so many yoga techniques are in that language. The easiest and most fun introduction to Sanskrit is *First Lessons in Sanskrit Grammar and Reading* by Judith M. Tyberg. Numerous other introductory workbooks are also currently available, thanks to the widespread interest of yoga practitioners.

1. Assume the preliminary version of the King Dancer Pose as described previously, holding your right foot behind you with your right hand and lifting your left arm straight in the air.

2. Exhaling, tilt your body forward from your hips. Your left arm now points upward at a steep diagonal angle. Keep your back straight if possible. Watch your balance!

3. Inhaling, lift your right foot with your right hand till your right thigh is parallel to the floor. Your torso may shift slightly to the side, but keep your face and gaze directed forward.

4. Hold the pose as long as you can without losing your balance, as long as 30 seconds. Pay attention to the shifts of energy in your body. Keep breathing!

5. Inhaling, lift your back up straight.

6. Exhaling, release your right foot and lower your left arm. Relax in the Mountain Pose for a moment.

7. Repeat the King Dancer Pose, lifting the left leg and right arm this time.

Students with petite-length arms and legs need to be particularly flexible in order to assume this posture correctly.

ARCHER POSTURE

Akarna Dhanurasana is the Archer Posture (not to be confused with the Arch Posture you learned in Hour 5). *Dhanu* means "bow," and *akarna* means "ear." The prerequisite for this pose is the Sitting Forward Bend, which you practiced in Hour 7. If you can't hold the Sitting Forward Bend comfortably yet, practice it some more before you attempt the Archer Pose.

This yoga posture increases the flexibility of the muscles and joints in your legs.

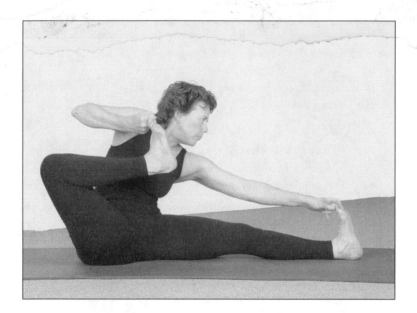

The Archer Posture.

(Photo credit: Alex Fernandez & Evolution Visual Services)

1. Sit on the floor in the Staff Pose.
2. Exhaling, lean forward from your hips and grasp your right big toe with your right index finger and your left big toe with your left index finger.
3. Inhaling, sit back up, pulling your right toe to your right ear. Keep your left leg straight on the floor. Your index fingers continue to grasp your toes.
4. Breathe diaphragmatically. Hold the pose for 15 to 30 seconds, or to your comfortable capacity.
5. Exhaling, bend forward, returning your right leg back to the starting position.
6. Inhaling, release your toes and sit back up straight. Relax for a few breaths. Be aware of how your body feels, especially your leg and lower back muscles.
7. Repeat the posture, bringing your left toe to your left ear this time.

GO TO ▶
If you find it difficult to lean forward far enough to grasp your toes, turn back to Hour 7 and spend some time practicing the Standing Forward Bend, the Sitting Forward Bend, the Symbol of Yoga, and Churn.

PROCEED WITH CAUTION

Never strain yourself in any new posture you're learning. You need to keep challenging yourself to continually improve in your yoga practice, but you don't need to hurt yourself! Avoid pulled muscles, strains, sprains, and falls by moving in and out of yoga postures attentively and by continually monitoring your body and breath while holding a pose.

If you can perform the Archer Pose comfortably, try this somewhat more challenging version.

1. Sit on the floor in the Staff Pose.

2. Exhaling, lean forward from your hips and grasp your left big toe with your right index finger. Now reach under your right arm with your left hand and grasp your right big toe with your left index finger.

3. Inhaling, sit back up, pulling your right toe to your left ear. Keep your left leg straight on the floor. You are still holding your left big toe with your right index finger.

4. Breathe smoothly and evenly. Hold the pose for 15 to 30 seconds, or to your comfortable capacity. Muscles in your body not directly involved in maintaining the posture should be relaxed.

5. Exhaling, bend forward, returning your right leg back to the starting position.

6. Inhaling, release your toes and sit back up in the Staff Pose.

7. Repeat the posture, bringing your left toe to your right ear this time.

In both poses you are imitating an archer who pulls a bowstring back to her ear before firing the arrow represented by your straight arm.

BACK BENDING MONKEY POSTURE

The Monkey Posture is called *Banarasana* by traditional yogis (*Banara* means "monkey"). Some yoga teachers call this the Crescent Moon posture because your arms, back, and backward-pointing leg form a crescent shape.

This pose stretches the pelvis as well as the thighs. It also gives a good stretching bend to the spine.

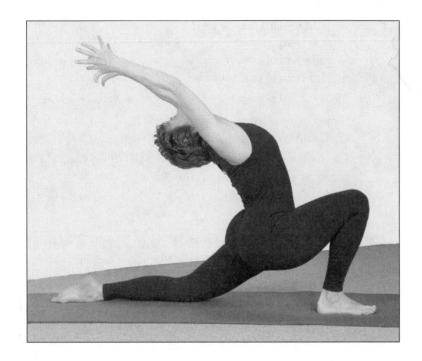

The Back Bending Monkey Posture.

(Photo credit: Alex Fernandez & Evolution Visual Services)

1. Begin on all fours with your hands and knees on the floor. Your arms should be straight, with your hands positioned beneath your shoulders. Your knees should be slightly apart, positioned beneath your hips.

2. Bring your right foot forward so that it rests between your hands.

3. Extend your left leg out behind you, resting your left knee on the floor.

4. Inhaling, lift your torso straight up and drop your head backward so that you are looking up at the ceiling. At the same time, stretch your arms straight out in front of you, then lift them straight up over your head. Press your palms together in the *Namaste* position.

STRICTLY DEFINED

Hindus greet each other with the phrase **"Namaste!"** which means, "I bow to the divinity in you." At the same time they press their palms together, fingers pointed upward, in front of their hearts to express affection and respect.

5. Hold the pose for a breath or two. Relax and adjust your body so that no part of it feels excessively strained.

GO TO ▶

The variation of the Monkey Posture you're learning here begins from the Lunge Stretch, which you practiced in Hour 2. Don't proceed to the Monkey Pose if you had difficulty with the Lunge Stretch. Instead, continue to work with other stretching and bending exercises till your legs develop more strength and flexibility.

6. Now arch your spine backward, lowering your head and neck backward as well. Your arms move backward, too, following your ears. Watch your balance! In the full pose, your spine will be flexed backward enough so that your arms point directly behind you.

7. Hold the full posture for 10 to 20 seconds. Keep breathing.

8. On an exhalation, raise your torso and head back to an upright position, with your arms and fingers pointing up at the ceiling.

9. On your next exhalation, lower your arms to the floor and return your legs to an all fours crawling position.

10. Repeat the posture with your right leg backward and your left foot forward this time.

In Hour 11, you'll learn some advanced Hatha Yoga postures that demand exceptional upper arm strength and flexibility.

HOUR'S UP!

Test your understanding of the content of this hour with the following quiz. Answer true or false to the following statements:

1. When holding the King Dancer and the Eagle Postures, it's helpful to keep your eyes focused on an unmoving object in your line of sight.

2. The Archer Posture is remarkably similar to the Arch Pose you learned in Hour 5.

3. Advanced hatha yogis can control their heart rate and respiration cycle.

4. The Camel Posture requires you to hunch forward.

5. The Back Bending Monkey Posture is closely related to the Lunge Stretch you learned in Hour 2.

6. It's important to allow your mind to wander during a Hatha Yoga session so that you remain in a relaxed state.

7. Yoga students should be gentle with themselves, but not complacent.

8. In the Archer Posture you should grasp your ears with your index fingers.

9. The Inclined Plane is an inverted posture, where your head is placed lower than your legs.

10. Your body forms a crescent shape in the Back Bending Monkey Posture.

HOUR 11
Advanced Hatha Yoga

CHAPTER SUMMARY

LESSON PLAN:
In this hour you will learn ...

- Advanced yoga poses require exceptional strength, coordination, and flexibility.
- It's possible to reap most of the benefits of yoga without mastering the hardest postures.
- The Crow and the Peacock are demanding balancing poses that require considerable upper body strength.
- The Wheel and the Scorpion are powerful backward-bending exercises.
- The Headstand is considered the foremost of all Hatha Yoga postures.

The most advanced of the Hatha Yoga postures are thrilling to behold. Some are poses you might not have believed a human being could twist into unless you'd seen it with your own eyes! Others demand advanced acrobatic skills and almost superhuman flexibility.

Fortunately, you don't have to master the most difficult poses in order to benefit from Hatha Yoga. In fact, a consistent program of beginning level poses can do as much to enhance your health as the sporadic practice of even the most challenging yoga postures. Keep in mind that "beginning," "intermediate," and "advanced" refer to the difficulty of accomplishing a pose, not to how much good that pose does for you. Comparatively simple postures like the Stomach Lift, which you learned in Hour 9, might be of far more value to a person who suffers from indigestion than advanced positions like the Scorpion or the Crow.

Find your skill level and enjoy the poses available to you at that stage. Yoga is good for your body and mind at every step of the journey, whether you can balance on your hands or not.

REACH BEYOND YOUR LIMITS

Some people seem born strong and supple. From day one they can almost effortlessly swing their bodies into complex advanced postures. For them, the poses in this chapter will be a delight. Other people will probably never be able to assume some of these advanced postures in the course of their natural lives. For them, this hour will be useful as a source of information only. They'll simply be getting a glimpse of the levels of achievement possible in the Hatha Yoga tradition rather than learning to do the postures themselves.

If you are reasonably strong and flexible, and have mastered most of the poses in the previous hours, you may be ready to reach beyond your previous limits and try these new postures. But take it easy. Don't push if you're not ready. If you think you may be prepared but still feel insecure, seek out a yoga teacher to help you move into the advanced pose the first time and to spot check to ensure you're holding it correctly.

MASTERING THE MORE CHALLENGING POSTURES

The Headstand is by far the best known of the postures illustrated here. Many Westerners have already been introduced to it in physical education classes in school. If, however, you are new to the Headstand, the Dolphin is one pose that may help prepare you both physically and psychologically for the ultimate inverted posture.

The Crow, the Scorpion, and the Peacock are not as difficult as they look if you have the strength in your arms to balance your weight on your hands. The Full Spinal Twist is accessible to flexible individuals with average or longer length limbs, but may be difficult for petite students. The Wheel is actually a relaxing and recharging posture for students who have worked on developing the flexibility of their spine.

 FYI *Path of Fire and Light* by Swami Rama introduces you to the advanced breathing exercises yogis really use in India. You'll be amazed at the techniques the yoga adepts master. Many are far beyond what physiologists in the Western world would have believed humanly possible until the yogis actually demonstrated them in laboratories.

DOLPHIN POSTURE

The *Matsyabhedasana* or Dolphin Posture (*matsyabheda* means "dolphin") looks easy but actually takes some strength to hold for any length of time. The version you're about to learn is sometimes called the Swimming Dolphin. (The Ganges River in India is filled with dolphins, although they are slimmer and harder to spot in the water than the bottlenose dolphins Westerners are familiar with.)

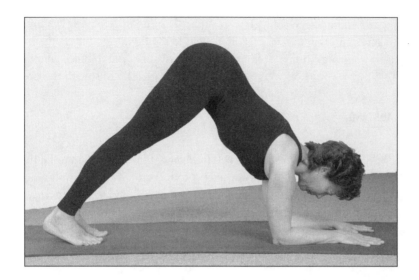

The Dolphin Posture.

(Photo credit: Alex Fernandez & Evolution Visual Services)

1. Begin in a crawling position with your hands, knees, and toes on the floor.

2. Lower your elbows, forearms, and hands, palms facing down, onto the floor. Your forearms should run parallel to your body and to each other.

3. Lower the top of your head to the floor between your elbows. At the same time straighten your legs, lifting your pelvis as high as you can into the air. Your body now forms an upside-down V shape with your head and forearms on the floor at one end and your toes on the floor at the other end.

4. Now shift your torso forward, lifting your head a foot or so. Your face should be parallel to the floor, staring down at your hands. Your upper arms form a steep diagonal angle to the floor. Your elbows, forearms, hands, and toes are now the only parts of your body in contact with the floor.

5. Bend your neck back, lifting your head farther and gazing up at the ceiling. Hold the pose for 10 to 20 seconds. Breathe diaphragmatically. Make small adjustments to the posture if you need to so that you're reasonably comfortable in the pose.

6. Lower your knees to the floor and come back up into a crawling position. Relax for a moment, then assume the Dolphin Pose one more time.

If you find it too difficult to continue holding the Dolphin Posture with your upper arms at a steep diagonal angle to the floor, try holding them at a 90-degree angle from the floor instead. This allows you to brace your upper body weight wholly on your elbows and makes it easier to stay in the pose longer.

HEADSTAND

In Hour 6, you learned the Shoulder Stand, which many yogis consider the "queen" of yoga postures. The Headstand, however, is said to be the "king." That's because the yogis consider it to be perhaps the most all-around beneficial posture in the Hatha Yoga tradition. It is said to benefit virtually every organ in the body. It increases blood flow to the brain and is reputed by yogis to strengthen your memory and help build your intelligence! It is intensely energizing when performed correctly. *Shirshasana* literally means "head posture" in Sanskrit.

Before attempting the Headstand, it would be helpful if you are already proficient in the Down Facing Dog Posture (which you learned in Hour 6) and the Dolphin Posture. These poses help you develop the arm and shoulder strength you need to master the Headstand.

Because the Headstand is so deep acting, it must be treated with respect. If you have never tried this posture before, do not attempt it by yourself. Have a friend on hand to steady your legs if you have trouble with your balance.

Do not attempt the Headstand if you have any of the following medical conditions:

- High blood pressure
- Glaucoma
- Osteoporosis
- Severe arthritis
- Severe obesity
- Weak neck
- Weak shoulders
- Weak back

Women: Do not attempt the Headstand when you are menstruating or while you are pregnant.

Avoid this posture if you tend to get dizzy or lightheaded easily. Also be cautious if you have a cold or earache or any other condition that might interfere with your inner ear's ability to keep you steady in a balanced position.

PROCEED WITH CAUTION

 If you have a serious back condition or if the vertebrae in your neck are weak, *under no circumstances* should you attempt the Headstand. Your cervical vertebrae will carry some of the weight of your body in this posture. They could become further damaged if there is already a problem in this area.

If you are new to the Headstand, work with this posture in two stages. Master this first variant, in which your knees remain bent not too far off the floor, before you proceed to the full position.

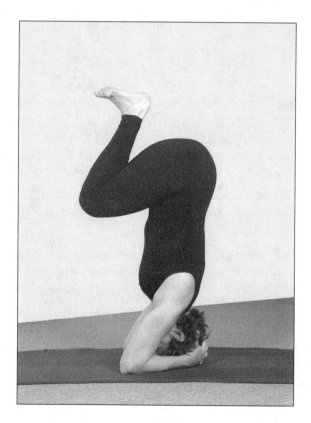

Preparation for the Headstand.

(Photo credit: Alex Fernandez & Evolution Visual Services)

1. Kneel on the floor. Interlace the fingers of your two hands. Place your hands, elbows, and forearms on the floor about six to nine inches in front of your knees. Your elbows should not be farther apart than the length of your forearm.

2. Lifting your hips a bit upward, put your head on the floor. It's not actually the very top of your head that lies on the floor but an area about two inches in front of the crown or top of your head. The back of your head should fit snugly against your interlaced fingers and palms.

3. Straighten your legs. Walk your feet toward your body until your back stands straight up from the floor.

4. Raise your right leg, bringing your right knee in toward your chest. Your right thigh is pointed downward near your torso while your right lower leg points upward from your bent knee.

5. When and if you are comfortable doing so, lift your left leg also, bringing your left knee against your torso and pointing your lower left leg upward next to your right leg. You will feel some pressure in your neck and head. However, most of your weight should be supported by your hands and arms.

6. Breathe diaphragmatically. Monitor your physical condition very closely. Try to stay relaxed and balanced. Don't hold this position longer than 15 seconds on your first attempt.

7. Lower your right foot to the floor, then your left foot. Return to a kneeling position. Relax in the Child's Pose (which you learned in Hour 3) for a few moments.

After you've developed a good sense of balance in this upside-down position, when you get to step 4, lift both legs at once rather than one at a time.

A common problem many beginners experience is placing their elbows too close or (more often) too far apart. This prevents you from being able to balance easily. This preliminary Headstand will help you work out any possible flaws in your technique before you go on to the more demanding full pose.

It is very important that you feel comfortable in this preliminary version of the Headstand before you attempt the next steps, which will carry you into the full pose.

JUST A MINUTE

You should be able to hold the preliminary version of the Headstand for at least half a minute without discomfort before you go on to the complete posture. You might be able to do this in your first session, or it may take weeks to build up to the full pose. Remember, in yoga there's no hurry. Your body is benefiting from the preliminary pose whether you achieve the full position or not.

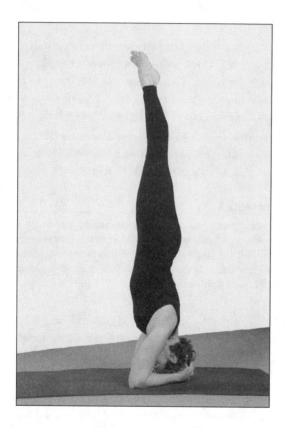

The Headstand.

(Photo credit: Alex Fernandez & Evolution Visual Services)

1. Assume the preliminary version of the Headstand, which was just described. Your body weight rests on your hands, arms, and the top of your head. Your knees are bent with your thighs pressed toward your torso and your lower legs pointing straight up into the air.

2. Keeping your knees bent, raise them until they point straight up in the air. Your feet should stay reasonably near your lower pelvis, which they pivot over as you make this move. When your knees are raised as far as they can go, your lower legs are hanging down behind your thighs. This will help you stay balanced.

3. Ready? Now raise your lower legs toward the ceiling and point your toes upward. Hold the posture, watching your balance carefully. Your back and legs should be straight.

4. Hold the posture only as long as you feel stable and comfortable. Monitor your physical and mental state continually. Breathe diaphragmatically. Do not hold the posture for longer than 15 seconds on your first try.

5. Come out of the pose by reversing your path in. Lower your lower legs behind you. Pivot your knees to your chest, keeping your heels fairly near your pelvis. Then swing your legs down to the floor. Come up into a kneeling position. Come out as slowly as you can practically, so that the extra blood in your head does not drain out too quickly.

6. Lie on your back in the Corpse Pose (which you learned in Hour 3) for at least a minute, until your breath and circulation return to normal. Allow your entire body to relax.

PROCEED WITH CAUTION

In the Headstand, your arms and hands should support the bulk of your body weight, not your head! If your head or neck start to feel uncomfortable, come out of the posture immediately. Most people do just fine in the Headstand, but some individuals occasionally injure themselves. Don't take chances. Build up to holding the full posture slowly and cautiously.

Gradually work up to holding the Headstand for a minute or so. Yoga adepts will hold the pose for 5 or 10 minutes, remaining mentally focused the entire time, listening for their body's inner signal that it's time to come out of the pose.

Just as some children find it easier learning to ride a bicycle with training wheels, some yoga students gain confidence in the Headstand by practicing it up against a wall. They gain the security of knowing the won't fall backwards because the wall will stop their fall. But they lose the ability to move their legs freely to adjust the posture. If you're insecure about falling, you're better off having a friend on hand who can steady you no matter which direction you teeter toward.

CROW POSTURE

The Crow or *Kakasana* strengthens your abdominal muscles as well as your shoulders, arms, and wrists. The crow is called *kaka* in Sanskrit, after the cawing sound it makes. The Crow Posture requires a lot of concentration, so it's said to improve mental abilities as well.

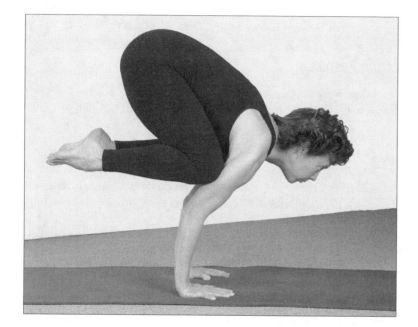

The Crow Posture.

(Photo credit: Alex Fernandez & Evolution Visual Services)

1. Squat on the floor with your feet about shoulder width apart. Your feet should be flat on the floor.

2. Bend forward so that you can place your palms on the floor directly below your shoulders. Spread your fingers apart like a bird's toes. This will help you balance in the Crow Pose.

3. Point your elbows slightly outward. You may need to accommodate this motion by shifting your fingers slightly inward.

4. Lifting yourself up on your toes, rest your knees on your upper arms. Feel your body weight shifting to your arms while you use your toes to balance.

5. Shift your weight farther forward until it rests primarily on your wrists and hands. Lift your toes off the floor and point your legs and feet straight out behind you. (Some people find this pose easier if they move their feet toward each other till their toes touch, while their knees or upper thighs continue to rest on their upper arms.)

6. Keep breathing! Monitor your balance and your general energy state. Stay in the posture for up to 15 seconds if you can do so comfortably.

7. Lower your feet and return to a standing position. Relax for a few moments in the Mountain Posture, which you learned in Hour 3.

PEACOCK POSTURE

Like the Crow, the Peacock is another pose in which you balance on your wrists and hands. In this pose, however, you will hold your body in a straight line parallel to the floor.

Because the Peacock Pose places so much carefully directed pressure on the abdomen, the pose is said to enhance the function of the stomach, intestines, and liver. It has a reputation as a powerful revitalizing exercise. This pose is called *Mayurasana* in Sanskrit (*Mayura* means "peacock").

FYI What's it like to actually live with a yoga master? *Radha: Diary of a Woman's Search* by Swami Sivananda Radha is the true story of Sylvia Hellman, a German dancer who traveled to Swami Sivananda's ashram in Rishikesh, India, to learn yoga from the world-renowned adept. She eventually went on to found her own yoga community, Yasodhara Ashram, in Canada.

The Peacock Posture.

(Photo credit: Johnathan Brown)

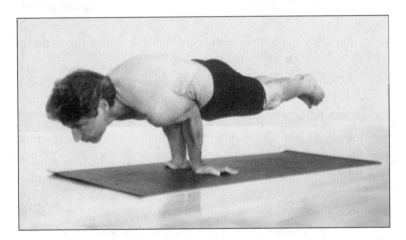

1. Sit on your heels. Space your knees wide apart.

2. Bring your elbows, forearms, and hands next to each other in front of your body, holding your arms forward, away from your torso. Your palms face upward.

3. Bend forward, putting your palms on the floor between your knees, with your fingers pointing back toward your body.

4. Rest your abdomen beneath your rib cage on your elbows.

5. Lean farther forward until your upper forehead reaches the floor. Stop at this point in the exercise if you find this position painful.

6. Stretch your right leg out behind you, then your left leg. At this point your weight is supported on your toes, wrists and hands, and upper forehead.

7. Lift your head off the floor. Keep your head, neck, and back in a straight, horizontal line above the floor.

8. Shift your weight forward till your body is resting entirely on your hands and wrists. Don't lift your legs, but allow them to rise naturally as your weight shifts forward. Except for your lower arms, which are perpendicular to the floor, the rest of your body is positioned horizontally.

9. Hold the pose for as long as you can comfortably. In the beginning, this should be for no more than 15 seconds. Breathe in a smooth and relaxed fashion.

10. To exit the posture, shift your weight backward until your toes touch the floor. Sit back up on your knees and relax.

The first time you get as far as step 5, when your forehead touches the floor, it's a good idea to stop and relax. Give your body time to adjust to the sense of pressure in the abdomen. Don't proceed further into the posture until you're comfortable in this position, even if it takes a few weeks of practice.

FULL SPINAL TWIST

You've already learned the Half Spinal Twist. Here is the advanced version of this deep-acting yoga exercise, called *Matsyendrasana* after the sage Matsyendra. This pose stretches the entire body, giving a particularly complete stretch to the spine. It's famous for its power to help heal a multitude of illnesses, strengthen the digestion, and heighten awareness. The pose's legendary ability to raise consciousness might be related to its profound effect on the nervous system through its powerful impact on the spinal column.

GO TO ▶
In Hour 8, you learned the Half Spinal Twist. Flexible students can now go on to the Full Spinal Twist. Go back to Hour 8 and make sure you're completely comfortable in both versions of the Half Spinal Twist taught there before you attempt the more difficult complete posture taught here.

The Full Spinal Twist.

(Photo credit: Alex Fernandez & Evolution Visual Services)

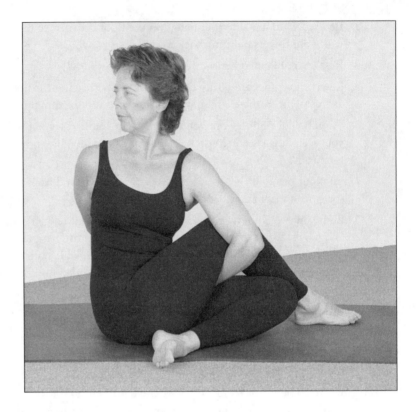

1. Sit on the floor in the Staff Pose, which you learned in Hour 6.

2. Place your left foot under your right thigh near your lower pelvis.

3. Lift your right foot over your left leg and position it against the outside of your left knee. Your right toes will just barely be extending beyond your left knee.

4. Position your body so that, while maintaining the leg lock described in steps 2 and 3, your right knee is pointed straight forward. Don't slump forward. You should be sitting straight up.

5. Exhaling, twist your torso to the right. Twist from the pelvis.

6. Your left elbow should be far enough to the right that it has passed your right knee. Take hold of your right foot with your left hand.

7. Wrap your right arm around behind you along your waist.

8. Breathe evenly, and hold the posture for 15 to 20 seconds.

9. Release the posture, return to the Staff Pose, and repeat the Full Spinal Twist, twisting in the opposite direction this time.

WHEEL POSTURE

Chakrasana or the Wheel Posture (*chakra* means "wheel") is a beautiful yoga pose advanced students love to show off. You may find posters on their walls of yogis modeling this posture.

This pose obviously stretches the spine, but also very effectively strengthens the arms and legs. According to yoga tradition, it's also especially good for the throat and brain, which it floods with fresh, nutrient-rich blood.

JUST A MINUTE

If you have not yet mastered the Arch Posture, which you learned in Hour 5, you are not ready to experiment with the Wheel Pose. Go back and work on the Arch first. When you can comfortably lift your pelvis quite high in that posture and hold it for at least half a minute, then you can begin thinking about trying the Wheel Pose.

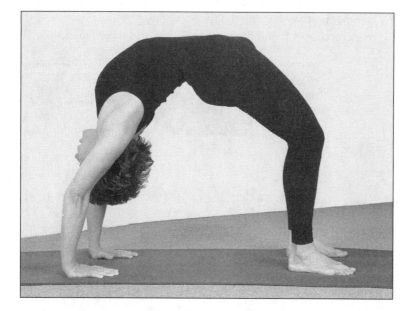

The Wheel Posture.

(Photo credit: Alex Fernandez & Evolution Visual Services)

1. Lie on the floor in the Corpse Pose. Stretch your arms overhead along the floor.

2. Bending your knees, pull your feet up to the bottom of your pelvis. Bending your arms, put your hands on the floor above your head, palms facing down, fingers pointing back toward your body.

3. Inhaling, lift your pelvis, abdomen, and chest up off the floor, one after another in that order, until your arms are nearly straight, holding your chest up off the floor. Your head hangs between your arms.

4. Hold the pose for 10 to 20 seconds. Breathe diaphragmatically. Be aware of the sense of lightness and energy in your body.

5. Exhaling, lower your body back down in reverse order, starting with your shoulders.

6. Relax in the Child's Pose, which you learned in Hour 3.

Very advanced students can raise one leg straight in the air while holding the Wheel or one of its variations. This is beautiful to see but it's a challenging move to master.

SCORPION POSTURE

The Scorpion or *Vrishchikasana* (*vrishchika* means "scorpion") is a very advanced posture which should not be attempted by anyone who hasn't already mastered both the Headstand and the Arch Pose. The Scorpion is another posture that you should not attempt for the first time without a yoga teacher or friend present to help you with your balance.

The Scorpion Posture.

(Photo credit: Alex Fernandez & Evolution Visual Services)

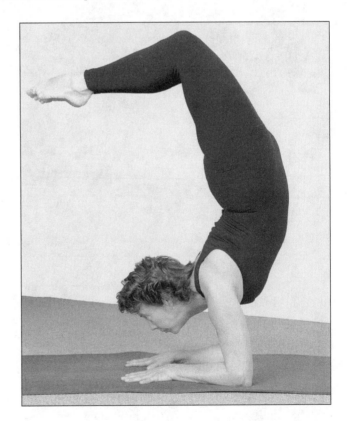

1. Begin in the full Headstand, which you learned earlier during this hour.

2. Slowly bend your knees, allowing your feet to move downward toward your back. At the same time, gently arch your back.

3. Unclasp your hands. Move your forearms along the floor until they lie parallel on either side of your head. Your palms should be on the floor. Be careful! If you feel discomfort in your head or neck, stop immediately. The bulk of your weight should still rest on your arms and hands throughout this step.

4. Shift your shoulders till they are directly above your elbows. Lift your head. Adjust the arch in your back and the position of your legs (which hang from the knees above your head) until you are balanced as comfortably as possible in this position.

5. Hold the pose for as long as you can without straining, but not for more than 10 seconds at the most during your first attempt. Keep breathing! Be sensitive to what's happening in your body so that you don't overexert yourself.

6. Reverse these steps to come out of the Scorpion.

7. Relax in the Child's Pose, which provides a counterposture to the Scorpion and will help relieve any tension in your back muscles and spinal column.

So far you've learned a lot of individual yoga poses. Now it's time to learn a series of postures that flow naturally into each other. This is the famous Sun Salutation, which you'll discover in Hour 12.

HOUR'S UP!

Take this quiz to see if you remember important material about the new yoga postures you've just learned. Answer true or false to the following statements:

1. The Wheel Pose is the "king" of all yoga postures.

2. The Dolphin Pose helps prepare you for the Headstand.

3. The Crow Pose requires you to make a cawing sound like a crow.

4. The Peacock Pose requires you to hold your body straight on a horizontal plane above the floor.

5. The Scorpion is a very advanced forward-bending posture.

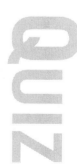

QUIZ

6. It's important to develop a mental attitude that, no matter what, you will master the advanced poses.

7. The advanced yoga poses provide much greater benefits than most of the beginning level postures.

8. Individuals with weak back and neck bones should not attempt the Headstand.

9. In the Headstand, most of your body weight should rest on the top of your skull.

10. The Peacock Pose is particularly good for the abdominal organs involved in digestion.

HOUR 12

Flowing Postures

CHAPTER SUMMARY

LESSON PLAN:

In this hour you will learn ...

- The Sun Salutation is designed to energize the body and focus the mind after getting out of bed in the morning.

- Saluting the Sun involves seven yoga postures that flow into each other in a continuous series.

- The Sun Salutation is commonly used as a warm-up before beginning a Hatha Yoga routine.

- Advanced students coordinate their breath with the 12 poses of the Sun Salutation.

- The Sun Salutation begins your day with an attitude of inward composure and respect for nature.

In India, most yogis rise before the sun. They quickly bathe, preferably in clean, flowing water such as the sacred streams of the Ganges River. (Most Westerners no doubt prefer to wash themselves in the shower, where they enjoy the option of hot running water.) Then the yogi puts on fresh clothes (or a single piece of cloth if a loin cloth is all the clothing he owns), and turns eastward to face the rising sun.

You are about to learn the 12-step exercise that many yogis then perform. This invigorating exercise gets the heart pumping, fills the lungs with fresh morning air, and stretches muscles still tight from a night of sleep. Called *Surya Namaskar* or the Sun Salutation (*Surya* means "sun," and *namaskar* means "I bow respectfully"), this Hatha Yoga technique prepares the body and mind for the day ahead.

MAKE THE POSTURES FLOW

The Sun Salutation is the perfect warm-up for the series of Hatha postures that many yoga students practice in the morning before sitting down for breakfast. And for those students who're too busy to fit in thirty minutes or an hour of yoga poses that day, the Sun Salutation is a quick and highly effective substitute.

So far you have learned a few dozen of the most important individual yoga poses. In this hour, as well as in Hour 13, you will learn how to put these poses together into a balanced format that works with every part of your body.

The Sun Salutation is particularly valuable for this purpose because it carries you gracefully from one position to the next in a flowing series of postures. Today, this exercise is practiced at *ashrams* and yoga studios around the world. It's like a meditative yoga dance.

STRICTLY DEFINED

An **ashram** is a community (often a house or complex of buildings) where spiritual students live together.

MASTERING THE SUN SALUTATION

The Indian tradition, out of which yoga grew, honors all of nature as sacred. The trees, the hills, the planets, and the stars are believed to be imbued with the all-pervading divine spirit. The sun is an especially appropriate symbol for divine being because it shares its light and warmth unfailingly and equally to all beings, great and small, saint and sinner. It is the perfect symbol for selfless giving and spiritual illumination.

To many of the ancient yogis who spent the night in bitterly cold caves or the dark jungles of India, a glimpse of the rising sun must have been a welcome sight. The Sun Salutation honors the radiant hearth at the center of the solar system, as well as the inner light it represents.

LEARN THE SUN SERIES

The Sun Salutation incorporates seven yoga postures arranged in a series of 12 poses (some of the postures are done twice). Yoga students who have learned the Sun Salutation in the traditional manner will carefully coordinate their breathing cycle with the poses. However, for the beginner this may entail too many factors to pay attention to at once. So don't worry about your breath at first. Instead, work on memorizing the series of postures and getting a feel for moving from one directly into another. Then you can experiment with adding breath awareness to your movements.

Traditionally, yoga practitioners face east to honor the sun as they practice this exercise.

SUN SALUTATION POSE 1

Begin the Sun Salutation by assuming the following physical and mental pose.

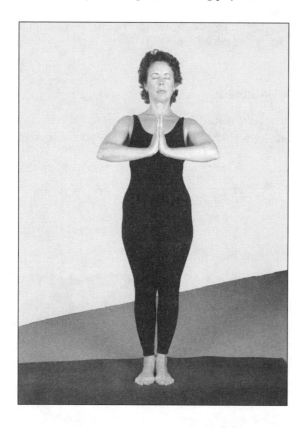

The Sun Salutation, position 1.

(Photo credit: Alex Fernandez & Evolution Visual Services)

1. Stand with your head, neck, and trunk straight. Place your feet a few inches apart. Press your palms together in the "namaste" or prayer position in front of your heart.

2. Close your eyes. Make sure your inhalations and exhalations are smooth, calm, and even. You should breathe through your nose, not your mouth, throughout this exercise.

3. Withdraw your mind from external sights and sounds, and from internal memories and plans. Bring your full attention into the present moment. Be conscious of the sacred space of your own silent inner awareness. Once your breath is tranquil and your mind is focused, you are ready to move on to the second position.

4. Open your eyes.

PROCEED WITH CAUTION

Don't rush through the Sun Salutation the first few times you try it. Take the time to get used to the feel of the postures and how they flow together, even if this means you spend several breaths in each pose. Once the series of positions begins to become automatic for you, you can speed up the exercise and coordinate it with your inhalations and exhalations.

SUN SALUTATION POSE 2

The second position is somewhat similar to the Standing Backward Bend you learned in Hour 7, except for the position of your arms and hips.

The Sun Salutation, position 2.

(Photo credit: Alex Fernandez & Evolution Visual Services)

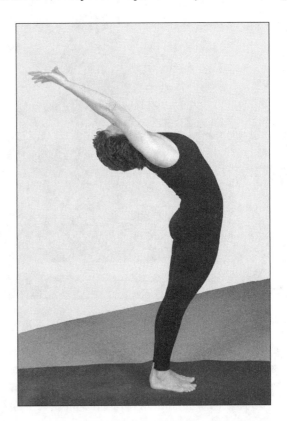

1. Inhaling, stretch your arms directly forward in front of you, with your palms facing down.

2. Continuing the inhalation, raise your arms up directly above your head. Stretch through your fingertips.

3. Continuing the inhalation, arch your back and bend backward as far as you can comfortably. Your arms follow your ears as you bend backward. Allow your hips to shift forward slightly in order to deepen your backward bend.

4. Do not hold the pose but continue directly into the next position.

SUN SALUTATION POSE 3

The third position is similar to the Standing Forward Bend you learned in Hour 7.

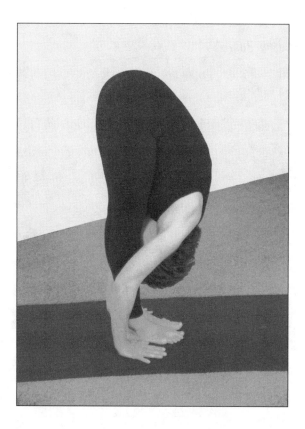

The Sun Salutation, position 3.

(Photo credit: Alex Fernandez & Evolution Visual Services)

1. Exhaling, return to an upright position with your arms extended directly over your head.

2. Continuing the exhalation, bend forward from your hips. Your arms follow your ears as you bend forward. Keep your knees straight.

3. As you finish your exhalation, place the palms of your hands on the floor directly to the side of your feet. If you can't reach your feet or the floor, reach down only as far as you can comfortably without bending your legs.

4. Do not hold the pose but continue directly into the next posture.

JUST A MINUTE

You might find it helpful to keep your hands on the same spot on the floor all the way from steps 3 through 10 of the Sun Salutation. This will ground you throughout the exercise and help you keep your balance.

SUN SALUTATION POSE 4

You will now move into a posture similar to the Lunge Stretch, which you learned in Hour 2.

The Sun Salutation, position 4.

(Photo credit: Alex Fernandez & Evolution Visual Services)

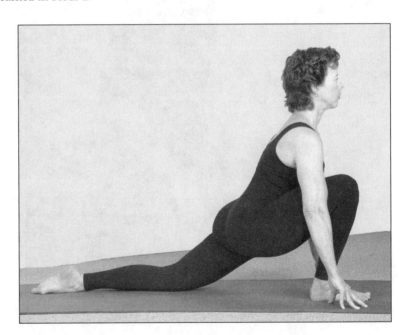

1. If you were not able to reach the floor in the last position, bend your knees slightly and place your palms on the floor. Your palms will not move from this spot until you reach position 11.

2. As you inhale, stretch your right leg out behind you as far as you can comfortably. Rest your right knee and the top of your right foot on the floor. Your left foot remains in the starting position.

3. As you continue inhaling, stretch your head backward and look up at the ceiling.

4. Move directly into the next pose.

You will repeat this pose later in the Sun Salutation cycle (position 9). However, the next time you will stretch your left leg backward and keep your right leg positioned forward, so both legs receive an equal stretch.

PROCEED WITH CAUTION

 Position 5 of the Sun Salutation is one of the few instances in your yoga practice where you are asked to hold your breath. You should not stop breathing in this pose for more than a short moment. In general, beginning level yoga students should not retain their breath but should continue to breathe diaphragmatically throughout their yoga routine.

SUN SALUTATION POSE 5

This pose looks somewhat similar to the Inclined Plane Posture you learned in Hour 10, except that your body is facing downward rather than upward.

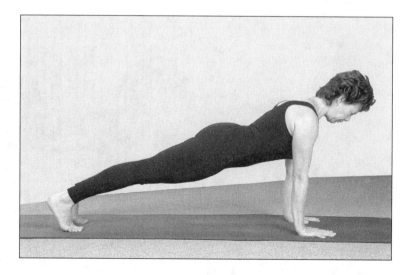

The Sun Salutation, position 5.

(Photo credit: Alex Fernandez & Evolution Visual Services)

1. Hold your breath! You should not exhale while moving through this position if you can hold your breath comfortably for a moment. Lower your head so that you are looking forward rather than upward.

2. Lift your right foot so that your right leg is now straight, resting on your right toes.

3. Extend your left leg backward and place your left foot a few inches from your right foot. You should now be supporting your body on your toes in the back, and on your wrists and hands in the front. Your arms, back, and legs are all straight. Your arms point directly down. The rest of your body points gradually upward from your toes.

4. Don't hold this position but move right on to posture 6.

SUN SALUTATION POSE 6

The next position is a transition pose leading into the Cobra. Your body will form a wavy line on the floor, much like a snake slithering forward.

The Sun Salutation, position 6.

(Photo credit: Alex Fernandez & Evolution Visual Services)

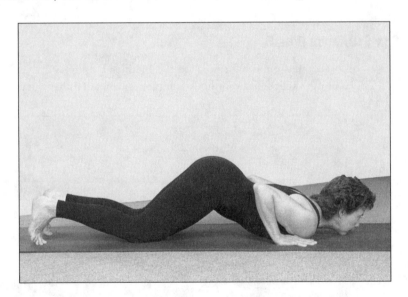

1. Exhaling, lower first your knees to the floor, then your chest. Rest your chin on the floor but keep your forehead up.

2. Your hands remain in the same spot as pose 5. Your elbows should stay close to your torso. Your pelvis is not touching the floor! Your hips are held a few inches above the ground.

3. Proceed directly to the next pose, without holding this posture.

FYI Interested in learning more about the amazing skills and abilities the yoga masters have demonstrated? *Walking with a Himalayan Master* by Justin O'Brien recounts the fascinating story of a Christian theologian's encounter with one of the greatest yoga masters of the twentieth century, and the numerous surprises and insights this great yogi had in store for him.

SUN SALUTATION POSE 7

The seventh position of the Sun Salutation is the Cobra Posture, which you learned in Hour 5.

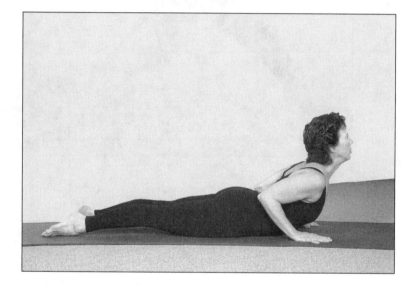

The Sun Salutation, position 7.

(Photo credit: Alex Fernandez & Evolution Visual Services)

1. Lower your hips and legs completely to the floor.
2. Inhaling, stretch your head backward as far as you can comfortably. Using only the muscles of your neck and upper back, lift your head off the floor.
3. As you continue inhaling, lift your upper chest off the floor. Arch your back backward as far as you can comfortably without using your arms to hold you up. The lift comes from your back muscles exclusively.
4. Students who have developed the flexibility of their spinal column may use their arms to push their upper torso up farther, but only after exerting their back muscles to full capacity in the lifting motion first. The pelvis and legs should remain relaxed. Your toes point backward.
5. Move directly into the next pose without holding this posture.

SUN SALUTATION POSE 8

The eighth position resembles the Down Facing Dog Posture you learned in Hour 6.

The Sun Salutation, position 8.

(Photo credit: Alex Fernandez & Evolution Visual Services)

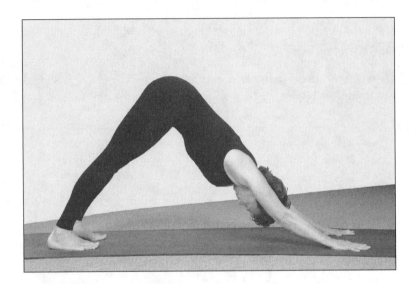

1. Exhaling, straighten your arms and push your pelvis up into the air. Your hands remain in place on the floor. As you lift your hips, shift the position of your feet so that they are now flat on the floor.

2. Only your feet, wrists and hands are now in contact with the floor. Your body forms an upside-down V shape.

3. Without pausing, proceed directly to the next posture.

SUN SALUTATION POSE 9

Position 9 of the Sun Salutation is identical to Position 4, except that you step forward with your right leg this time instead of your left.

1. As you inhale, take a giant step forward with your right leg, without shifting your hand position on the floor. Try to step so that your right foot is placed between your hands. Lower your pelvis toward the floor. Your right knee now juts out in front of you.

2. Your left leg, from the knee downward, should now be stretched out behind you along the floor. As you continue inhaling, press your torso against your right thigh.

3. Bend your head backward and look up at the ceiling.

4. Move right into the next pose.

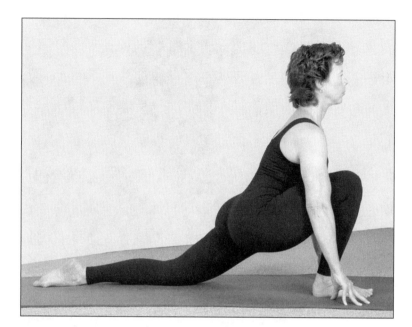

The Sun Salutation, position 9.

(Photo credit: Alex Fernandez & Evolution Visual Services)

JUST A MINUTE

The Sun Salutation is a superb aerobic conditioning exercise. After you gain familiarity with the postures, try moving through the series several times fairly rapidly. You're guaranteed to work up a sweat!

SUN SALUTATION POSE 10

You will now move back into the Standing Forward Bend.

1. Exhaling, lift your pelvis upward enough so that you can swing your left leg forward. Place your left foot next to your right foot on the floor between your hands.

2. As you continue exhaling, straighten your legs while bending forward from your hips. Your hands should not leave the floor. You should now be in a standing position with your head hanging downward and your palms flat on the floor. If you can't reach the floor in this position, don't bend your knees. Instead keep your legs straight and extend your hands down as far as you can comfortably.

3. Don't hold this pose. Go directly to the next posture.

The Sun Salutation, position 10.

(Photo credit: Alex Fernandez & Evolution Visual Services)

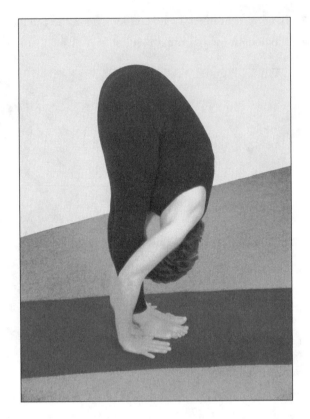

SUN SALUTATION POSE 11

You will now return to a Standing Backward Bend.

1. Inhaling, raise your torso, extending your arms outward and upward, following your ears as you return to a standing position.

2. As you continue inhaling, arch as far backward as you can comfortably, thrusting your hips slightly forward to deepen the bend. Your arms are stretched back following your head.

3. Don't pause in the posture. Move immediately to the last pose.

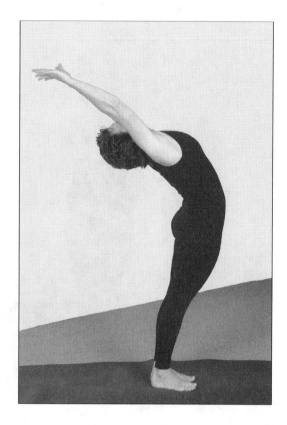

The Sun Salutation, position 11.

(Photo credit: Alex Fernandez & Evolution Visual Services)

SUN SALUTATION POSE 12

You will now return to your starting position, refreshed and invigorated.

1. Exhaling, stand up straight with your arms stretched over your head.

2. As you continue exhaling, reach forward with your arms, then bring your palms together at the center of your chest in the "namaste" or prayer position.

3. Close your eyes. Turn your attention to your inner state. Watch your breath until it slows to its normal resting rate. Feel your heart rate slow down as you relax. Your mental state will reflect both alertness and tranquility.

The Sun Salutation, position 12.

(Photo credit: Alex Fernandez & Evolution Visual Services)

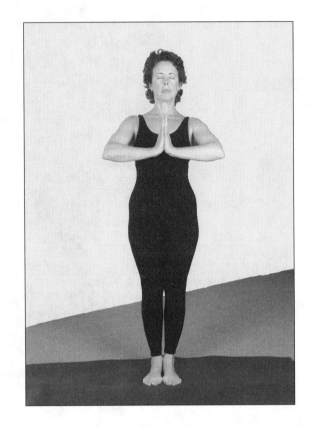

GO TO ▶
The Gayatri mantra is an inner version of the Sun Salutation. Repeated mentally, it aligns your thoughts with the inner light. Working with mantras is an important part of the yoga tradition. In Hour 15, you will learn how mantras are incorporated into concentration and meditation techniques. You will also learn a number of mantras and affirmations yoga students often work with.

You might wish to repeat the Sun Salutation cycle two or three more times, alternating which leg you bring forward first in positions 4 and 9. As you become more adept at this exercise series, you will be able to move through it fairly quickly, so several complete cycles will not take very long.

At first, coordinating your breath with the movements might seem awkward. After you have practiced the cycle a number of times, the breath and the movements will flow together naturally, the breath actually supporting your motions as your lungs expand and contract.

The Sun Salutation begins and ends in a meditative mood. It is based on a respectful attitude toward all nature and toward one's own body and Inner Self. Practiced early in the morning, it roots the day in sacred silence and reverence.

Congratulations! By now you've learned many of the most important postures taught in the Hatha Yoga tradition. Some of these poses may have been easy for you. Others may be too demanding for you to attempt at this time. Yet adding even a few of these wonderful postures—those postures you can hold comfortably—to your daily routine can made a big difference in the way you feel.

You've also learned the Sun Salutation, a favorite flowing series of poses that many yoga students practice enthusiastically. It puts several of the yoga poses together in a graceful sequence that increases your heart and breathing rates while toning your muscles and exercising your internal organs.

Now it's time to set up a Hatha Yoga routine you can practice several times a week. Hour 13 will show you how to put all this information together to design a program that's uniquely right for you and will introduce you to some products that might help you through your session.

HOUR'S UP!

Quiz yourself on the material contained in this hour. Answer true or false to the following statements:

1. The Sun Salutation is commonly used to warm up the body before beginning a Hatha Yoga routine.
2. The Sun Salutation requires you to hold each of twelve positions for a minute each.
3. Traditionally, yoga practitioners face west at sunset to thank the sun for its light and warmth that day when they perform the Sun Salutation.
4. Advanced yoga students coordinate their inhalations and exhalations with their movements through the Sun Salutation.
5. The Gayatri Mantra invokes the blessings of the inner light.
6. The Sun Salutation begins and ends in a meditative mood.
7. The Cobra Posture is incorporated in the Sun Salutation.
8. There is one pose in the Sun Salutation during which you are asked to hold your breath.
9. The Sun Salutation incorporates 7 yoga postures arranged in a series of 12 poses.
10. The position of your hands on the floor changes constantly throughout the Sun Salutation cycle.

QUIZ

HOUR 13

Your Hatha Routine

CHAPTER SUMMARY

LESSON PLAN:
In this hour you will learn ...

- Signing up for a Hatha Yoga class is a smart investment that pays dividends for your health and well-being.

- You can easily create a Hatha program suitable for your unique level of strength and flexibility.

- A yoga session should include postures and counterpostures that work each section of your body in a balanced manner.

- Special tools are available to help you create a conducive atmosphere and aid your progress in your yoga practice.

- Yoga retreat centers are an especially healthful and relaxing way to spend a vacation.

By this time you have a pretty good sense for what Hatha Yoga is all about. You've already learned many of the most important postures in the yoga system. Now it's time to put all the elements together into a program that works for you.

Keep in mind that advanced postures are not necessarily more beneficial than beginning poses, they're just harder to do. Begin where you are, not a step or two ahead of yourself. The simplest postures can have profound healing and conditioning effects if you practice them correctly and regularly.

DESIGN YOUR SESSION

There are six basic principles you need to know in order to set up a personal practice:

- Every stretch and bend in yoga calls for a countermovement. Yogis know that the path to health is fundamentally simple. It involves maintaining a state of balance, the dynamic equilibrium of a healthy, creative life. This is perfectly illustrated in Hatha practice. For every forward stretch, there must be a backward stretch. Every posture that requires you to bend to the right also requires you to bend to the left. Don't do more than two or three of a particular type of posture in a row, such as the Cobra, Locust, and Bow, all back-bending exercises, without introducing a forward-bending posture like the Child's Pose. Keep your Hatha routine balanced!

- The time best spent in yoga balances not just your physical body but also your energy state and your mental processes. Therefore, a good yoga workout includes breathing exercises and concentration techniques. Breathing exercises work your respiratory organs while both stimulating and soothing your nervous system. In Hatha Yoga, concentration farther activates portions of your brain—providing a workout for your gray matter as well as your muscle tissue.

FYI Does your back ache? You might want to have a look at *Back Care Basics: A Doctor's Gentle Yoga Program for Back and Neck Pain Relief* by Mary Pullig Schatz, M.D. Dr. Schatz will help you understand why your back hurts and how yoga can help solve the problem.

- After exerting yourself, you should take the time to relax. As you practice relaxation poses like the Corpse Posture or the Child's Pose, you'll learn how to let go of stress and tension more quickly and more deeply. This is a valuable skill to master, particularly if you've got a high-stress job or if you find meeting life's daily challenges especially draining. Take a moment to relax after every posture, even if it means simply remaining in the standing or sitting position you're already in for two or three breaths as your body releases the posture you just held. After doing several mildly strenuous poses in a row (again, such as the Cobra, Locust, and Bow), take a little more time in a full relaxation posture such as the Child's Pose or Crocodile to allow any residual tension to melt out of your body. Don't skip the relaxation phase at the end of each posture. Return to equilibrium before exerting yourself in the next pose.

- Sequence your routine so that you begin a number of poses from the same starting position (standing, sitting, kneeling, prone, supine). This way you won't be continually interrupting the flow of your session by abruptly standing up or sitting down.

- Commit to doing your Hatha Yoga practice regularly. This point is particularly critical. Decide how much time you're willing to spend on your yoga routine (a half-hour, hour, 90 minutes), and how many days per week you can devote to the practice. Three times a week is the minimum in order to sustain the momentum of your practice and begin to see fairly rapid improvement in the mastery of the postures. Four or five times a week is ideal for most people. This gives you a few days of rest, while allowing you to experience the maximum benefits from the postures. Advanced and strongly committed students may do a Hatha routine seven days a week. They find they feel so much better after their yoga workout that they'd rather not start the day without it.

- It is definitely preferable to do your yoga at the same time each day. Try to adjust your daily schedule to accommodate this, if possible. In choosing a time of day for postures, bear in mind that you'll want to do yoga before, not after, a meal. When you go through your Hatha program at 7 each morning or at 6:30 each night, the postures become integrated into your *diurnal biorhythms*. You will find that if you start your yoga practice with diaphragmatic breathing, for example, then your body automatically begins breathing diaphragmatically even before you begin the exercise. Your subconscious "knows" that it's time to start your Hatha routine and unconsciously gears up for the session.

STRICTLY DEFINED

Your **diurnal biorhythms** are the natural cycles your body goes through during a typical day. You wake up, feel hungry, and get sleepy at about the same time each day. More subtle cycles, such as your blood pressure and body temperature, also fluctuate with the time of day. Expert yogis take advantage of these cycles to maximize their yoga practice.

This hour contains five sample yoga routines you can follow step by step or modify according to your needs. They are designed to suit four fitness levels: unfit (Gentle routine), average fitness and flexibility (Beginning routine), above average fitness and flexibility (Intermediate routine), and superb physical condition (Advanced routine).

DESIGN YOUR GENTLE ROUTINE

The Gentle Hatha Yoga routine can be particularly helpful for the following types of individuals:

- Beginning students who are extremely stiff and inflexible
- Elderly students with a limited range of motion
- Patients recovering from an illness or injury
- Pregnant or menstruating women
- Students who have only a few minutes to spare
- People who suffer from chronic tension

In the following lists, next to each exercise you'll find the hour where the posture or technique is described in detail, if you need to go back and refresh your memory.

TIME SAVER

 Looking for websites that will put you in touch with the major Hatha Yoga traditions being taught in America today? You can learn more about B.K.S. Iyengar's style of yoga at www.iyengar-yoga.com. For information about T.K.V. Desikachar's Viniyoga, log on to www.viniyoga.com. Richard Freeman's brand of Ashtanga yoga is presented at www.yogaworkshop.com.

1. Diaphragmatic Breathing (Hour 4) in the Crocodile Pose (Hour 3)
2. Head Roll (Hour 2)
3. Shoulder Roll (Hour 2)
4. Wrist Roll (Hour 2)
5. Knee Roll (Hour 2)
6. Ankle Roll (Hour 2)
7. Standing Stretch (Hour 2)
8. Tip Toe Stretch (Hour 3)
9. Cat Stretch (Hour 2)
10. Reclining Stretch (Hour 2)
11. Diaphragmatic Breathing (Hour 4) in the Corpse Pose (Hour 3)

The Tip Toe Stretch should be performed only by students who can keep their balance standing on their toes for five seconds or more. Work up to the Cat Stretch gradually if you are physically weak. This is a mild exercise that can be ideal for helping you rebuild your strength.

Begin and end each Gentle session with a few minutes of Diaphragmatic Breathing. This will help you get in the habit of breathing the way nature intended. It will help you feel both tranquil and lightly energized.

By the way, it's a great idea to actually attend a formal Hatha Yoga class before setting up your own yoga program, if at all possible. A certified Hatha instructor can check to ensure that you are holding the postures properly, and can make suggestions based on his or her own personal experience to help you get the most benefit out of your practice.

DESIGN YOUR FIRST BEGINNING ROUTINE

The first Beginning routine is ideal for most people with normal health and average flexibility. Begin with breathing exercises to calm and center your mind. Next, warm up with a few stretches and bends. Then move into classic yoga postures like the Cobra and the Half Fish Pose.

Don't be intimidated by the number of yoga poses in this list. You will be holding most of these postures for only 15 to 30 seconds, so you'll move through the sequence fairly rapidly. To make your yoga session last longer and to increase the physiological benefits, repeat each pose three or four times.

1. Diaphragmatic Breathing (Hour 4) in the Mountain Pose (Hour 3)
2. The Complete Breath (Hour 4) in the Mountain Pose (Hour 3)
3. Standing Stretch (Hour 2)
4. Cat Stretch (Hour 2)
5. Lunge Stretch (Hour 2)
6. Reclining Stretch (Hour 2)
7. Stomach Lift (Hour 9)
8. Standing Side Bend (Hour 7)
9. Standing Backward Bend (Hour 7)
10. Standing Forward Bend (Hour 7)
11. Sitting Forward Bend (Hour 7)
12. Churn (Hour 7)
13. Butterfly (Hour 7)
14. Symbol of Yoga (Hour 7)
15. Cobra Pose (Hour 5)
16. Locust Pose (Hour 5)
17. Bow Pose (Hour 5)
18. Child's Pose (Hour 3)
19. Half Fish Pose (Hour 5)
20. Arch Pose (Hour 5)
21. Bridge Pose (Hour 5)
22. Knees to Chest Pose (Hour 3)
23. Tension and Relaxation Exercise in the Corpse Pose (Hour 3)

Don't rush through the program. Remember to pause and relax a moment after each pose.

PROCEED WITH CAUTION

Don't begin any yoga program without first reviewing the precautions listed in Hour 2. Remember: If you have a serious medical condition, check with your doctor before starting an exercise routine. Pregnant and menstruating women also need to use extra caution.

Design Your Second Beginning Routine

Here is a second yoga session also designed for the average student. Once again you'll begin with a breathing exercise and move through some stretches to limber you up. This session ends with the 31 Points concentration exercise.

1. Alternate Nostril Breathing (Hour 4) in the Easy Posture (Hour 14) or Chair Posture (Hour 14)
2. Standing Stretch (Hour 2)
3. Cat Stretch (Hour 2)
4. Lunge Stretch (Hour 2)
5. Reclining Stretch (Hour 2)
6. Stomach Lift (Hour 9)
7. Tree Pose (Hour 3)
8. Angle Pose (Hour 8)
9. Triangle Pose (Hour 8)
10. Revolving Triangle (Hour 8)
11. Torso Twist (Hour 8)
12. Half Spinal Twist (Hour 8)
13. Reclining Twist (Hour 8)
14. Rocking Chair Roll (Hour 8)
15. Staff Pose (Hour 6)
16. Shoulder Stand (Hour 6)
17. Plow Pose (Hour 6)
18. Pigeon Pose (Hour 6)
19. Down Facing Dog Pose (Hour 6)
20. Warrior Pose (Hour 6)
21. Horse Riding Pose (Hour 6)
22. Leg Lift (Hour 9)
23. Balance Pose (Hour 9)
24. 31 Points (Hour 3) in the Corpse Pose (Hour 3)

Take your time. Remember to relax for at least a few breaths between each posture. If you find yourself pressed for time, skip a few of the postures rather than skipping your moment of relaxation between poses.

JUST A MINUTE

Many yoga students fit their Hatha practice in first thing in the morning, before breakfast. If you find it most convenient to do your yoga routine early in the day, spend a few extra minutes doing the rolls and bending exercises before launching into the formal yoga poses. This will help limber your muscles, which might still be stiff from your night of sleep.

Design Your Intermediate Routine

The Intermediate Hatha Yoga routine is for students with somewhat above average flexibility and ability to balance. It's a good idea for Intermediate students to start with a few Beginning level sessions before launching into this more challenging program. However, the more demanding postures required here will keep the session interesting for individuals progressing beyond the Beginning stage.

The Intermediate session begins with a mentally stabilizing breathing exercise. You might wish to do Alternate Nostril Breathing either seated cross-legged on the floor or sitting upright in a chair. The routine then moves into the Sun Salutation, which will help warm up your body for the following yoga exercises.

1. Alternate Nostril Breathing (Hour 4)
2. Two to six repetitions of the Sun Salutation (Hour 12)
3. Stomach Lift (Hour 9)
4. Revolving Triangle (Hour 8)
5. Locust Pose (Hour 5)
6. Bow Pose (Hour 5)
7. Child's Pose (Hour 3)
8. Arch Pose (Hour 5)
9. Bridge Pose (Hour 5)
10. Shoulder Stand (Hour 6)
11. Plow Pose (Hour 6)
12. Camel Pose (Hour 10)
13. Knees to Chest Pose (Hour 3)
14. Inclined Plane Pose (Hour 10)
15. Eagle Pose (Hour 10)

16. King Dancer Pose (Hour 10)

17. Archer Pose (Hour 10)

18. Back Bending Monkey Pose (Hour 10)

19. Half Spinal Twist (Hour 8)

20. Leg Lift (Hour 9)

21. Balance Pose (Hour 9)

22. 61 Points (Hour 3) in the Corpse Pose (Hour 3)

Add extra relaxation poses as needed. It's important to allow your circulation to return to normal between postures, so don't neglect the relaxation phase following each pose.

FYI   *Asana Pranayama Mudra Bandha* by Swami Satyananda Saraswati is an excellent yoga book from India that will help you understand the postures, breathing exercises, hand positions, and body "locks" used in the yoga tradition. The Bihar School of Yoga is one of the premier yoga teaching and research institutions in the world.

DESIGN YOUR ADVANCED ROUTINE

The Advanced Hatha Yoga routine is suitable for individuals with superb flexibility as well as superior upper body strength. You will need good concentration and the ability to hold your balance in some of the difficult postures included in this session.

1. Glowing Face Breathing (Hour 4)

2. Bellows Breathing (Hour 4)

3. Humming Breath (Hour 4)

4. Six to ten repetitions of the Sun Salutation (Hour 12)

5. Stomach Lift (Hour 9)

6. Stomach Roll (Hour 9)

7. Angle Pose (Hour 8)

8. Triangle Pose (Hour 8)

9. Revolving Triangle Pose (Hour 8)

10. Shoulder Stand (Hour 6)

11. Plow Pose (Hour 6)

12. Fish Pose (Hour 5)

13. Knees to Chest Pose (Hour 3)

14. Dolphin Pose (Hour 11)

15. Headstand (Hour 11)

16. Corpse Pose (Hour 3)

17. Crow Pose (Hour 11)

18. Peacock Pose (Hour 11)

19. Wheel Pose (Hour 11)

20. Scorpion Pose (Hour 11)

21. Full Spinal Twist (Hour 11)

22. 61 Points (Hour 3) in the Corpse Pose (Hour 3)

Add extra relaxation postures if necessary.

 FYI The Yoga Alliance is devoted to upgrading and standardizing training for yoga teachers. For more information, log on to www.yogaalliance.com.

CREATING AN ATMOSPHERE

Some students find it helpful to create an atmosphere in their home that promotes yoga practice. You might wish to allot a room or the corner of one room in your house exclusively to yoga practice. If this isn't practical, you can still psychologically cordon off a portion of your living quarters by keeping that area neat and clean, and putting up pictures, paintings, or posters that inspire you to continually return to your yoga practice. For some people, this means photographs of saints and adepts from the yoga tradition. For others it might be pictures of an inspirational spiritual figure such as Jesus Christ, Krishna, or Buddha, or an image of the Divine Mother. Pictures of yoga practitioners holding Hatha Yoga or meditation postures can also do the trick.

You may find it helpful to light a candle when you begin your practice, and put it out when you end your session. This gives your yoga routine a pleasant sense of inauguration and closure, and sets this special time off from the rest of the events of the day.

Other individuals prefer to burn incense or an aromatic oil, or to play soft music, to enhance the atmosphere during their yoga practice. Traditionally, however, music and fragrances are not recommended. This is because pleasing sounds and smells may distract you from your inward focus. Remember

GO TO ▷
In Hour 16, you will learn a number of techniques for drawing your awareness inward and improving your concentration. The ultimate purpose of yoga is to acquire self-knowledge. This requires turning your attention momentarily away from the busy outer world into the inner universe of your soul.

that while you're holding the Hatha Yoga postures, your attention should be centered within. You should be attuning yourself to your body and energy level, not to your external environment. It's best to create an atmosphere of light, spaciousness, and tranquility, then turn your concentration from the room around you to the inner space of your body and mind.

AIDS TO HATHA PRACTICE

What equipment do you need to maximize your Hatha Yoga session? Provided that the room where you are doing your practice is carpeted, you don't actually need to spend any money on yoga paraphernalia at all. However, if you must do your postures on a bare floor or very thin rug, you should invest in a yoga mat. A yoga mat will provide just the amount of cushioning you need to avoid injuring or bruising your back while doing postures on the floor. It also provides traction to keep you from slipping as you move through the poses. Look for a yoga mat that's long enough to allow you to lie on it full length. Most yoga mats are portable so you can tuck them away after your Hatha routine, or easily carry them with you to a yoga class.

If you're not sure that you're doing Diaphragmatic Breathing correctly, or if you want help perfecting your practice of this natural form of breathing, you may want to invest in a yoga sandbag or breath pillow. These pillows generally weigh between 5 and 10 pounds, and are designed to fit over your upper abdomen (just below your rib cage) while you lie on the floor in the Corpse Posture. You can feel confident you're breathing diaphragmatically if you notice the pillow gently moving up and down while your chest and shoulders don't move at all.

If you page through a yoga magazine or visit a well-stocked book stall at your local yoga center, you will discover a host of yoga products. These include props to hoist different parts of your body during Hatha postures, and large balls or curved tables for you to lie on backward to increase the flexibility of your spine. You'll find straps to hold your legs or arms together during poses in which you might be tempted to move out of the correct position. There are belts short-limbed students can use in postures where the short length of their arms prevents them from reaching all the way. There are even slings you can hang from to deepen yogic stretches. The vast majority of yoga practitioners are able to do just fine without these items, however.

For several hundred dollars, you can purchase biofeedback equipment that measures the level of tension and relaxation you achieve during a yoga pose. For people who are not particularly introspective, this can be helpful.

However, once you begin getting the hang of the postures and developing a fuller sense of your body state, your own awareness will do the job just as well.

Many traditional yogis in India own nothing but one change of clothing, a rosary, and a water pot. Hatha Yoga was developed by individuals committed to self-reliance. No doubt many of the ancient masters would be astonished at the variety of products and devices available to yoga students today.

It is important, however, that you wear loose, comfortable clothing during your yoga session. You need to be able to move freely! So no tight pants, and no shirts or blouses that constrict the movement of your arms. A T-shirt and elastic-waist shorts or pants will do just fine.

YOGA RETREAT CENTERS, CLASSES, AND EVENTS

Yoga helps you look and feel so much better that, once you start your program, you may not be able to imagine a day without it. The way you feel after beginning a consistent yoga program is ample proof of the system's effectiveness. No wonder Hatha Yoga has been around for at least a thousand years and has spread all over the world!

Signing up for a yoga class is not only a wonderful way to enhance your own yoga practice, it's also a great way to meet people with similar interests in health and self-development. Check in the Yellow Pages under "Yoga" for the classes nearest you.

Have you considered taking a yoga vacation? Numerous spas and yoga retreat centers around the country offer getaway programs where you can work on honing your yoga skills under the guidance of experienced teachers, while also enjoying massage, Ayurvedic medical treatment, and often great vegetarian food as well. You can sign up for courses in yoga philosophy, meditation, vegetarian cooking, yogic cleansing, and holistic health practices. Yoga vacations are rejuvenating and educational. Wouldn't it be great to come home from a vacation relaxed, centered, and spiritually energized? See Appendix C for a list of yoga retreat centers. Many of the larger yoga organizations, such as the Ananda Community near Nevada City, the Mount Madonna Center south of San Francisco, and the Himalayan Institute in eastern Pennsylvania, offer yoga vacation options.

If you'd rather spend two days than two weeks immersing yourself in the yoga lifestyle, consider attending a yoga conference. You'll get to meet

GO TO ▶
Check Appendix C for yoga organizations that supply yoga mats, breath pillows, clothing appropriate for doing Hatha postures, and other yoga-related supplies. Or log on to www.yogapro.com for information about Hatha mats and other tools you can use to enhance your experience of Hatha Yoga.

some of the most knowledgeable and skilled Hatha teachers in the Western world who will be happy to answer your questions and concerns. Check your local bookstore for yoga magazines like *Yoga Journal* and *Yoga International*, which list upcoming conferences and events.

By now you know the most important yoga poses and have selected the postures you want to incorporate in your Hatha practice. In the upcoming section of this book you'll go on to learn about the next level of yoga practice: meditation. Having begun to work with your body and energy stage, you'll now go on to work at increasingly subtle levels with your mind and spirit.

HOUR'S UP!

Here's your quiz for Hour 13. Check to see how many of these statements you can answer correctly. Answer true or false to the following statements:

1. A breath pillow is designed to provide a workout for your diaphragm.

2. Playing soft music and burning incense during your Hatha session is highly recommended in the yoga tradition.

3. If you have learned Hatha Yoga postures from a book like this one, there isn't much point in attending a formal yoga class.

4. The relaxation portion of your yoga session is the least important part of the program, and should be skipped if you're pressed for time.

5. Breathing exercises help strengthen your respiratory organs and both soothe and stimulate your nervous system.

6. Each bend and twist in one direction should be balanced with a counter-posture requiring you to bend or twist in the opposite direction.

7. Doing yoga at the same time each day is one way yogis work with their body's biorhythms.

8. Doing the advanced yoga routine provides far more physiological benefits for your body than one of the beginning level routines.

9. Doing the Sun Salutation near the beginning of a Hatha session is an excellent way to warm up your body before starting the formal yoga postures.

10. Yoga retreat centers offer classes in Hatha postures, meditation, and vegetarian cooking.

QUIZ

PART IV
Mastering Meditation

HOUR 14   Introduction to Meditation

HOUR 15   Learn to Meditate

HOUR 16   Create Inner Focus

HOUR 17   Overcome Obstacles

HOUR 18   Ignite Your Energies

HOUR 19   Awaken Your Awareness

HOUR 14

Introduction to Meditation

CHAPTER SUMMARY

LESSON PLAN:

In this hour you will learn …

- The original purpose of Hatha Yoga was to prepare the body for inner exploration and a rich spiritual life.

- Meditation connects us with an infinite inner reservoir of guidance, healing, and creativity.

- Meditation stimulates the parasympathetic nervous system, reducing the symptoms of stress.

- Meditation creates a safe, enjoyable "high" without the use of drugs.

- There are five basic sitting postures traditionally used in meditation.

In the spiritual tradition of India, mastery of the Hatha Yoga postures is considered just one rung on the ladder to personal fulfillment and well-being. Working with the body leads to working with the mind. If inwardly you're unfocused, angry, depressed, or anxious, then no matter how fabulous the hatha exercises help you look or how physically healthy they help you become, you're still miles away from the balanced and tranquil state yogis aspire to.

The ancient seers of India developed a methodical system of meditation exercises to help people confront and release their anxieties, defuse their frustrations, and connect with their inner guidance. In Hours 14 through 19, you'll be introduced to the inner world of meditation as it was mapped by the great yoga masters. Yoga is ultimately about the expansion of consciousness, and that means traveling the hidden paths of the world within to your innermost core.

GO BEYOND YOUR BODY

Originally, the purpose of Hatha Yoga was to develop a body that was healthy, supple, and strong, so that the yogi could sit in a stable, upright posture comfortably for hours of meditation at a time. Hatha, together with a balanced yogic diet, a moderate amount of physical activity, and a positive frame of mind, helped build a healthy body. This contributed to freedom from disease, injury, and premature death—all obstacles on the path to enlightenment that yogis sought to avoid.

FYI *Meditation and Its Practice* by Swami Rama is one of the clearest and most practical introductions to the process of meditation available in English. It lays out a month-by-month series of exercises to guide you along the inner path, and explains how yogis use mantras and breath awareness to dive deeper within their spirit.

For the yogis of the Himalayas, meditation was the pathway to enlightenment. Since the early 1970s, when medical researchers in the West began studying the effects of meditation, numerous reasons for learning to sit quietly and turn the mind inward have been extensively documented.

BENEFITS OF MEDITATION

A few of the physiological and psychological benefits of meditation include:

- Meditation slows your breathing rate and metabolism by as much as 50 percent. This allows your body to relax deeply and begin to regenerate itself.

- The effect of meditation on your internal systems slows down the aging process, which may be one reason why advanced yogis often look years, even decades, younger than they actually are.

- Meditation alleviates the biological effects of stress, and may help relieve some stress-related diseases such as hypertension (high blood pressure).

- Meditation increases your peripheral blood flow, promoting muscular relaxation and enhancing healing and vitality.

- Meditation stimulates the parasympathetic nervous system, the part of your nervous system that promotes physical calmness and mental tranquility.

- Meditation helps you face your inner conflicts with objectivity and compassion.

- Meditation helps allay worry and anxiety, promoting instead serenity and self-confidence.

- Meditation increases mental focus, enhancing your ability to act effectively in the world.

- Meditation promotes insight, fostering self-awareness.

While psychoanalysis introduces people to the psychological dynamics behind their neurotic feelings and actions, meditation puts them in touch with the highest part of themselves. When you learn to meditate you contact the wisest and most serene aspect of your inner self, and open the channel to your intuitive powers.

As your ability to move into a meditative state deepens, you begin to see through your problems to practical solutions. You stop identifying with the most fearful, irritable, or depressed aspects of your personality, and begin to experience yourself as a balanced, creative, and joyful spirit fully capable of meeting life's challenges. You learn to draw on inner resources you may not even have been aware you possessed.

FYI *The Wellness Tree* by Justin O'Brien, Ph.D., explains how yoga and meditation can lead you to the Tree of Life, your inner source of energy and vitality.

A Natural High

Today many Westerners deal with their problems—or avoid dealing with them—by turning to drugs and alcohol. Let's compare the effects of popular drugs with meditation.

Throughout the world, people use alcohol to help them relax, loosen up, and forget their cares. Unfortunately, alcohol is one of the most toxic substances you can buy without a prescription. Long-term excessive use has debilitating effects on the liver, brain, heart, pancreas, stomach lining, and immune system. Binge drinking has proven fatal on many a college campus. Drinking is also a leading cause of driving fatalities.

Hatha Yoga and meditation also help you relax and loosen up. Hatha Yoga tones and invigorates the same physical organs that alcohol attacks, while meditation provides the focus and objectivity that help people face their problems in life, rather than running away from them.

PROCEED WITH CAUTION

Contrary to the popular myth, meditation is not for everyone. Traditionally, meditation teachers would screen their students carefully before initiating them in the powerful techniques of the inward journey. Psychotics and seriously fearful, neurotic individuals will probably benefit more from psychotherapy or medication than meditation.

Many people work and play extremely hard, living insanely busy lives that don't allow their bodies and minds time to recharge. Often they turn to stimulants to keep them going. These range from caffeine and nicotine to cocaine or prescription drugs such as amphetamines. These work by cranking up the body's production of brain chemicals such as dopamine and norepinephrine, which produce a hit of energy and elevate the mood. But the brain quickly becomes depleted, and when it does, its signals of distress create the symptoms of withdrawal.

Meditation induces a deep state of relaxation that allows the tensions draining your life force to melt away. It innervates your body, providing the stamina you need to stay the course of your busy schedule, and does so without any harmful side effects.

Today, pharmaceutical depressants are among the most commonly prescribed drugs. These include Atavan, Valium, Xanax, and Dalmane. They can reduce anxiety and help people sleep better. For some people, these are lifesavers. However, they don't really help people resolve the problems causing their anxiety in the first place.

Meditation empowers you to confront, control, and release your fears. It puts you, not the drug, in control of your life, and helps you address the bad habits that are sabotaging your happiness.

Mood- and Mind-Altering Drugs

Some of the most common street drugs are opiates such as heroin. Opiates have been used for thousands of years to treat pain and increase endurance. These are seductive drugs because they produce a sense of euphoria. Unfortunately, even small doses can quickly lead to addiction. Yet a blissful sense of peace and well-being is one of the most commonly reported effects of meditation. People emerge from their meditation healthy and refreshed, not shaky and ill as drugs addicts do from their latest fix.

Some people turn to hallucinogens such as LSD, peyote, and magic mushrooms in order to explore the phenomena of consciousness. Unfortunately, bad trips and overdoses can lead to illness and in some cases even death. Meditation is the premier method for exploring consciousness. It's a safe and time-tested path to the expansion of awareness.

Mastering the Meditation Postures

Before you learn to meditate, you have to learn to sit still. Sounds easy, right? Unfortunately, few people in the West know how to do this. Adults often try to force children to sit quietly. Kids usually find the experience excruciatingly difficult, particularly if they're overstimulated by the caffeine in the soft drinks they drink instead of water, or by the massive amount of sugar in the typical

American diet. And because most adults spend their days in near-constant motion, it may feel strange to sit completely still for any length of time.

Throughout the day you're running here and there on one errand or another. A meditation session is the one time of day when both your body and your mind stop running. It is not a passive, almost vegetative state like the one you may experience while watching television. Your mind will be alert and attentive, but in a relaxed way. Sitting up straight optimizes nerve function in the spine and brain, which leads to clarity of consciousness. It also facilitates the free movement of your diaphragm, leading to a fuller, smoother breathing cycle.

Try the following experiment:

1. Sit up with your head, neck, and trunk in a straight line. Breathe diaphragmatically for a moment or so.
2. Now slump forward for a moment. Let your head hang forward slightly.

You probably noticed a very distinct difference in the way you felt. The upright pose helped you feel more energized and alert. In the hunched posture, even though your back muscles were more relaxed, you probably felt more sluggish and mentally dull. Compare the two postures again and see if you can also feel how much more freely you can breathe in the upright posture.

The great yoga master Patanjali (author of the *Yoga Sutras*, which you'll learn more about in Hour 22) defined the perfect meditative posture as "that posture which is steady and comfortable." It allows you to sit up straight without slumping, swaying, jerking, or fidgeting for a half-hour or more. Neither your back nor your legs should feel strained.

If you've never sat in a meditative posture before, you may find that after a few minutes your legs start to "fall asleep." They start to ache or feel prickly, then become numb. Adjust the placement of your legs slightly to minimize this problem. Keep your first meditation sessions short to allow your knees and ankles a chance to adjust to this new position. You'll find that if you persist in practicing these poses, in a short time this difficulty will disappear. However, if you still feel discomfort after several attempts to sit on the floor, use a chair instead!

See which of the following five poses you feel most comfortable sitting in. This will be the posture you'll hold for the meditation exercises you'll practice in Hours 15 through 19.

GO TO ▷
Many Westerners start slumping forward after a few minutes when they sit for meditation. Due to a lifetime of poor posture, the muscles that are supposed to support their spine are underdeveloped. To help strengthen these important muscles, spend extra time working with the Staff Pose you learned in Hour 6. The Churn from Hour 7 and the Half Spinal Twist from Hour 8 will also help.

You'll eventually want to work up to meditation sessions of 20 to 30 minutes at least once a day (there's more on when to meditate and on timing your meditations in Hour 16). As you begin experiencing the benefits of meditation, you may find that these few minutes are a highlight of your day!

JUST A MINUTE

If you've been sitting in chairs and sofas all your life, sitting on the floor can be hard on your back and knees. Use a meditation cushion to ease the strain on your lower back. It will lift your pelvis a few inches off the floor, increasing the angle between your spine and thighbones.

EASY POSTURE

The enormous advantage of sitting in the Easy Posture or *Sukhasana* (*sukha* means "easy" or "pleasant") is that the majority of people can sit in this pose fairly effortlessly. The disadvantage is that it's not as stable as the next three postures. Because it doesn't lock your lower back into place, it's easy to unconsciously slump forward.

The Easy Posture.

(Photo credit: Johnathan Brown)

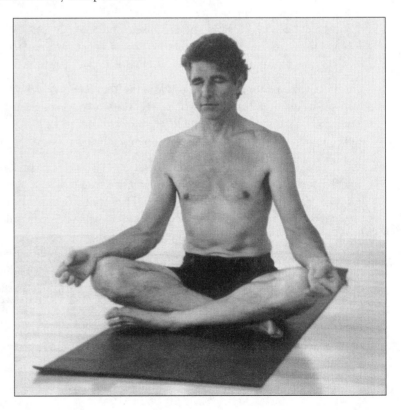

1. Sit down cross-legged on the floor. Your left foot should be beneath your right knee and your right foot beneath your left knee.

2. Rest your right hand on your right knee, and your left hand on your left knee. Your palms should face upward. Let the tips of your index fingers lightly touch the tips of your thumbs.

3. Sit up straight with your head, neck, and back in alignment.

4. Relax all the muscles in your body except those involved in holding your back, neck, and head up in a straight line.

If your arms are petite in length, your hands may not reach your knees without your tilting forward. In this case, rest your hands farther up your thighs so that you can sit up straight without leaning forward.

If it feels too unnatural to rest your hands with your palms turned upward, leave them turned downward in the beginning.

The vast majority of people raised in Western cultures are unused to sitting on the floor. This may be because their ancestors hail, for the most part, from northern European latitudes where for much of the year it was too cold to sit on the ground. In those cultures, people began sitting on chairs in order to conserve body heat during the long, cold winters. Today sitting on chairs is taken so completely for granted that Americans are startled when they visit India or other countries where much of the population routinely sits on the ground.

Centuries of sitting on stools, chairs, and sofas has created an epidemic of lower back problems in Western civilization. Back pain is one of the leading causes of employee illness in America. Hatha Yoga is excellent for helping strengthen the muscles of the lower back, as well as increasing their suppleness. But until the muscles in your back and thighs are strong and flexible enough for you to sit comfortably on the floor for a half-hour or more, using a meditation cushion is a good idea. These cushions are called *asanas* in Sanskrit, the same word used for a Hatha Yoga posture.

There are numerous types of meditation cushions on the market. The tall, Zen-style zafu cushions are not recommended for this purpose, as they lift your pelvis too high, exaggerating the angle between your spine and thigh bones, and increasing the pressure on your knees. Look for the lowest cushion you can sit on comfortably. Cushions filled with buckwheat hulls are ideal because you can adjust their height depending on how increasingly flexible you become over time. They also conform to the shape of your body,

GO TO ▶
If you have a hard time stabilizing yourself in a meditation posture because your knees ride far up off the floor, spend a few extra minutes each day working with the Butterfly and the Symbol of Yoga Postures you learned in Hour 7. These will help you develop the flexibility you need to sit on the floor comfortably.

providing firm but not hard support. They are probably the most comfortable cushions available. You can order one for between $18 and $35; log on to www.himalayaninstitute.org or call 1-800-822-4547.

TIME SAVER

 A folded blanket can serve just as well for sitting on the floor as a meditation cushion. Use a blanket made of natural material like wool or cotton rather than one made of synthetic fabrics that, according to the yogis, block the currents of subtle energy between your body and the earth. Pillows are generally not a good idea because they're too soft and, since they bulge in the middle, they distribute your weight unevenly.

AUSPICIOUS POSTURE

The Auspicious Posture is called *Swastikasana* in Sanskrit because in this pose your legs cross each other in a swastikalike design. For thousands of years, the swastika has been a symbol of good luck and auspiciousness in the Hindu, Buddhist, and Jain religious traditions. Unfortunately, since the advent of the Third Reich in the 1930s, the swastika is now indelibly associated with Nazi Germany in the minds of most Westerners. You'll notice that when the swastika appears in Eastern spiritual art, the top and bottom bars run horizontally. When Adolph Hitler adopted this symbol, he distorted both its appearance and its meaning, flipping it to the side so that the top and bottom bars run diagonally.

In the Auspicious Posture the ankles lock at the groin. This helps stabilize your trunk in an upright position.

1. Sit down cross-legged on the floor. Position the sole of your right foot against the underside of your left thigh.

2. Tuck your left foot between your right calf and right thigh. Your left big toe can be seen over the top of your right calf but the other left toes are now hidden inside your bent right leg.

3. Your right foot should now be sandwiched between your left calf and thigh. Only your right toe should be visible above your left leg.

4. Rest your right hand on your right knee, and your left hand on your left knee. The tips of your index fingers lightly touch the tips of your thumbs.

5. Sit up with your head, neck, and trunk straight.

6. Except for the muscles holding your back, neck, and head upright, the rest of your body should be relaxed.

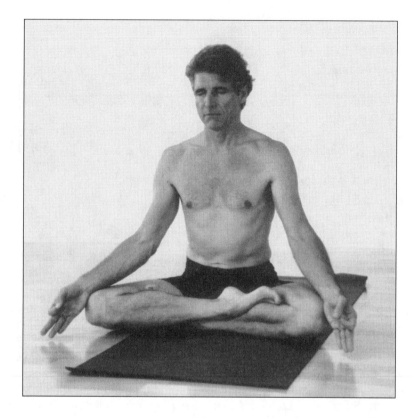

The Auspicious Posture.

(Photo credit: Johnathan Brown)

If it feels more comfortable to do so, try this posture with your legs reversed: Tuck your right foot between your left calf and thigh first.

Notice that your body weight is better distributed in this posture than the Easy Pose. This is because your entire legs, including your knees, are on the floor, forming a solid foundation for the rest of your body.

ACCOMPLISHED POSTURE

The Accomplished Posture or *Siddhasana* (*siddha* means "mastery," "perfection," or "accomplishment") is the meditation pose preferred by celibate male yogis. The pressure it applies to the perineum (the area between the anus and genital organs) was believed to inhibit the sexual drive in males. You will often see yoga masters and advanced students in this posture, so it's being presented here, but generally Indian yogis advise Westerners to avoid this sitting position unless personally instructed in how to hold it by a knowledgeable teacher.

*The Perfect
Posture.*

*(Photo credit:
Johnathan Brown)*

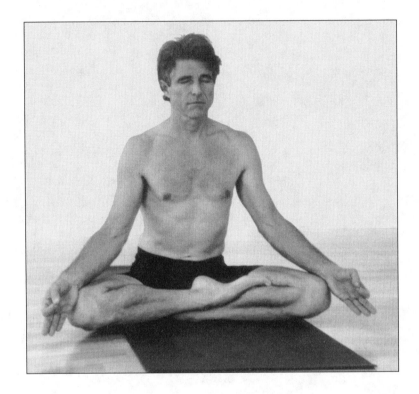

1. Sit cross-legged on the floor. Then position your left heel against your perineum.

2. Tuck your right heel against your pubic bone. Your right ankle now rests directly over or directly in line with your left ankle.

3. Tuck your right foot in between your left thigh and calf. Only your right big toe should remain visible. Pull your left foot up slightly so that only your left big toe is visible from between your right thigh and calf.

4. Place your right hand on your right knee, and your left hand on your left knee. The tips of your index fingers should lightly touch the tips of your thumbs.

5. Sit upright with your head, neck, and trunk straight.

6. Relax your entire body, except for the muscles holding you up in a sitting position.

LOTUS POSTURE

Padmasana or the Lotus Posture (*padma* literally means "lotus") is the meditation pose most closely associated with yoga in Western minds. Ironically, this posture is not preferred for use in meditation in the Indian tradition. There are technical reasons for this having to do with the way yogis manipulate their internal energies during advanced practices.

While supple-bodied students can hold this posture fairly easily, most Westerners find this pose painful in the beginning. Don't hold this position for more than half a minute on your first attempt. This is an excellent posture for locking your body into an upright position, but if it's too uncomfortable, work with one of the other poses described here instead.

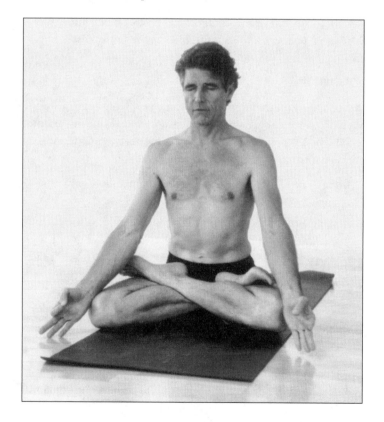

The Lotus Posture.

(Photo credit: Johnathan Brown)

1. Sit cross-legged on the floor. Place your left foot on the uppermost portion of your right thigh. Your left sole should point upward.

2. Place your right foot on the uppermost portion of your left thigh with your right sole pointing upward. At this point both your heels are pressed against your lower abdomen.

3. Place your right hand on your right knee, and your left hand on your left knee, with your index fingertips lightly touching the tips of your thumbs.

4. Sit up straight with your head, neck, and trunk in a line.

5. Relax your body, except for the muscles holding you in the sitting posture.

Some individuals find that starting with putting the right foot on the left thigh is more comfortable than beginning with the left foot on the right thigh.

Advanced students form several hatha postures, including the Fish Pose and Symbol of Yoga, with their legs folded in the Lotus Pose.

CHAIR POSTURE

Due to illness, infirmity, or injury, some people just can't sit on the floor. *Maitri Asana* or the Chair Posture (*maitri* actually means "friendship" or "good will") is perfect for them. There are several important steps to ensuring that you're sitting correctly in this pose.

1. Select a chair with a firm seat angled parallel to the floor. Avoid soft, heavily cushioned, or diagonally angled seats.

2. Sit down on the chair, placing your feet flat on the floor. This may mean that you have to sit forward on the chair in order for your feet to be positioned squarely on the floor directly in front of the chair. Your feet will be a foot or so apart.

3. Straighten your back. Imagine that there is a small hook attached to the top of your skull and someone is pulling up on it. This will help you pull your spine into a vertical position.

4. Place your hands in your lap with your palms turned upward. The tips of your thumbs and index fingers should lightly touch.

5. Scan your body to ensure that you're relaxed and comfortable, while maintaining a fully upright position in the chair.

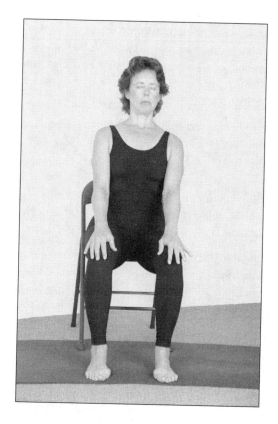

The Chair Posture.

(Photo credit: Alex Fernandez & Evolution Visual Services)

If you experiment with the five meditation postures listed here, you'll probably find that sitting in a chair is the least conducive to an upright posture. Most chairs are not designed for you to put your feet squarely on the ground while you sit straight at the same time. You will need to find a chair that works best for you. Resist the temptation to lean forward or backward, or to slump downward.

COMFORTABLE BUT STEADY

A very few people, either due to a back injury, paralysis, or extreme weakness, simply cannot sit up straight, or can't sit up at all. In preparing for meditation, these students should use pillows to prop themselves up as nearly vertically as they can without experiencing discomfort. The more your sitting posture moves from the vertical, the more likely you are to become distracted, and the more easily you may find yourself falling asleep during meditation.

Patanjali explained that the perfect meditation posture is steady and comfortable. Although the postures illustrated in this hour are classic, they are by no means your only alternatives. If they don't feel right to you, explore a variety of different poses until you find one that works for your body. The point is to be able to sit upright without strain.

Now you're ready to begin your inward journey. Hour 15 will teach you how to meditate.

HOUR'S UP!

Here's a quiz to help you measure your mastery of the material presented in Hour 14. Answer true or false to the following statements:

1. Traditionally, the purpose of Hatha Yoga was to prepare students for the inner journey of meditation.

2. Meditation increases your respiratory rate, making you far more mentally alert.

3. Meditation enhances insight and self-awareness.

4. If your doctor has prescribed a pharmaceutical depressant for you, you should not attempt to meditate.

5. Peace and well-being is a commonly reported side effect of meditation.

6. The ideal meditation posture is steady and comfortable.

7. The Accomplished Posture is the best general-purpose meditation posture.

8. The thicker and harder the meditation cushion you use, the better.

9. Sitting up straight allows the nerve fibers in your spine to work optimally.

10. Sitting up straight allows your diaphragm to pump used air out of your body most efficiently.

HOUR 15

Learn to Meditate

LESSON PLAN:

In this hour you will learn ...

- Meditation helps you sort through the material in your unconscious mind.
- Ultimately, meditation introduces you to your super-conscious mind.
- Breath awareness is one of the yogi's most effective tools for deepening meditation.
- Mantras are important tools for deepening your state of inner awareness.
- Meditation defuses the emotional charge associated with painful memories.

When you learn to meditate, you begin an inward journey that carries you past the part of your mind you're most familiar with—your routine conscious awareness—to aspects of yourself you may barely be acquainted with at all, your subconscious and superconscious awareness. Remember that the Sanskrit word *yoga* actually means "union." The yoga practice of meditation unites you with all aspects of your personality, and integrates them into a unified whole.

Meditation begins by narrowing the range of your awareness, making you focus intently on one feeling, sound, or image. It ends by expanding the limits of your awareness indefinitely, to the point that advanced yogis actually experience themselves connecting with the unified field of all reality.

In Hour 4, you learned yogic breathing. In Hour 14, you learned to sit in a yogic posture. In this hour, you will put those skills together, and learn how to enter the world within you, the hidden dimensions of your own being. With regular practice, you'll learn how to align yourself with the vast resources of your Higher Self.

ENTER THE INNER WORLD

Yogis recognize three distinct stages of the inward journey. The first is called contemplation or *dharana* in Sanskrit. If you've ever been in love, you know this state well. You think intently about your lover, how he or she looks, what he or she said, what you did the last time you were together. All your thoughts focus around one theme as you contemplate the person you're so attracted to.

Meditation (called *dhyana* in the yoga tradition) takes this process to the next level. Now instead of thinking many different thoughts about one thing, you hold only one thought about that object in the field of your awareness. Imagine being so in love that you see nothing in your mind's eye but your lover's smiling face. Traditional yogis believe that by learning to hold your focus so intently that no other thoughts interrupt your meditation (not even other thoughts about that same thing), you gain tremendous mental power. You will begin practicing this level of awareness in this hour.

Advanced yogis move on to a third level of total mental absorption called *samadhi*. In this state you become so completely absorbed in one single thought or image that even your consciousness of yourself as the person thinking the thought vanishes. You experience a state of complete yoga or union with the object of your attention. If you're deeply in love, for example, you would experience yourself actually merging as one with your beloved.

STRICTLY DEFINED

Dharana means contemplation, or to think about one subject exclusively. **Dhyana** means meditation. In this state there is only one object in the mind. **Samadhi** is the state of full mental absorption in which even the sense of one's own existence apart from the object one is focused on disappears.

Yoga adepts in India teach that mastering this third state can lead to extraordinary psychic powers. Yoga lore is full of stories of great saints who use their advanced yogic skills to rescue, heal, or transform others who urgently need their help. In Hour 19, you'll discover some of the amazing experiences said to be available to yoga masters who can enter very deep states of meditation at will.

But even the greatest yoga master had to begin at the beginning. In yoga you begin with your breath.

CHECKING YOUR BREATHING CYCLE

Several times each day, take a moment to perform the following exercise in breath awareness:

1. Sit up with your head, neck, and trunk in a straight line.

2. Bring your full awareness to your nostrils. Focus intently on the sensation of air passing in and out of your nose. Notice that the air you breathe feels a bit cool as it enters your nostrils, but seems warmer when it passes back out of your nostrils.

3. Focus very closely on your breath. You are almost certainly breathing predominantly out of one nostril rather than the other. Pay close attention till you can tell whether you're mostly breathing through your right nostril or your left, or (though this is less likely) you're breathing through both nostrils equally.

4. If you can't tell which nostril you're breathing through predominantly, close off your left nostril with your fingers and check how fully you're breathing through your right nostril. Now use your fingers to close off your right nostril and check how fully you're breathing through your left nostril. Generally, you'll find you're breathing more through one nostril than the other.

GO TO ▶
Breath awareness is fundamental both to Hatha Yoga and meditation practice. Breath is the key yogis use to unlock the controls of their involuntary nervous system—the part of the nervous system that functions automatically and that people ordinarily can't regulate consciously. Review Hour 4 for information about this process.

Taking this inventory several times a day is not at all an idle exercise. It's an important way to monitor brain function, which yogis discovered thousands of years ago. If you're breathing mostly through your right nostril, your brain is geared up to be active. This is the best time to begin an aggressive aerobic exercise routine, for example, or to digest a heavy meal. If you're breathing mostly through your left nostril, however, your brain is primed for a passive activity such as listening to a lecture or watching television.

When you begin to meditate regularly, you'll be amazed at how useful this information is. If you're breathing predominantly through your right nostril when you sit down to meditate, you may find it difficult to focus on your practice. Instead, your mind will tend to race off to activities you're planning for the future. You'll probably feel restless and impatient. Your logical, analytic mind will be active and will resist your attempt to focus on one meditation object only.

If, on the other hand, you're breathing predominantly through your left nostril, you may find yourself having the opposite problem. You might feel dreamy or mentally inert. You might meditate for a moment but then in an instant, so quickly you don't even catch yourself doing it, you slip off into a reverie. You're tempted to daydream rather than focus your mind in meditation.

As you learned in Hour 4, your body cycles back and forth between right and left nostril predominance throughout the day. Yogis in India watch their nostril dominance very closely, and time their activities in accord with this natural cycle. Yogis will begin a journey when their right nostril is predominant, for example, or will sit down to relax when their left nostril is flowing.

FYI *How to Meditate Using Chakras, Mantras and Breath* by Dennis Chernin, M.D., provides an excellent introduction to the mechanics of meditation. It leads readers systematically through a beginning level practice. Dr. Chernin is a leading American homeopath and holistic physician who incorporates yoga and meditation in his medical practice.

Focus on Your Breath

Understanding your respiratory cycle provides vital clues that can help you maximize the time you spend sitting for meditation. Yogis who receive traditional training in India learn how to work with their breath and consequently often make very rapid progress in their inner work. Westerners are generally not initiated in this aspect of meditation. Consequently they waste enormous amounts of time fidgeting or fantasizing when they're supposed to be meditating. Western students are often quite good at holding a meditation posture, but holding their minds in meditative focus is another story.

The secret to meditating well is to open your sushumna. You might remember from Hour 4 that the sushumna is the central canal that runs down the middle of the back, and through which kundalini or the awakened power of consciousness is said to flow. Yogis say the sushumna is in the subtle body, not the physical body, though it corresponds to the center of the spinal column. Whether or not you believe the sushumna or kundalini or any subtle bodies actually exist, you can definitely feel the changes in the quality of your mental processes when you do the exercises that yogis claim activate the central canal.

Experiment with the following technique to get a sense of what opening the central canal actually feels like. Not everyone will experience the full result on the first try, but the majority of students who conscientiously work with this exercise on a daily basis achieve success within about two weeks.

1. Sit down in your favorite meditation posture from Hour 14. Sit upright with your head, neck, and trunk in a straight line. Close your eyes.

2. Bring your full awareness to your breath. Check to see whether you're breathing predominantly through your right or left nostril, or more or less equally through both.

3. Make sure you're breathing diaphragmatically (as described in Hour 4). Breathe diaphragmatically for about a minute. Don't let your mind wander, but keep it focused on your breathing process. Your breath should be smooth and even, with no jerks or pauses. Your breath should not be shallow, but shouldn't be so deep, either, that you feel a sense of strain toward the end of your inhalation or exhalation. Your breathing should feel easy and natural.

4. Now do the Alternate Nostril Breathing exercise described in Hour 4. It's important to keep your mind focused on your breath because your mental focus activates nerves that regulate your respiratory cycle. If your thoughts start to wander off, gently guide them back to your breath. Breathe slowly in a relaxed manner, but not so slowly that you feel like you're not getting enough air.

5. By now the Diaphragmatic Breathing and Alternate Nostril Breathing exercises will have made you begin to feel calm and centered. Your sense of mental clarity is greatly heightened. Notice that you now feel fully present in the moment.

6. Bring your full awareness to your nasal septum, the bridge of cartilage between your two nostrils. Focus intently on this point inside your nose as you continue breathing diaphragmatically. If you feel that you are still breathing predominantly through one nostril, shift your awareness to the opposite side of your nasal septum. Keep your attention there until you begin to feel that nostril start to open and clear.

7. When the nostril that seemed more closed begins to open, shift your awareness back to the center of the nasal septum. Focus intently on that point, feeling the air very gently pass in and out of both nostrils equally.

8. When air flows through both nostrils equally, slowly, gently, and smoothly, without jerks or pauses, you have opened the central channel called sushumna, and are experiencing the state yogis call "joyous mind." Remain in this state for a minute or two, enjoying the sense of clarity and tranquility it produces.

9. Open your eyes, stretch, and get up.

JUST A MINUTE

If you're feeling bored, you're not meditating. Meditation is a state of one-pointed mental concentration in which there's no room for distracting thoughts and feelings, including boredom. You can develop greater enthusiasm for your practice by reading inspirational books and spending time with more advanced meditators. This will help you stay more focused during meditation.

Regulate Your Nervous System

Congratulations! You have just experienced your first meditation session! Notice that while you were fully engrossed in your breathing process, intense concentration was fairly easy and distracting thoughts were few. You were deeply focused on one sensation, the feeling of air passing in and out of your nose. For those few moments, your mind was in a state of meditation.

Don't be concerned if this yogic process seems a bit mechanical right now. This preliminary exercise is a shortcut to the meditative state, and will give you a small taste of the sense of peace and presence that deep meditation provides. Remember that when students learn to play the piano, they're often asked to learn the scales first. Once they've mastered the mechanical-seeming process of playing the scales, playing favorite tunes becomes easy. When you master your breathing process, you are learning to "play the scales" of your nervous system, working with the nerve currents in your brain and spine to create a highly focused yogic state. Your body is now in such a state of balance that your body awareness starts to slip away, and a new, much richer, awareness of your mental status—your status as a spiritual being—begins to unfold inside you.

You have learned to use two valuable tools, a comfortable and steady sitting posture and breath awareness. These will help you on your inner journey. Now it's time to introduce an important third element, the special sound yogis call a *mantra*.

STRICTLY DEFINED

A **mantra** is a sound used in the yoga tradition to deepen the state of inner awareness.

Chant Your Mantra

When you are in a state of meditation, two things will *not* be happening. First, you should not be thinking. Thinking involves using the part of your brain involved in forming words and sentences. When this happens, you have slipped out of the state of meditation into the lower state of contemplation. Instead of holding just one object of awareness in your mind, you are thinking a number of different thoughts about it, or about something else. The laserlike beam of awareness you need to remain in a meditative state has become unfocused and your mental process begins to be scattered.

Secondly, you should not be trying to "empty" your mind and think of nothing. You'll only create frustration for yourself if you mistakenly believe "emptying" the mind is meditation. It is the nature of the mind to pay attention to some object—that's its job. If you try to shut down the mind by forcing all content out of your awareness, control of your mental process will slip away from you like a bar of soap slipping out of your wet fingers.

If both thinking and not thinking are unhelpful, how exactly do you meditate? The sages of antiquity came up with an amazingly clever device that allowed them to control the flow of their thoughts relatively easily. This way they could remain in a state of meditation for long periods, even hours or days at a time. This device is a mantra.

The benefits of mantra meditation are as follows:

- Physical well-being
- Emotional stability
- Mental clarity
- Spiritual growth

GO TO ▶

In this hour, you're learning how to use sacred sounds in meditation. In Hour 16, you'll learn how to use visual images. Some people find it easier to focus on images rather than sounds. Hour 16 will also introduce you to advanced mantras designed to help you go beyond sights and sounds altogether.

CONTROL THE GENIE

Yogis in India like to tell their students about the poor villager who discovered a magic bottle in the forest. When he uncorked the bottle, a powerful genie popped out. "You helped me escape from the bottle, so I have to do anything you command," the genie explained. "But you have to keep me busy. If you run out of work for me to do, in that moment I'll regain my freedom. And the first thing I'm going to do when I get loose is eat you for dinner!"

The villager was delighted to find himself in control of such a powerful servant and quickly set about fulfilling his dreams. "Build me a beautiful mansion, the largest one in South India!" Within a few moments, the mansion had been built. "Bring me all the gold and silver, and all the delicacies, and all the fashionable clothing I've ever wanted. And make all the women fall helplessly in love with me!" Within minutes, each project was completed. Soon the villager started running out of things to ask for. Realizing that he was about to be eaten for dinner, he ran to his guru to ask for help.

"Order the genie to build a tall pole. Command him to climb to the top and when he reaches it, to climb back down to the bottom. Tell him that when he gets to the bottom, he must climb back up to the top again," the guru suggested.

The villager quickly followed these instructions. Soon the genie was completely preoccupied climbing up and down the pole. He was no longer a threat to the villager or anyone else.

The genie, of course, represents your mind, which is constantly obeying your commands for better or worse, whether to create castles in the air or to complete real life projects. However, if you don't keep your mind constructively engaged it can turn on you and create all sorts of havoc: jealousy, greed, self-doubt, worry, depression. When you sit for your spiritual practice it will constantly interrupt your meditation with one concern, desire, or plan after another.

The mental equivalent of ordering the genie to climb up and down a pole is to ask your mind to chant a mantra. As your mind sounds out the mantra again and again, an astonishing phenomenon occurs. You experience yourself as a conscious entity separate from your mental process. You are the awareness that commands the genie of your mind to say the mantra, and you are the consciousness that listens to the sound of the mantra as your mind obeys you. The mind is your instrument; you are its master. The mantra is the tool you give your mental instrument to work with while you step back inside yourself and observe the process of your mind at work.

Once you have access to this "witness" consciousness within yourself, you will be in a position to explore both the subconscious and superconscious components of your inner being. Working through the material in your subconscious is like going through your basement and throwing out the junk that has collected there. You become able to let go of old fears and misconceptions, to see through your self-created limitations and delusions. Contacting your superconscious helps you gain the clarity, willpower, and inner guidance you need to make your way more cheerfully and effectively through life.

PROCEED WITH CAUTION

It's always best to learn meditation from an experienced teacher. He or she can help you distinguish between inspired guidance from your superconscious and unhelpful promptings from your subconscious. Most of the "voices" and "visions" particularly imaginative beginners experience in meditation are illusions, not divine revelations.

CHOOSE A MANTRA

The mantra or sound you use to help you deepen your meditation can be a meaningless sound like *hreem* or *hring*. It can be the name of a deity, or a short, inspiring phrase. Most mantras used by meditators in authentic yogic lineages come from the Sanskrit, and are considered highly sacred. They were originally conceived by great saints in high states of meditation. Because these mantras have been repeated trillions of times down through the ages by millions of meditators, yogis consider them to be very potent. The mantras are believed to have been energized by the conscious attention of so many sincere practitioners.

In traditional yoga lineages, students need special authorization to begin a mantra practice, and don't choose their own mantra. Instead, an experienced teacher selects a mantra for them based on their personality traits and spiritual inclinations. Yogis believe a mantra is most effective when it's given by a guru who has connected with its inner power and is able to transmit its subtle energy. The moment a guru first whispers a sacred mantra in a disciple's ear is called *diksha* or initiation in the tradition. It's considered a highly sacred moment, a second birth.

If you have already received a mantra from a spiritual mentor, you may wish to use that sound in the meditation exercise that follows. If you don't have a mantra, you can use *So Hum*, a well-known mantra that means "I am one with Divine Spirit." It's pronounced as if you were saying, "Can't remember the words to the song? *So hum* it."

WORK WITH INNER SOUND

Meditation is a living experience. Reading about it can point you toward an inward state or teach you the philosophy behind it, but only by sitting down and actually trying it will you begin to reap its many benefits. Here is a beginning level mantra practice:

1. Assume your meditation posture. Sit up comfortably with your head, neck, and spine straight.

2. Close your eyes and allow your body to relax. Your back stays straight but it should feel at ease, not forced or strained.

3. Pay attention to your breath for a few moments. It should be even, slow, and smooth. If it's jerky or shallow, relax another minute until your breathing is a little deeper and flows without jerking or stopping. Focus on your nasal septum, the bridge between your nostrils. If you are able to do so, allow your breath to flow smoothly and evenly through both nostrils equally.

4. Begin to mentally repeat your mantra or the sound *So Hum*. Listen attentively to the syllables as you mentally sound them out. Don't worry about coordinating the sound of the mantra with your inhalation or exhalation. Just keep repeating the mantra as quickly or slowly as feels natural.

5. If thoughts or mental images interrupt your meditation, simply dismiss them. Don't fight with your uninvited thoughts. Just keep turning your attention back to your mantra.

6. After a few minutes, stop consciously repeating the mantra. Enjoy the silent, pure awareness you are experiencing.

7. Open your eyes and sit quietly for a moment. Assimilate the tranquility and mental clarity you experienced in your meditation.

PROCEED WITH CAUTION

Some beginning meditation students experience bright lights and swirling colors when they close their eyes and focus within. In most cases, these are the result of neurons firing in your brain or optic nerve, not of divine visitations. Advanced yogis generally advise beginners to ignore this internal imagery.

MASTERING YOUR MIND

Beginners are frequently distracted by extraneous thoughts that rush into their minds, demanding attention. Anger, regret, or delight about events that occurred in the past may flash in your mind. Worries and plans about the future might arise. The desire to fantasize about romance, professional success, an exciting adventure, or some other theme may present itself very forcefully. The contents of your mind, particularly those that contain an emotional charge or sense of urgency, may constantly present themselves to you. Material from just below the surface of your ordinary awareness, and ultimately thoughts and feelings from deep in your unconscious, will impinge on your awareness. During meditation, you will definitely get to know your own mind!

The key to successful meditation is to master the contents of your mind, and not allow them to master you. So when you assume your meditation posture, make a mental resolution, "While I'm sitting in meditation, I will not allow myself to be distracted from my practice. I will deal with any concerns that arise in my mind only after my meditation is over." When thoughts appear such as "I need to wash my hair" or "I was going to turn on the TV and watch the news," don't worry about them or act on them. Instead just watch your thoughts go by, just as you disinterestedly watch traffic go by at an intersection.

When thoughts try to capture your attention, return your awareness to the sound of your mantra. Stay with the mantra! You can deal with your dirty hair or the news report later.

If you practice mantra meditation regularly, you'll begin having an amazing experience. Particularly emotionally charged or disturbing thoughts such as "I hate my sister-in-law!" might recur again and again. However, if you keep returning to your mantra rather than getting caught up in the train of your thoughts, remembering the snide remark your sister-in-law made last Thursday or how unattractive her new hairstyle is, then after a while the thought begins to lose its emotional impact. The mere thought of your sister-in-law no longer makes you angry or upset. You gain the ability to watch thoughts about emotionally distressing experiences dispassionately, as if you were watching birds flying around outside your kitchen window. Instead of being caught in mental melodrama, you begin to experience life with clarity and calmness. Instead of obsessing about certain topics, you become able to direct your thoughts toward or away from those subjects at will. Instead of just reacting to events occurring in your life on the basis of your past conditioning, you begin to make conscious, proactive decisions affecting your future.

Remember that if, during meditation, you're able to open your central channel so that the breath flows equally through both your nostrils as described earlier in this hour, you'll experience far fewer distracting thoughts during your meditation.

Use a Mala

If you visit India you'll often see yogis wearing malas, rosaries usually containing 108 beads. There is almost always a noticeably larger 109th bead called the guru bead. The beads are often made of rudrashaka seeds, sandalwood, or crystal. Many yoga centers around the world sell malas in their bookshops.

JUST A MINUTE

It's helpful to use a mala to keep track of the amount of time you've spent in meditation. You can purchase a Japa Kit at 1-800-822-4547 or at www.himalayaninstitute. org which includes a sandalwood mala, 10 gemstones for keeping track of completed rounds, an instruction booklet, and a log to keep track of your mantra practice.

Malas serve two main purposes in the yoga tradition. The first is to help meditators keep count of how many times they've repeated their mantra. This is especially helpful if a student has made a vow to chant it a certain number of times during each meditation session. (This kind of vow is called *purascharana* in Sanskrit.) The second reason is that the physical act of handling a rosary helps to keep the mind focused on the mantra.

If you own a mala, you might wish to make a mental resolution to repeat your mantra 100 times the next time you sit for meditation. Assume your meditation posture and begin breathing diaphragmatically. Open your central channel if you are able to do so. Then take out your mala and hold it in your right hand. (Malas are traditionally held in the right hand, although if you are left-handed you may wish to use your left hand should you find this easier.) Start with the bead right next to the larger guru bead and chant your mantra, slipping one bead between your fingers for each mantra until you come back to the guru bead after 108 repetitions.

Yogis usually rest the mala on their middle finger or ring finger and push the beads away from them, using their thumb. You can push or pull the beads in whatever manner feels most comfortable and natural to you. If you wish to recite your mantra several hundred times, when you get to the guru bead, don't skip over it. Instead flip the mala around in your hand and begin counting the next hundred beads in the opposite direction.

Don't give yourself credit for 108 repetitions when you finish your mala. Instead only count 100 repetitions, even though you actually chanted the mantra 108 times. The extra eight repetitions are offered for the welfare of the universe.

A mala symbolizes the connection between human consciousness and the cosmos. In yoga astronomy, the moon is said to take 108 steps, called *padas*, around the ecliptic. Stopping at the guru bead and turning back represents the sun changing its northward and southward courses at the summer and winter solstices. When you use a mala, you are replicating the movements of the two greatest lights in the sky.

Malas are not worn for decoration, like a necklace. If you look closely you'll see advanced yoga students often do wear malas around their necks, but they're concealed under their shirts and blouses. This is because in the yoga tradition it's considered inappropriate to advertise the fact that you're doing a spiritual practice.

Yogis believe that a mala becomes "charged up" with spiritual energy if a practitioner repeatedly chants a sacred mantra using it. The mala then acts like a secret talisman, blessing and protecting its wearer. Malas should only be handled by their owners. Don't let anyone else touch yours.

PRACTICE JAPA

Chanting your mantra continuously is called *japa* in the yoga tradition. Japa can be practiced at three levels:

- The mantra is recited out loud.
- The mantra is whispered, or merely thought but the lips still move as if forming the sound.
- The mantra is sounded only in the mind.

Speaking the mantra out loud is usually best for beginners because it helps them learn the pronunciation and also helps them stay focused. If your mind starts to wander, you may find yourself mispronouncing the mantra. In this way you get instant feedback that your attention drifted away from your spiritual practice. However, your mantra is for you alone, so you should not chant it out loud if others are sitting nearby and can overhear you. Mantras that are only repeated mentally are considered the most potent, however. So as soon as you feel comfortable that you've mastered the pronunciation of your mantra, chant it in your mind only.

Japa is a very highly regarded practice in the yoga tradition. Many yogis practice japa not only during formal meditation sessions but whenever they have a chance during the day—for example, when they're out walking or waiting in line. Most of us fill our minds with trivial mental chatter that only winds up cluttering the unconscious mind. Yogis fill their minds with the sacred vibrations of their mantra instead. Their goal is to chant the mantra so many millions of times that its blessing force permeates their unconscious mind, purifying and illuminating their entire personality.

QUIZ

HOUR'S UP!

Test your grasp of the information in Hour 15 with the following quick quiz. Answer true or false to the following statements:

1. You should pay close attention to visions and words you see and hear in your mind during meditation—these are almost always the promptings of your Higher Self.

2. If you breathe predominantly through your right nostril during meditation, you're likely to float off in a daydream.

3. When you breathe predominantly through your left nostril, it's a good time for a passive activity like listening to a lecture.

4. Breathing through both nostrils equally helps produce a tranquil, balanced frame of mind.

5. A mantra is a special sound yogis use to help keep their minds focused during meditation.

6. Emptying your mind is the essence of meditation.

7. A mala is a rosary yogis use to help keep track of the number of times they've said their mantra.

8. It's important to respond to the issues that arise in your mind during meditation immediately, while they're still fresh in your awareness.

9. Watching the contents of your awareness dispassionately helps to defuse the emotional charge of painful memories.

10. Traditionally, a mantra is given by a guru who selects the right sound based on the disciple's character and special needs.

HOUR 16

Create Inner Focus

CHAPTER SUMMARY

LESSON PLAN:

In this hour you will learn ...

- Meditation entails the exploration of a whole new world: the universe of inner awareness.
- Yogis use visualization to improve their concentration.
- Meditators contemplate inspiring ideals to expand their sense of self.
- The Gayatri mantra is a favorite for connecting with one's inner light.
- Because the mind can play tricks on a meditator, it's important to beware of common pitfalls on the inner path.

In the West we idolize great explorers like Christopher Columbus, Ferdinand Magellan, Leif Ericksen, and Neil Armstrong. It's fascinating to read about adventurers like Marco Polo and the whole new parts of the world they opened up for our ancestors—for better or worse.

In Eastern cultures however, there is also a tremendous respect for explorers of the inner worlds—the Taoist masters in China, the shamans of northern Asia, and especially the yogis of India who have been famous throughout the East for their profound insights into the nature of consciousness, as well as their seemingly magical powers and abilities, since time immemorial.

In the West, though, we ignore the inner dimensions of our being. While the existence of a Higher Self and the importance of the quest for self-knowledge are taken for granted in many Eastern cultures, we in the West tend to focus almost exclusively on outer goals: a successful career, fulfilling relationships, an attractive body, a beautiful home, and so on. At no point—not in our schools, not usually even in our churches and synagogues—are we taught to travel inward or to value quiet time spent sitting alone by ourselves.

The meditation techniques developed in the yoga tradition provide a vital and long-neglected service in the Western world. They systematically guide us through the final frontier that few Western adventurers have yet explored: our own inner being.

ESTABLISHING A MEDITATION ROUTINE

Setting aside time each day to sit and meditate is an exciting commitment to inner life. When you make the decision to begin this inward journey, you are like a treasure hunter setting off for parts unknown on a grand quest. The ultimate reward, according to the yogis, is enlightenment. Yet every step along the way is full of illuminating power because it allows you to get to know yourself intimately.

Whatever time of day you sit down to meditate, resolve in advance how long you want to sit. Five minutes is plenty your first few tries. But increase the amount of time you spend meditating to 10 or 15 minutes by your fourth or fifth session. Fifteen to thirty minutes twice a day is ideal for a new student. If your schedule is extremely busy, keep in mind that 10 minutes of focused meditation once a day does more good than a full hour of listless meditation twice a day. If 10 minutes is all you can spare, then make those minutes count!

PREPARE TO SIT

Meditating shortly after eating is a bad idea, though it's better than not meditating at all. For two or three hours after a meal much of the energy in your body is directed toward digestion. You need fresh, oxygenated blood in your brain, not in your stomach, to meditate well.

It's best to wear loose, comfortable clothing when you sit for meditation. Loosen your belt and tie, if you're wearing them, or better yet, take them off. You don't want to be wearing anything that constricts your abdominal movement, preventing you from breathing diaphragmatically. Tight pants may obstruct your respiration, forcing you to use your chest muscles to breathe. Wear clothes that allow you to sit upright comfortably and breathe easily.

In India, yogis usually bathe before meditation. This may mean submerging themselves in a river for a complete bath, or simply sprinkling water on their face, rinsing out their mouth, and washing their hands and feet. You might want to wash your face and hands and brush your teeth if you have the time. This refreshes the body and also creates a symbolic sense of purity that facilitates the mental cleansing that occurs in meditation.

Remember to use the bathroom before you sit down to meditate. Beginning meditators face enough distractions without also having to contend with the call of nature!

FYI *The Power of Mantra and the Mystery of Initiation* by Pandit Rajmani Tigunait, Ph.D., introduces readers to the mysterious spiritual forces at work in mantra meditation as they are understood in the cave monasteries and forest hermitages of India. This amazing book offers a fascinating glimpse into the inner world of advanced adepts in the East.

BEGIN YOUR MEDITATION ROUTINE

Here is a sample meditation session you might want to work with:

1. Wash your face and hands.

2. Sit in your meditation posture with your head, neck, and trunk in a straight line. Close your eyes.

3. Resolve that for the next 15 minutes, you will devote your attention exclusively to your meditation practice. Or if you have a mala, resolve that you will recite your mantra for three full rounds of the mala (or however many rounds you feel comfortable doing).

4. Bring your full awareness to your breath. Make sure you're breathing diaphragmatically. Your breath should be smooth and even, with no jerks or pauses.

5. Bring your full awareness to the bridge between your nostrils. Focus intently on this point inside your nose as you continue breathing diaphragmatically. If you feel that you are breathing predominantly through one nostril, shift your awareness to the opposite side of your nasal septum. Keep your attention there until you begin to feel that nostril beginning to open and clear.

6. When air flows through both nostrils equally, slowly, gently, and smoothly, without jerks or pauses, it is time to begin your mantra practice. If you have difficulty reaching this state of respiratory equilibrium, simply continue focusing on breathing diaphragmatically.

7. Repeat your mantra mentally (or out loud, if this helps you concentrate). If you have a mala, slip one bead between your fingers for each mantra you say. Pay close attention to your mental process. Be aware of the part of you that is willing your mind to chant the mantra, to the part of you that is listening to it, and to the syllables of the mantra itself.

8. If thoughts or images appear in your mind during meditation, don't engage with them. Don't fight them or try to force them to disappear.

But don't get completely caught up in them and lose your meditative focus, either. Just let them pass by like the traffic outside your home. Return the focus of your attention to the mantra.

9. Don't react to noises in your environment (unless an emergency arises you must respond to). You don't need to feel angry or frustrated that sounds around you cause distractions. There will always be noise. If the room were absolutely still, you would hear the sound of yourself breathing and of your blood pumping through your veins. Allow the sounds around you to continue, but pay attention only to the sound of your mantra.

10. Be aware of your awareness of the mantra. That pure awareness is not your body, not even your thoughts. It is the one who thinks, breathes, and recites the mantra, but it is more subtle than your body or mind. It is deeply peaceful but also intensely lucid. It effortlessly commands your mind to repeat the mantra and effortlessly listens to the sound. This pure inner awareness is your Higher Self.

11. Gradually the sound of your mantra will fade away. The mantra has led you to the perfect stillness and clarity within yourself. Enjoy this sense of lucid tranquility for a few moments.

12. When your 15 minutes are over or you are finished with the rounds of your mala, slowly open your eyes. Don't get up immediately, but give yourself a minute to bask in the sense of calmness and refreshment. Then stretch your limbs and rise.

Intermediate level meditators find that they no longer have to will themselves to chant the mantra during meditation. Rather, the mantra begins repeating itself as soon as they sit down on their meditation cushion. Traditional yogis continue chanting their mantras throughout the day, whether they're sitting for formal meditation or going about their business. They consider it a great blessing if they keep hearing the mantra in their dreams. This indicates the blessing vibrations of the sacred sound are permeating their unconscious mind.

Don't confuse the relaxed and focused condition you experience in meditation with hypnosis or a trance state. You should not be in a passive mental state when you are meditating. On the contrary, although you are deeply physically relaxed, you are also very mentally alert and in full conscious control of yourself during the meditative process.

TIME SAVER

The first few times you sit for meditation, it's extremely helpful to have someone guide you through the process. *Learn to Meditate* by Rolf Sovik, Psy.D. (Himalayan Institute, 1-800-822-4547 or www.himalayaninstitute.org), is a particularly useful audiocassette that teaches you the rudiments of meditative practice. It includes an easy-to-follow relaxation exercise and a guided meditation.

VISUALIZE AN OBJECT

Mantra meditation is one of the easiest and most highly recommended forms of meditation. However, some people aren't as oriented to sounds as they are to sight. For them, holding a visual object in the field of their awareness is easier than reciting a sound.

In India, many yogis visualize a deity as they meditate. These visualizations involve so much detail that holding the entire vision in one's mind requires a great deal of concentration. Every component of the image has symbolic meaning. For example, the many weapons held by the warrior goddess Durga represent the Higher Self's capacity to offer protection and to destroy negative aspects of the meditator's personality such as hatred or greed. The huge bulk of the elephant-headed god Ganesh represents the indomitable strength and immense majesty of the Higher Self.

You might want to try meditating on a spiritual image that has special meaning for you, such as the loving face of Jesus Christ or his mother Mary if you are a Christian. A great saint or spiritual teacher you feel close to might do just as well. You should hold the saint or deity's face or entire body clearly in your awareness, visualizing it in great detail. The figure doesn't move or speak, but simply radiates unconditional love and wisdom.

MEDITATING ON AN IMAGE

You might want to experiment with using a visual image in meditation. Try the following exercise and see if it suits you better than working with a mantra:

1. Wash your face and hands.
2. Sit upright but relaxed in your meditation posture. Close your eyes.
3. Resolve that for the next 15 minutes, you will devote your attention solely to your meditation practice. This time is not for external distractions or random thoughts.

4. Breathe diaphragmatically. Focus intently on the bridge between your nostrils until the air flows through both nostrils equally. If this doesn't happen, continue focusing on breathing diaphragmatically.

5. Visualize a great saint or deity sitting directly in front of you. Imagine that they're sitting completely still, but their face is glowing with love. If there is no special sage or deity you feel close to, imagine a brilliant white light in front of you, radiating unconditional love.

6. If thoughts or other images appear in your mind, don't get caught up in them. Just let them pass out of your awareness without provoking any interest or emotion. Keep your focus on the image you are using for meditation.

7. Become aware of your awareness of the image. That pure awareness is more than just your body and mind. It is deeply peaceful but also intensely lucid. It effortlessly commands your mind to visualize the mental image before you and effortlessly gazes at the image. This pure inner awareness is your Higher Self.

8. Gradually the image will fade away. It has led you to a place of perfect serenity and clarity within yourself. Enjoy this sense of lucid tranquility for a few moments.

9. When your meditation session is complete, slowly open your eyes. Don't get up right away but give yourself a minute to bask in the sense of calmness and refreshment you feel. Then stretch your limbs and stand up.

GO TO ▶
Mantras, mandalas, and yantras are important tools used in the tantric tradition. In the West, many beginning students mistakenly think tantra means the yoga of sex. In reality, tantrics use sophisticated methodologies to harness the energies of their subtle body and mind in the quest for enlightenment. For insight into the way yogis work with tantric techniques, see Hour 24.

VISUALIZING A COSMIC PATTERN

Religions such as Judaism and Islam discourage adherents from working with anthropomorphic images and require you instead to focus on abstract designs like the Star of David. Yogis work with two types of abstract images: mandalas and yantras.

Mandalas are usually round or square geometric patterns that represent the way different grades of consciousness operate within a whole. These are powerful centering devices that direct your attention to the center of the visual pattern and simultaneously to your own inner core.

FYI

Tools for Tantra by the famous twentieth-century yogi and scholar Harish Johari is one of the finest treatments of mantra and yantra available in English. The book contains beautiful full-page color plates of some of the most important yantras in the yoga tradition, suitable for home meditation.

Yantra is a Sanskrit word that literally means "machine." A yantra is a mandala that has been "turned on" through the meditator's one-pointed concentration. Each angle, triangle, petal, line, and dot in the yantra has special significance for the meditator—it's no longer just a visual abstraction but a living mechanism that carries the meditator to his or her innermost essence.

The famous Sri Yantra (see the following figure) represents the Mother of the Universe in the yoga tradition. (Traditional yoga honors the divine spirit in both male and female forms.) The innermost triangle represents the cosmic matrix from which the universe emerges. The geometric forms that surround it stand for the cosmic energies that radiate out from this primordial womb. The dot at the very center stands for consciousness itself. When yogis meditate on Sri Yantra they enter at the outermost gates of the design, and follow the angles to the center of their own inner awareness.

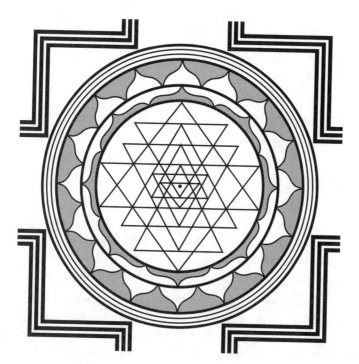

Sri Yantra, the best-known yantra.

Yogis always use mantras together with yantras, although you don't need a yantra to work with a mantra. Sound energy is considered more primal and powerful than visual forms in the meditation tradition, perhaps because when most people think they use words rather than images.

CONTEMPLATION OF AN IDEAL

Holding one sound or image in your awareness for 15 minutes, or even for 5 minutes, is not necessarily an easy task, particularly for Westerners who are trained from childhood to direct their attention exclusively outward toward the objects of the world. For yoga students who find the leap to meditation too big a jump to start with, the practice of contemplation might be an easier first step on the journey to inner understanding.

There might be an affirmation or a verse from the Bible, Torah, or Koran, or a line of poetry that especially inspires you and elevates your spirit. From "God is love" to "Thy will be done," there is no shortage of mind- and heart-expanding aphorisms ideal for contemplation.

In the tradition of India there are four "great sayings" (*maha vakyas*) that are often used for contemplation. These four short sentences have been used by yoga and philosophy students in India for at least 1,200 years to expand their awareness. They are as follows:

- *Aham Brahmasmi:* I am one with Divine Being.
- *Ayam Atma Brahma:* My Inner Self is one with the Self of all beings.
- *Prajnanam Brahma:* The supreme reality is illumined awareness.
- *Tat Tvam Asi:* You (my soul) are that (all pervading spirit).

FIND YOUR INNER CORE

If you've studied Western psychology, you know that psychologists and psychiatrists work with the complex knot of conflicts, neuroses, repressed memories and desires, and self-loathing that lie just under the surface of conscious awareness. Eastern psychology, on which yoga is based (you'll learn more about it in Hour 21), is radically different.

The yoga view is that if you look deeply enough, you can see beneath the turbulent waves of your subconscious mind to the calm depths of your superconsciousness. Many yogis report that from the superconscious perspective, everything in the universe is literally "all one." Everything is interconnected through a vast underlying network of consciousness called *mahat*. It's because of mahat that telepathy works (which connects mind to mind) and precognition works (which connects the future with the present), according to the yogis.

STRICTLY DEFINED

Mahat literally means "the greatness." It refers to the cosmic consciousness connecting all things.

In the deepest meditative states, some yogis have reported that the distinction between the individual soul and the soul of the universe begins to dissolve. They experience union with the underlying intelligence of the entire cosmos. The four "great sayings" are reminders that your essence is one with the essence of the universe, just as a drop of water is in a sense one with the entire ocean.

EXPAND YOUR SENSE OF SELF

Here is a sample contemplation based on this principle of unity. It gives an expanded sense of oneself, an appreciation for life everywhere, and respect for the vast intelligence that, yogis claim, connects and directs all aspects of nature.

1. Wash your hands and face.

2. Relax in your meditation posture but keep your back, head, and neck straight. Close your eyes.

3. Resolve that the next 15 minutes will be devoted to your inner work only. Extraneous thoughts and images may come and go, but will not hold your attention.

4. Focus intently on the bridge between your nostrils until you find yourself breathing through both nostrils equally. If this doesn't occur, simply keep breathing diaphragmatically.

5. Call one of the four great sayings (for example, "My Inner Self is one with the Self of all beings")—or any other inspiring statement or affirmation you prefer—into your awareness. Carefully ponder what the saying actually means. How have you experienced its truth in your life? Do you feel it to be true not only in your mind, but in your heart and in your gut?

6. If other thoughts interrupt your contemplation, gently turn your attention away from them, back to the affirmation you are contemplating.

7. Now imagine your skin no longer forms the boundary of your consciousness. Imagine your consciousness expanding outward, filling the room, the house, the neighborhood, and on out till it embraces the whole universe. Allow yourself to feel your unity with all of creation.

8. Gradually return to body consciousness. Slowly open your eyes. Pause a moment to enjoy the sense of expanded awareness you felt during your contemplation. Then stretch your limbs and rise.

 FYI Westerners usually think of the divine as a god, not a goddess. Yet the goddess plays an enormous role in traditional yoga. My book *The Living Goddess: Reclaiming the Tradition of the Mother of the Universe* provides detailed information about how goddess spirituality is integrated into yoga.

CONNECT WITH INNER GUIDANCE

It's usual for meditators in the yoga tradition who have an especially strong desire for mystical experience to perform a purascharana. You might remember from Hour 15 that a purascharana is the commitment to recite a certain mantra a given number of times. Advanced yogis have often recited particular mantras many millions of times.

One of the most common and most highly regarded purascharanas involves meditating on the famous Gayatri mantra. This is one of the most honored mantras in the yoga tradition. In Sanskrit the Gayatri goes:

Om bhur bhuvah svaha

Tat Savitur vareniyam.

Bhargo devasya dhi mahi

Dhiyo yo na prachodayat.

The meaning is, "With loving reverence, I bow to the Inner Sun, the most splendid light in all the worlds. Please illuminate my mind."

Often before initiating a disciple in more advanced practices, a guru will recommend that a student recite the Gayatri mantra 10,000 times or more. This is considered the preeminent mantra for awakening your intuitive powers and putting you in touch with divine guidance. It's also said to "remove curses," which is to say it clears out blocks and complexes in the subconscious mind that may be preventing inner growth. Savitur or the "Inner Sun" is the light within that helps you find your way through life. It leads to external fulfillment and internal illumination.

The Gayatri mantra is incredibly old. It first appeared in the *Rig Veda*, a text composed 6,000 years ago in Pakistan. Because it is so ancient and because it's been chanted trillions of times by so many sincere souls, including many thousands of great saints, it's believed that the mantra has enormous blessing power.

If you're interested in doing a purascharana of the Gayatri mantra, you need to meet with a teacher at your local yoga center who can teach you the rhythm and pronunciation and help you determine how many repetitions it would be helpful for you to do. Your teacher will also explain a few minor restrictions that come with the practice. These are not too difficult but they do include making some adjustments so that you can meditate at the same time each day and maintain a vegetarian diet for the duration of the practice. (See Hour 20 for some vegetarian dishes.)

PROCEED WITH CAUTION

It is very tempting to chant a mantra mechanically, while another part of your awareness drifts away and thinks about other things. Successful meditation, however, demands your full concentration. The moment you notice your attention has shifted from your meditation practice, bring it back to your mantra or yantra. This develops willpower and inner focus.

GUIDANCE OR GARBAGE?

There is one important potential problem in particular that you need to watch out for when you begin a meditation practice. It is very important not to confuse the garbage coming from your subconscious with the guidance coming from your superconscious. It sometimes takes time to learn to differentiate between true intuitive insight and simple wishful thinking. This is one of the reasons the role of the guru is emphasized in the yoga tradition. He or she can help you steer clear of the shoals of self-delusion that may be brought on by mistaking miscues from the subconscious for valuable insight.

Generally speaking, beginners should beware of "voices" or "visions" that spontaneously occur in meditation. In the majority of cases, these are the work of your imagination. When in doubt, go ahead and doubt!

Some students take to meditation like ducks to water. But most beginning meditators, particularly in the West where no aspect of the culture encourages people to search out the center of their own awareness, find it difficult to sit quietly at first. In Hour 17, you'll learn about common problems students face in meditation and how to overcome them.

HOUR'S UP!

It's time to quiz yourself on the material you've just learned in Hour 16. Answer true or false to the following statements:

1. Eating right before meditation improves your digestion and enhances your meditative focus.

2. Meditation and hypnosis are closely related mental states.

3. A mandala is a symmetrical geometric design used to deepen meditation.

4. Yogis commonly practice the Gayatri mantra to help awaken their intuitive powers.

5. The yoga tradition speaks of both subconscious and superconscious aspects of the personality.

6. Contemplating inspiring sayings has never been a valued part of the yoga tradition.

7. Yantras provide a visual path to the center of consciousness.

8. You should get up immediately after meditation so that your blood circulation can return to normal.

9. The four great sayings of the contemplative tradition are designed to remind us that each man is an island.

10. Bathing before meditation helps create a sense of inner purity.

HOUR 17

Overcome Obstacles

CHAPTER SUMMARY

LESSON PLAN:

In this hour you will learn ...

- Ancient yoga masters addressed the difficulties beginning yoga students have when they start meditating.

- Meditators in the West face a unique set of problems when starting a spiritual practice.

- Traditionally, disciples were required to meet high standards before being initiated in mantra meditation.

- Meditation is not a "cult" activity but a foundation stone of all religious traditions.

- Some beginners find that meditating in a group helps create a deeper meditative state.

Yoga lore is full of stories about demons and deities who rush forward to obstruct yogis' success in meditation. From the Buddha and the great Hindu sages to the most innocent beginning students, everyone who sits for meditation at some point or another (usually sooner rather than later) encounters problems that block their ability to enter or maintain a meditative state.

Because these difficulties are so common, a vast literature grew up in the Hindu, Buddhist, and Jain traditions offering advice about how to deal with them. Nine of the most frequent impediments are listed in the great yoga classic the *Yoga Sutras*, composed by the sage Patanjali in or before the second century B.C.E.

INNER ROADBLOCKS

The first major problem Patanjali mentions is that some people just aren't suited to inner life. When meditation was introduced to the West on a mass scale in the 1970s, enthusiastic proponents gave the impression that meditation was an ideal technique that can be practiced by anyone. Unfortunately, this isn't really true.

Traditionally, would-be meditators were required to demonstrate both emotional stability and psychological maturity before they were given a mantra. Gurus would redirect beginners who showed no aptitude for focusing their mind to other less internalized forms of yoga.

Before a guru accepted a new disciple, the student had to exhibit the following characteristics:

- Personal ethics
- Emotional equilibrium
- Mental clarity
- Ability to concentrate
- Motivation toward enlightenment

It was a serious breach of the yogic code to teach meditation to people of unfit character. Meditation was believed to confer many extraordinary powers that naturally arise when the latent abilities of the mind are awakened and focused. Therefore, the secrets of inner life were carefully guarded and passed on only to disciples a guru felt he or she could trust.

People who are seriously neurotic or psychotic can actually be damaged by meditation. Turning inward puts you in touch with the contents of your subconscious mind, which might be a harrowing experience for those who are mentally unbalanced. People like these need to be working with a psychotherapist or physician, not with a meditation technique.

Some people simply can't focus inward. The ability to turn the mind in on itself just isn't there. For others, the desire to make the inner journey is absent. People turn to inner life when they're ready. Trying to foist a meditative lifestyle on others prematurely is like expecting a fruit to ripen out of season.

In Hour 23, you'll learn about other forms of yoga, such as Karma Yoga and Bhakti Yoga, which may be more appropriate for people who have difficulty turning their minds inward.

PROCEED WITH CAUTION

If you're enthused about your meditation practice, you may be tempted to try to make your friends or family meditate with you. This is a bad idea. Meditation is not for everyone and was never meant to be forced on others. The best you can do is work on your own inner development. When people see the positive changes in you, they may become curious and inquire about your practice. This is a more appropriate point to begin discussing meditation.

Let's take a look at the other eight obstacles to success in meditation that Patanjali identifies in the *Yoga Sutras*.

DOUBT

Doubt, the second obstacle Patanjali mentions, takes two forms. First there is the doubt that meditation really works. Second, even if you're fully aware that meditation really does deliver as promised, you may doubt your own ability to master the technique.

If you're unsure about the value of meditation, you would do well to read any of the numerous studies that have been done on the technique by Western scientists confirming its power, as well as biographies of the great meditation masters of past and present, and what they've achieved through their inner practice. A few of these books are listed in Appendix D.

Ultimately, the proof of the pudding is in the eating. Yoga and meditation have proven their effectiveness so many times that their techniques have spread around the globe. If you're following the instructions closely and practicing sincerely, you should begin experiencing some of the benefits of meditation practically from your first sitting.

SLOTH

Laziness is the next obstacle on Patanjali's list. If you can recall the concept of *tamas* from Hour 1, you'll remember that one of the three fundamental forces of the universe is inertia. An object at rest tends to stay at rest!

Getting it together to meditate regularly and overcome tamas requires marshalling the second fundamental force of nature, *rajas*. Rajas is the active, dynamic potency of the universe that is essential in developing self-discipline. Rajas is most easily activated by enthusiasm. Learning about the great saints and sages, or spending time with more advanced meditators is an excellent way to increase your desire to practice. When you do sit for meditation you will be cultivating the third of the three fundamental forces of nature, *sattva*, or balance and harmony.

POOR HEALTH

The fourth obstacle is illness. Fever, fatigue, nausea, headache, and other physical ailments prevent your brain from functioning with the clarity it needs in order to meditate. But persistent problems such as back pain, chronic fatigue syndrome, low thyroid function, and other such long-term difficulties can present a continual challenge to successful meditation.

GO TO ▶
Eating meat will not prevent you from having a successful meditation, but it won't help you, either. A balanced vegetarian diet is considered optimal for improving the clarity of consciousness. In case you're interested in experimenting with this effect, Hour 20 introduces you to a yogic diet.

For this reason, yoga is intensely health-oriented. The yoga postures, along with a yogic diet, yogic cleaning techniques, and yoga psychology, are all geared to keep you in as good shape physically as you can possibly be. These topics are all covered in this book.

DELUSION

Self-delusion is another typical problem with potentially awful consequences. There is a tendency for overly imaginative students to mistake the contents of their subconscious minds for the promptings of the superconscious. An image flashed from the unconscious may be taken for a divine vision, or a fanciful thought or desire such as "Yoga masters from the Himalayas are contacting me telepathically" or "I'm the messenger of God" may be misunderstood as a reality.

Numerous Sanskrit yoga texts emphasize that the first requirement on the inner path is *viveka*, or the ability to tell the difference between what's real and unreal, what's true and untrue. This isn't always easy, perhaps especially in the modern West where so many people have been cut off from spiritual and psychic experience their entire lives until they begin to meditate.

In the East, meditators had thoroughly trained teachers on hand to help them discriminate between healthy and unhealthy inner experiences. Working with an experienced spiritual mentor is always a good idea, provided the guru figure is authentic and capable. In any case, it's good to maintain an attitude of humility and be on guard against any inner "message" that increases your sense of egotism. Real intuitive flashes from the superconscious carry with them a sense of definiteness and self-validity. They also help you transcend, not bloat, your vanity.

CRAVING

The value of desire is fully acknowledged in the yoga tradition. *Kama* (desire for sensual pleasure, especially for sex) and *artha* (desire for wealth and the good things money can buy) are important motivating factors that help keep the world going 'round. But it can be extraordinarily difficult to focus on your mantra for even five minutes if your mind is totally dominated by romantic fantasies or by obsessive preoccupation with the things you own or want to buy.

FYI My book *Meditation Is Boring? Putting Life in Your Spiritual Practice* deals with problems new meditators face in their practice, and offers advice from leading saints and yogis on how to deepen your spiritual practice. It also describes my experiences with some of the greatest yoga masters of our time.

One of the ways yogis work with craving is to cultivate charity. Giving to those in need is an excellent way to begin letting go of the things you cling to mentally, as well as learning to make the needs of others a higher priority. If a person is obsessed with making money, for example, his guru might recommend making large donations to the poor or to worthy organizations. If another person is preoccupied with overeating, her guru might suggest that she devote a certain amount of time each day to feeding others.

Many yogis living in caves or forests own literally nothing to give away. If they still are distracted from their meditation by the desire for money or material possessions, their gurus sometimes have them visualize having huge amounts of gold and offering it all to God. If the desire for sex is the distraction, the guru might have them visualize God or the Goddess as their lover and meditation as their tryst. There is always a way to redirect desire to make it work for instead of against your spiritual practice.

Misunderstanding

The seventh major problem Patanjali noted was failure to understand or follow instructions properly. If you attend a meditation class you'll quickly note that this is still a problem today. Your instructor will always ask the beginning meditators in the room to breathe silently, because noisy breath is usually an indication that a person is tense and unconsciously forcing air through his or her nostrils. No matter how many times the teacher explains how to breathe properly, there's always at least one student in the room who'll continue to breathe noisily and erratically. The student might be completely sincere but the instructions are just not sinking in.

In the yoga tradition, the antidote to this problem is first to monitor yourself carefully. Second, it's helpful to request the guidance and support of a qualified teacher who can check your practice. The guru introduces you to your Inner Self and carefully watches over your progress. For this reason, the spiritual mentor is tremendously respected in the yoga tradition.

FAILURE

Occasionally, you'll meet a yoga student who has been practicing meditation for some time but claims not to have experienced any benefits. The sage Vyasa addressed this eighth complaint in a famous commentary on the *Yoga Sutras*. He said that if you are doing the practice correctly, in short order you will definitely begin to see the effects. Yogic meditation is a time-tested technology based on the science of consciousness, developed by great masters of the past who devoted their lives to understanding the nature of the mind. The vast majority of students who follow the instructions properly and with full attentiveness will see results quickly.

In the unlikely event that you practice meditation for a few months and still are not feeling its effect in your life, you should check in with a qualified meditation teacher. He or she can provide insight into the block that is slowing your progress. Once students get the feel for doing meditation correctly, they often make rapid progress.

FYI Want to read Patanjali's *Yoga Sutras* yourself? Numerous English translations are now available. Perhaps the easiest to read is *How to Know God* by Swami Prabhavananda and Christopher Isherwood. For more advanced students, *Yoga Philosophy of Patanjali* by Swami Hariharananda Aranya is a superb introduction to the real spiritual depth of this yoga classic.

INCONSISTENCY

The ninth and last concern mentioned by Patanjali is sometimes raised by intermediate-level meditators. They complain that although they have seen dramatic benefits from their meditation, these results aren't consistent. Sometimes they can enter a meditative state easily, and its uplifting force stays with them all day. Other times it's a struggle to find their meditative focus, or the serenity and clarity they feel during their practice fades away as the day progresses.

Whenever you learn a skill it takes time to stabilize your new ability. When you first learned to walk, sometimes you made it across the room, other times you stumbled. As with any other skill, practice makes perfect. Advanced yoga masters are able to shift their awareness into deep states of meditation— states barely accessible to most humans—in a matter of seconds. The results of their practice are consistent and reliable. Yours will be, too, if you persist with patience and determination. The benefits of meditation are immense, ranging all the way from a light relaxation to enlightenment itself. It's worth the effort!

WESTERN CONCERNS

Students learning meditation in Western cultures today face a unique set of concerns Patanjali could hardly have envisioned 2,200 years ago. He grew up in a civilization that recognized the value of inner work. Full-time meditators were financially supported by Indian society, and people felt lucky to have meditators in their midst. They recognized the tremendous blessing force that emanated from saints and yogis.

Students in the West don't have that luxury. They live in a culture where some people may even regard meditation practice as a quirky kind of thing to do. Occasionally family members or friends may be amused or even irritated by your desire to meditate. They may want to know why you don't join them in front of the TV or get up and "do something constructive."

In some areas of modern America, parts of California being a prime example, there is substantial encouragement for people's meditation work. In other parts of the country, the lack of support may be complete. Meditators may feel lonely and isolated. The solution to this problem is *satsang* or spiritual fellowship. It literally means "the companionship of truth."

Look in the Yellow Pages under "Yoga" for a yoga center near you. You may or may not feel comfortable with the people in the yoga group nearby or the style of yoga they practice, so shop around. Having someone to share your enthusiasm for meditation with will help make the inner journey easier. Although meditation is the most private of all activities, it's also a fascinating journey that you can travel with other pilgrims on the inner path.

STILLING THE MIND

It's important to recognize that taking time to be with your self and to explore the inner reaches of your awareness is not a waste of time. In fact, it's one of the best uses imaginable for your time. When you make contact with a deeper reality, you directly experience that being alone with yourself is an amazing and worthwhile endeavor. In fact, it's the ideal antidote to the sense of shallowness and meaninglessness many people experience, even many individuals who on the surface of their lives appear to be prosperous and successful.

Meditation adds a sense of purpose and perspective to live by, helping you live more consciously, with deeper self-awareness and greater appreciation for the wonder of self-existence.

PROCEED WITH CAUTION

 Meditation is one of the most valuable assets you can have in life. However, it is not a substitute for life itself. Occasionally beginners become so enthusiastic about their meditative practice that they neglect their relationships and responsibilities. Meditation helps you become more effective in dealing with duties and with other people. It's not meant to make you run away from them.

FACING FEAR

Because inner life is unknown to most Westerners, a small percentage of new meditators experience fear when they begin their inward journey. The familiar world of tangible objects drops away and ghosts from the subconscious may appear. Yoga literature speaks of the types of uninvited visions that may play before the mind's eye, or the uneasy sense of not being alone that a small percentage of new meditators feel when they finally are alone in meditation.

Yoga literature offers three bits of advice for beginners who find themselves feeling anxious when they sit to meditate:

- Recognize that the uneasiness you experience is wholly a projection of your mind. Most fears are not rooted in reality but in the imagination.

- If you begin feeling unsettled during your meditation practice, return your attention to your breath at once. Feel yourself breathing in and out at a slow and natural pace. Watching the breath transports you out of the past and future, bringing you back to the present moment and a sense of calm lucidity. It also helps the nervous system relax.

- If a sense of anxiety persists during your meditation, it's time to seek counseling. An experienced meditation teacher or competent therapist can help you deal with uncomfortable feelings arising from your unconscious.

When people—often for the first time in their lives—become intensely aware of their core of consciousness, some suddenly experience a disconcerting sense of their own mortality. Generally, people push the thought of death out of their minds for most of their lives. When they become acutely aware of their own consciousness, some meditators feel themselves vividly confronted with the possibility that it may end some day.

The yoga tradition claims that consciousness is eternal, without beginning or end. That core of consciousness you experience as most fundamentally who you are is your Higher Self, according to the yogis, and that Higher Self never dies. Deep meditation puts you in touch with your immortal soul. Learning to abide in this inner essence is equivalent to immortality, yoga texts say. So ultimately meditation carries you beyond the greatest fear of all, the fear of death.

Whether you are just interested in learning to relax and let go of stress, whether you want to develop enough inner tranquility to face the crises and inevitable losses of life with serenity, or whether you seriously desire enlightenment, beginning a meditation routine is a major step in the direction of your goal. Patanjali assures his readers that the more intense and motivated the student, the more rapid the progress in meditation.

GO TO ▶
Advanced meditators often focus on subtle centers in their body called chakras. In Hour 18, you'll learn the seven major chakras, the abilities and emotional states associated with them, and how they're used in the yoga tradition.

GROUP MEDITATION

Western students often imagine the great yogis of history as solitary masters living by themselves somewhere in the vast Himalayan mountain range. In reality, most yogis lived in ashrams (spiritual communities) or at home. Yogis recognize the value of sharing their meditation practice with others.

Many yoga centers and ashrams offer group meditations. If you are experiencing a block in your meditation, it's not unlikely that another member of a meditation group has encountered the same problem. You might find their advice on how they dealt with the difficulty illuminating. Likewise, if you have trouble disciplining yourself to meditate regularly or to sit through your full session, consider organizing a group meditation. Even a once-weekly group sitting can be helpful.

Some students find group meditations irritating. They are distracted by the sound of other meditators sniffing, fidgeting, or even breathing or swallowing. But if you're not super sensitive to noise, you may find group meditation a powerful experience. When each of the participants is focused and sincere, a powerful group dynamic emerges that creates an inward current each member can feel. That flow of energy helps to carry even students who ordinarily have a difficult time with meditation very quickly into deeper states.

FYI Meditation is preeminently about withdrawing your awareness from memories of the past or concerns about the future, and placing you instead squarely in the moment. *The Power of Now: A Guide to Spiritual Enlightenment* by Eckhart Tolle is perhaps the best account in English of the inestimable value of living in the present.

In Hour 18, you will learn about the centers of consciousness within the body and the latent powers of awareness that yogis say can be awakened through meditation.

HOUR'S UP!

Here's a quiz to see how well you've absorbed the information in Hour 17. Answer true or false to the following statements:

1. Everyone can benefit from meditating.

2. Traditionally, an ethical character and personal maturity were prerequisites for meditation practice.

3. Yogis do not consider poor health an obstacle to success in meditation.

4. Meditators must take care not to confuse images from their subconscious minds with real intuitive insights.

5. Desire is considered the worst of all evils in the yoga tradition.

6. Paying attention to your meditation teacher's instructions is not really that important.

7. Meditating in a group is a technique used only by beginners.

8. Meditators need to practice regularly in order to achieve consistently good meditations.

9. The Desert Fathers of early Christianity practiced a type of meditation.

10. Patanjali, the author of the *Yoga Sutras*, was not concerned with the problems beginner-level meditators sometimes experience.

HOUR 18

Ignite Inner Energies

CHAPTER SUMMARY

LESSON PLAN:

In this hour you will learn ...

- Advanced yogis work with *kundalini*, the energy of consciousness, to heighten their awareness.

- Yogis typically concentrate on seven chakras or vortices of energy in the subtle body.

- Exceptional abilities sometimes develop as a consequence of intense meditative focus.

- Enlightenment is said to occur when kundalini permanently activates the highest chakra in the brain.

More than 2,500 years ago, Buddha made up his mind that he would either become enlightened or die. He sat down under a tree at Bodh Gaya and meditated without stop for 40 days and 40 nights. Even today yogis go on retreats in the Himalayas, walling themselves up in mountain caves where they sit in meditation, without light or heat, for months on end.

Few practitioners in the West have that level of commitment to their meditation routine! But they have to admit that India's determined inner explorers might well have uncovered secrets about the mind and internal energy states that Western scientists have yet to discover.

Advanced meditators of the Eastern traditions—whether their background is Hindu, Buddhist, Sikh, Jain, or even atheist as some Indian yogis are—share a common inner frame of reference. They all talk about kundalini, an inner force that greatly magnifies a meditator's consciousness, and about an internal system of chakras or vortices of subtle energy that govern your emotional state and creative potential.

In this hour, you'll learn about the inner framework of consciousness, the subtle energies that adepts work with in meditation. Bear in mind that kundalini and the chakras are not biological realities, but vectors of consciousness and energy that operate in the subtle body. You can sense their activity during meditation, but they won't show up in a CAT scan.

THE POWER WITHIN

If you attend a meditation class, you might overhear some new students claiming they feel their *kundalini* rising. Perhaps they felt a prickly sensation in their backs or a flush of heat rising up their torso. Eastern yogis most often dismiss these reports as resulting from a beginner's overactive imagination or inability to tell the difference between ordinary physiological phenomena and genuine spiritual experience. When kundalini really rises it has a profoundly energizing and reorganizing effect on consciousness.

STRICTLY DEFINED

Kundalini is the energy of consciousness in the human organism. It has been called the "serpent power" because in most individuals it lies coiled at the bottom of the spine like a sleeping snake. When it awakens and streaks up the spine it produces dramatic mystical experiences.

In reality, the full activation of the kundalini is an extremely rare experience that usually only occurs after years of advanced yogic practice. Chapter 11 of a famous Hindu classic called the *Bhagavad Gita* describes this experience in detail. It is a staggering, mind-shattering event that throws open the soul's doors to cosmic consciousness.

Although Western scientists have been slow to recognize the existence of kundalini, this force produces real effects that have long been noted in more inwardly focused cultures. Take a moment to become conscious of this power within your own body by doing this exercise:

1. Sit upright in your meditation posture. Relax your body but keep your back straight. Close your eyes.

2. Inhale deeply, imagining that your breath is rising from the very bottom of your torso. Feel it filling up your body to the very top of your skull.

3. Exhale deeply, imagining that your breath is sinking from the top of your head to the bottom of your torso. Repeat these deep, whole body breaths for half a minute or so.

4. Now focus your full awareness in the center of your brain. How alive do you feel? How lucid do you feel? Are you fully awake? Are there parts of your body that feel sluggish? Are there parts of your mind that still feel asleep?

5. Be aware of your own awareness. How focused is your attention? Is your consciousness clear and one-pointed, or scattered and easily distracted? How long can you hold your attention on your experience of pure consciousness without mental wavering? Take stock of how fully conscious you really are.

6. Shift your attention to your breath. Make sure you are breathing diaphragmatically. Open your eyes and stand up.

The yogis claim that when great adepts like the Buddha experience the full awakening of their kundalini, their consciousness expands exponentially, and they become aware of all dimensions of reality past, present, and future.

Your Degree of Awareness

According to the yoga tradition, most people sleepwalk through life. They're not really completely awake or fully self-conscious. They simply react to the events happening around them out of habit and conditioning, rather than evaluating each unique event on its own merits, and responding in a direct, conscious manner.

This is because, yogis claim, in most people kundalini or the force of consciousness is largely dormant. They only experience themselves as truly conscious beings when they sit down to perform a meditative exercise like you did in the last exercise, and even then they can only hold a fully conscious state for a very short period of time, sometimes even for just a few seconds.

When kundalini begins to awaken, remarkable changes might occur in the personality. Depending on how it moves through the subtle body and which chakra it activates (more about chakras in a moment), an individual might suddenly develop extraordinary charisma. The person can't walk into a room without everyone else instantly sensing their presence.

Some people may develop such extraordinary love and empathy that they gain the ability to heal or they might display exceptional artistic or intellectual gifts. The focused power of their awareness allows them to solve scientific or mathematical problems that have stumped others for centuries. Or it gives them the ability to create breathtaking music, paintings, or poetry seemingly effortlessly. Kundalini is activating parts of their inner psychic mechanism that are asleep in most people.

In the yoga tradition, kundalini is deliberately aroused in order to produce full-blown mystical experiences. The yogi transcends the limitations of his or her ordinary awareness and moves into a state of cosmic consciousness.

FYI Although many Western yoga students are fascinated by the topic of kundalini, only a few books on the subject written in English represent the yogic tradition authentically. Reliable books include *Kundalini: The Arousal of the Inner Energy* by Adjit Mookerjee, and *Layayoga: An Advanced Method of Concentration* by Shyam Sundar Goswami.

THE ENERGY OF CONSCIOUSNESS

Once a yogi has purified his body through Hatha Yoga and a yogic diet, purified his character by ethical behavior, and purified his mind through meditation, he is ready to begin intensive work with kundalini. Yogis have pioneered a number of ways to arouse this energy. They work with hatha postures, vigorous breathing exercises and breath retention, specific mantras and advanced meditation exercises in order to fully activate the force of their awareness and the many powers and abilities it stimulates.

Kundalini work must always be performed under the careful guidance of an experienced teacher. There is a hospital in Bangalore, South India, that specifically treats cases of kundalini gone bad. When the power is aroused prematurely, too rapidly, or without proper supervision, it can cause serious psychiatric and physiological problems.

The kundalini master Swami Satyananda Saraswati of the Bihar School of Yoga emphasizes that work with this force must be slow, sensible, and systematic. Then the energy can be raised safely and directed for the benefit of all humankind.

EXPERIENCE YOUR CHAKRAS

Kundalini is believed to lie largely dormant in most people at the base of the spine. In men it's said to be concentrated at the perineum, between the genital organ and the anus. In women it's located near the root of the uterus at the cervix. Yogis awaken the power, then carefully lead it up the spine through seven major way stations called *chakras*.

STRICTLY DEFINED

A **chakra** is an energy center in the subtle body. Chakra is Sanskrit for "wheel," because the chakras are often visualized as wheel-shaped whirling vortices of consciousness and energy. It is incorrect to pronounce chakra *shakra*, as some New Agers do. The correct pronunciation is *chuck-ruh*.

As each of the chakras in turn is stimulated, extraordinary mental abilities associated with that chakra may be activated. Yogis deliberately meditate on particular chakras to gain these powers.

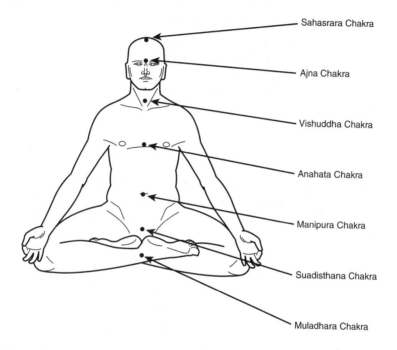

— Sahasrara Chakra

— Ajna Chakra

— Vishuddha Chakra

— Anahata Chakra

— Manipura Chakra

— Suadisthana Chakra

— Muladhara Chakra

The seven chakras.

Take a moment to see if you can sense the chakras in your own body and the feelings and powers associated with each one.

1. Sit upright in your meditation posture. Relax your body but keep your back straight. Close your eyes.

2. Breathe diaphragmatically. Focus your awareness on the bridge between your nostrils until your breath begins flowing equally in both nostrils. When this occurs the central channel in your subtle body is said to be opening. It is through this channel that kundalini can flow at its maximum rate.

3. Bring your full awareness to your sacrum, the very bottom portion of your spine. Shift your attention slightly forward to your perineum if you are male, or to your cervix if you are female. Be intensely aware of this area. What feelings do you associate with it? Are you aware of any energy being held in this region?

4. Draw your attention back to your spine and, as you inhale, shift it upward a few notches. Shift it slightly forward to the root of your penis if you are male, or to your uterus if you are female. What do you feel here? Is the energy here healthy or distorted, flowing or blocked? Breathe diaphragmatically.

5. Draw your attention back to your spine and, as you inhale, shift it upward until you reach the vertebra just behind your navel. Shift your concentration forward into your solar plexus, the knot of nerves in your navel area. Focus intently. Does the area feel hot or cold, tense or relaxed, sluggish or active? What emotions does this area trigger in your awareness?

6. Draw your attention back to your spine and, as you inhale, shift it upward till you reach the vertebra just behind your heart. Shift your awareness forward into your heart region at the center of your chest. Pay close attention to this area. Does it feel open and flowing like a river, still and placid like a lake, or clogged and muddy like a sewer? What feelings are you experiencing here?

7. Draw your attention back to your spine and, as you inhale, shift it upward till you reach your throat. Shift your awareness forward to the hollow of your throat. Focus intensely. Do you sense any energy in motion here? Are any emotions associated with this region?

8. Draw your attention back to your spine and, as you inhale, shift it upward into your head. Focus at the point between your eyebrows. Then shift your awareness backward from that point about three inches. You are now positioned in the forward-central portion of your brain. Concentrate carefully. What are you experiencing here? Don't be distracted by thoughts. Simply be aware of the sensations that arise spontaneously at this center of consciousness.

9. Now inhale, drawing your full attention upward toward the top of your skull. Hold your awareness as high up within the center of your brain for as long as you can without straining. (If you notice the muscles around your eyes spontaneously tensing, relax them.) Pay close attention. What are you experiencing in this area?

10. As you exhale, allow your awareness to slip back downward toward your nostrils. Breathe diaphragmatically. Open your eyes and stand up.

The seven centers you have just visited are the seven major chakras of the yoga tradition, the gears of consciousness through which your personality operates. Knowingly or unknowingly, you are shifting up and down through these gears throughout the day. They provide the framework of your conscious experience.

> **FYI** There is a lot of talk in New Age circles about activating or clearing your chakras. But what is a chakra really, and how did the meditation masters of antiquity work with them? An excellent introduction to this often misunderstood topic is *Chakras: Energy Centers of Transformation* by the yogi/scholar Harish Johari.

THE SEVEN CENTERS

In yoga, each of the chakras or seven gears of consciousness is visualized in a specific symbolic manner. It's as if every chakra is a round or square flower with a certain number of petals. Each has a certain shape and color, and a certain seed syllable or special mantra associated with it. Each also relates to a particular element and sense. When kundalini rises through the chakras, they blossom like flowers in full bloom.

YOUR SACRAL CENTER

The first chakra forms the foundation of the personality.

Chakra:	Muladhara
Meaning of name:	Root, foundation
Location:	Bottom of spine
Shape:	Square
Color:	Yellow
Number of petals:	Four
Seed syllable:	Lum
Element:	Earth
Sense:	Smell
Body correspondence:	Sacro-coccygeal plexus

The *muladhara* or root chakra (*mula* is Sanskrit for "root") is located near the bottom of the spine, and is the seat of kundalini. It's no coincidence that the word "sacrum" (the fused vertebrae at the base of the spine) sounds like "sacred," because the sacred energy of consciousness is said to be coiled at the bottom of the spine like a snake coiled in a pot (*kunda* is Sanskrit for "pot"). In Latin, *sacrum* actually meant "the sacred bone."

The energy of consciousness or "serpent power" rests in the muladhara chakra for years, even for an entire lifetime in most people, releasing just enough energy to keep the body active and the mind functioning at an ordinary level. But when it is activated through yoga practice, the kundalini begins to surge upward through the central channel in the subtle body (corresponding to the spinal column in the physical body), to some degree stimulating each of the chakras it passes through on its way up to the top of the head. When the kundalini reaches the *sahasrara* or topmost chakra, it is said to produce cosmic consciousness. If the yogi can hold this awesome power in the highest chakra, she enters a condition of permanent enlightenment.

The emotional issues associated with the root chakra have to do with your fundamental sense of security. Fear and panic arising from a primal sense of insecurity, or a deep sense of groundedness and being comfortable with physical reality manifest at this level. Usually children up to the age of about seven function primarily out of this chakra.

Yogis associate the root chakra with levitation and the psychic ability to manifest any odor at will.

PROCEED WITH CAUTION

If you try holding your breath for any length of time, you'll find that besides feeling extremely uncomfortable, your consciousness will become incredibly concentrated. Advanced yogis took advantage of this principle and gradually trained themselves to slow their breath rate dramatically, so they could more easily control their kundalini. Breath retention is not recommended for beginners and should *never* be practiced without advice from a qualified teacher, as it can result in brain and heart damage.

Your Sex Center

The second chakra is primarily associated with sexuality.

Chakra:	Svadhisthana
Meaning of name:	Seat of the self
Location:	Genital organs
Shape:	Circle
Color:	Light blue
Number of petals:	Six
Seed syllable:	Vum

Element:	Water
Sense:	Taste
Body correspondence:	Pelvic plexus

The second or *svadhisthana* chakra relates to the astral world—the world of daydreams and imagination in the waking state and dreams and hypnogogic imagery in the sleep state. As such, it's deeply connected with fantasy, the world of the imagination children live in from about the age of eight to fourteen. During this period puberty usually occurs, and the proper functioning of this chakra is closely connected with a healthy expression of sexuality.

When this chakra functions ineffectively, the imagination may be underactive or warped, and one's sexuality may be overactivated or stifled.

Yogis associate the second chakra with a working knowledge of the astral plane and the ability to walk on water.

YOUR NAVEL CENTER

The old saying "meditating on your navel" comes from yogis who meditate on their third center, the *manipura* chakra, which is located at the navel.

Chakra:	Manipura
Meaning of name:	City of jewels
Location:	Navel
Shape:	Downward pointing triangle
Color:	Red
Number of petals:	Ten
Seed syllable:	Rum
Element:	Fire
Sense:	Sight
Body correspondence:	Solar plexus

The third chakra controls issues related to domination and submission. A strong third chakra makes a person indomitable; in fact, this chakra is related to the *hara* center that Chinese martial artists focus on in their quest for invincibility. If the manipura chakra functions inefficiently, a person "lacks backbone," is "spineless," and can easily be controlled by others. Young people between the ages of 15 and 21, who are establishing their place in their social hierarchy, often operate out of this level of consciousness.

GO TO ▶
The primary focus of this book is to give you a practical understanding of beginning-level yoga and meditation techniques. However, a fuller understanding of these methods is possible only if you have some grasp of yoga philosophy and psychology. Hour 22 will introduce you to the psychology behind the practices you've been learning here.

Yogis associated the gut chakra with excellent health and indomitability, the acquisition of wealth, and control of the element fire.

Your Heart Center

The fourth center or *anahata* chakra is located in the center of your chest between your breasts.

Chakra:	Anahata
Meaning of name:	Uncaused sound
Location:	Heart
Shape:	Six-pointed star
Color:	Gray
Number of petals:	Twelve
Seed syllable:	Yum
Element:	Air
Sense:	Touch
Body correspondence:	Cardiac plexus

Faith, charity, and harmony are the positive qualities of the heart center. Male and female energies, spiritual and material impulses, all balance here when the chakra is operating optimally. However, if heart energy is skewed, anger and ill will can emanate from this region.

Between the ages of 22 and 28, most people make a commitment to their life partner, and adult friendships are cemented. As the individual grows more mature, the desire to help and support others becomes increasingly strong. This has to do with the activation of this heart-oriented level of consciousness.

Yogis associate the heart chakra with unconditional love, the ability to heal others, blessing power, and selfless service.

JUST A MINUTE

The shapes and colors associated with the chakras are symbolic in nature only. The actual chakras don't exist in physical matter so they don't actually have a form the eyes can see. In reality, they're made of pure energy. However, they do correspond to certain nerve centers and glands in the physical body.

Your Throat Center

It's not unusual for yoga students to report they have the most difficulty sensing the presence of the fifth or *vishuddha* chakra. This is in part because it's associated with ether, an element even more subtle than air. While feeling this chakra in the pit of the throat can be tricky, its effects in people's lives are usually quite obvious.

Chakra:	Vishuddha
Meaning of name:	Stainless
Location:	Throat
Shape:	Crescent
Color:	Purple
Number of petals:	Sixteen
Seed syllable:	Hum
Element:	Ether
Sense:	Hearing
Body correspondence:	Pharyngeal plexus

Vishuddha literally means "purity." When this chakra is acting optimally, thoughts are pure, free from hostility or greed. The power of discrimination is enhanced, allowing one to think clearly and act on the basis of good judgment. Artistic creativity and the ability to speak in an uplifting and inspiring manner are sometimes connected with a flowering fifth chakra. When this chakra is weak, a person may be inarticulate or foul-mouthed, foolish, or uninspired.

This chakra is naturally activated when a normal person reaches the age range of 29 to 35. By this time he or she has begun to develop more mature judgment based on ample life experience.

Mastery of the vishuddha chakra is said to give supernormal knowledge of the past, present, and future, as well as telepathic powers. Saints who live for years without taking any food are said to be absorbing nutrients directly from the atmosphere through this chakra.

FYI *Mantra and Meditation* by Pandit Usharbudh Arya, D. Litt., takes you inside the tradition of the Himalayan masters to introduce you to meditation as it's actually practiced by the yogic adepts. It explains the field of mantra and how this energy operates in the depths of your unconscious as you sit for meditation.

Your Eyebrow Center

The pituitary gland is one of the main command centers of the physical body. The chakra associated with it, the sixth or *ajna* chakra, actually means "command."

Chakra:	Ajna
Meaning of name:	Command center
Location:	Point behind the eyebrows
Shape:	Circle
Color:	White
Number of petals:	Two
Seed syllable:	Om
Element:	Source of matter
Sense:	Intuition
Body correspondence:	Pituitary gland

Contrary to popular misconception, the sixth chakra is not actually right between the eyebrows. It is behind that point a few inches, closer to the center of your brain. It may be a useful exercise for you to try to find this center inside your skull right now. You'll find that if you close your eyes and focus intently inside your head, there are portions of your brain where your consciousness seems to "click" into gear, automatically becoming clearer and more focused. These are the various chakras within the cranium. One of the two most important chakras in the brain is the ajna or "command center" of consciousness.

Intellectual genius and penetrating insight are generated at this chakra. From the age of 36 to 42 the adult brain is normally operating optimally. The conscience is fully formed and willpower is strong if this chakra is well energized. If not, the person has difficulty making decisions, lacks a sense of ethics, or is mentally dull.

Yogis associate the sixth chakra with divine knowledge and a host of psychic powers. It is the portal into transcendent states of consciousness beyond normal human awareness.

YOUR BRAIN CENTERS

The second of the two most important chakra in the cranium is the *sahas-rara*. *Sahasrara* literally means "a thousand," referring to the thousand petals of this most powerful of all centers of consciousness.

Chakra:	Sahasrara
Meaning of name:	A thousand petals
Location:	Top of the skull
Shape:	Circular
Color:	Rainbowlike spectrum
Number of petals:	1,000
Seed syllable:	Silence
Element:	Beyond physical and mental elements
Sense:	Superconsciousness
Body correspondence:	Pineal gland

All the other chakras are said to be contained within the seventh or sahas-rara chakra. Very few people ever reach this level of consciousness, which is directed upward and outward beyond the human realm. However, in ancient times, when people were more spiritually oriented, it was felt that by the age of 43 a person should have arrived at this level of maturity.

It is through this exit that yogis are said to consciously leave and re-enter their bodies. When kundalini reaches and permanently activates this center, a person is said to become fully enlightened. Yogis claim that at this point the soul can return to her body to serve humanity, or leave this world altogether for much higher dimensions of reality.

FYI *The Serpent Power* by Sir John Woodroffe was one of the earliest and best introductions in English to the subject of kundalini. Sir John (who also wrote under the pen name "Arthur Avalon") was a High Court Commissioner for the British Raj in Calcutta in the early twentieth century. He was so impressed by yoga science that he studied with an Indian guru for years—unusual for a British gentleman of that period. His books on yoga remain classics in the field even today.

There are three more important chakras in the brain between the eyebrow center and the thousand-petaled center at the top of the skull. The *guru* chakra is used to connect with inner guidance and the wisdom of the lineage of sages. Yogis focus at the *soma* chakra in order to experience extraordinary states of inner bliss. The *jnana* chakra is used to burn away karmic complexes that may be stunting spiritual growth.

There are numerous other chakras in the subtle body. The chakras in the palms of the hands, for example, are used to deliver blessings and healing power in the yoga tradition. The chakras in a guru's feet are said to be so resonant with spiritual energy that disciples vie to touch them!

In the next hour, however, you'll learn more about higher states of consciousness you might begin experiencing as your meditation deepens, as well as about the psychic powers associated with the evolution of human consciousness.

HOUR'S UP!

Ready for your quiz covering the material you've been introduced to in Hour 18? Answer true or false to the following statements:

1. Kundalini lies dormant in the bottom chakra in most people.
2. No yogi is able to meditate for longer than 24 hours at a time.
3. Kundalini or "the serpent power" is a biological force that acts through the nervous system.
4. The heart chakra governs emotions such as fear and the sense of security.
5. Superior physical health and indomitability are associated with the navel chakra.
6. A guru's guidance is absolutely essential before attempting the advanced breathing exercises that can awaken the serpent power.
7. Activation of the topmost chakra produces extraordinary mystical experiences.
8. Generally, people's attention naturally ascends through the chakras as they mature.
9. The throat chakra is the command center that contains all the other chakras.
10. Meditation is the only way to awaken the force of kundalini.

HOUR 19

Awaken Your Awareness

CHAPTER SUMMARY

LESSON PLAN:
In this hour you will learn ...

- Yogis have catalogued a series of increasingly advanced stages of consciousness that gradually become accessible to meditators.

- Yogic adepts maintain heightened states of consciousness even while they're asleep.

- There is a fourth state of consciousness beyond waking, dreaming, and deep sleep that most people are unaware of.

- Psychic powers are a byproduct of advanced meditative processes, according to the yoga tradition.

Yogis of all traditions describe a series of increasingly deeper states of meditation leading to full superconsciousness. Mastering some of these states, according to the yogis, can unlock hidden abilities of the mind called *siddhis* or "accomplishments." These are commonly called psychic powers in the West.

Advanced meditators also describe an experience they call *yoga nidra*. In this condition a yogi's body remains in a state of deep sleep while his or her mind stays fully awake. It was through the practice of yoga nidra that a great adept like Buddha could meditate continuously for nearly 40 days and nights. His body might have slept but he was still fully mentally alert, wholly engaged in his quest for enlightenment 24 hours a day.

In this hour, you'll be introduced to a few of the remarkable phenomena that very advanced meditators sometimes encounter in their spiritual practice. You'll also learn about the levels of samadhi, deep meditative absorption, in which you transcend the ordinary functioning of your mind and experience actual superconscious states.

LATENT MENTAL POWERS

Most people experience extrasensory perception (ESP) at some point in their lives. Suddenly they simply know what someone else is thinking or doing, even though there is no physical way they could acquire this information. Or they might sense what's about to happen before it actually occurs. For the most part, Western science refuses to accept the legitimacy of these phenomena. However, the existence of ESP is fully acknowledged in yoga science. In fact, yoga texts mention that as the inner windows of your awareness become more transparent due to meditative practice, psychic phenomena are likely to begin occurring. This will happen only occasionally for beginning-level meditators, but some advanced adepts are said to have developed truly extraordinary psychic powers which they use to help their disciples and rescue people in distress.

SPECIAL YOGIC ABILITIES

In the *Yoga Sutras*, the sage Patanjali devotes one whole chapter to the subject of psychic abilities. He includes a long list of extrasensory powers that some advanced meditators are said to have demonstrated, and mentions the specific meditation technique that leads to each power. A few of the yogic powers he describes are as follows:

- Telepathy
- Clairvoyance
- Knowledge of the future
- Visions of past historical events
- Memory of previous incarnations
- The ability to leave the body at will
- Superhuman physical strength
- Understanding the language of animals
- The ability to manipulate matter and energy through the force of will

Patanjali lists five ways in which you can acquire supernormal powers. The first is to be born with them as a consequence of having developed them in a previous incarnation. Second, some people have flashes of supersensory experiences when they use certain psychoactive herbs. Third, extreme forms of asceticism can lead to extrasensory experience. (Fasting in the wilderness for 40 days in order to have a divine vision is even mentioned in the Bible.)

The last two methods the sage notes are mantra and meditation. The yoga tradition has preserved many mantras that are said to release hidden powers of consciousness. Meditation stills the thought waves and focuses the mind, allowing intuitive insight to flow into one's ordinary awareness. This happens frequently enough that Patanjali felt compelled to bring up the subject in his classic introductory work on yoga.

BEWARE OF PSYCHIC POWERS!

It's hard to read Patanjali's list of psychic powers without getting excited. If they really do exist, who wouldn't want to have these paranormal abilities? But Patanjali is not cataloging these powers in order to inspire you to pursue them. On the contrary, in the *Yoga Sutras* he goes out of his way to *warn* meditators about them.

What Patanjali specifically says is, "Psychic powers seem exciting and desirable to the average person. But in reality they get in the way of developing even higher states of consciousness, which are the real goal of yoga. Having psychic abilities can lead to an inflated ego and many other undesirable consequences."

When psychic powers are used without first having purified the mind through ethical practices (see Hour 22), the meditator may be tempted to use his supernormal abilities to manipulate others. If the powers appear before the person connects with her inner wisdom, well-meaning attempts to use these skills in order to help others may in fact just make matters worse.

PROCEED WITH CAUTION

The greatest yoga classic of all time, Patanjali's *Yoga Sutras,* emphatically warns yoga students against becoming preoccupied with attaining psychic powers. These are seen as potential obstacles to the development of still higher states of consciousness that are the actual goal of yoga and meditation.

INNER MESSAGES

Yogic lore is brimming with stories of amazing, superhuman-seeming powers displayed by great adepts. Yet the yoga lineages teach that the masters don't chase psychic powers. Rather, psychic powers chase the masters.

What the tradition is saying is that individuals who pursue psychic powers are usually motivated by self-interest, and their quest can easily turn into a form of sorcery. But a yogi who is motivated by the desire for spiritual awakening or the sincere longing to benefit others continually purifies her mind and deepens her ability to connect with her Higher Self through meditation. Then psychic abilities appear unbidden. When there is an emergency or someone needs special help, the Higher Self acts spontaneously to resolve the problem. Grace showers down from a higher power and the situation automatically reorganizes itself to provide the best possible outcome.

One out of many thousands of such true stories is about Anandamayi Ma, the great yogic adept born in 1896 in East Bengal. One day she got up in the middle of a festival and started walking toward the train station. Her disciples ran after her, asking where she was going. "Sarnath," she replied.

The disciples explained that the train didn't stop at the Sarnath station but Anandamayi Ma got on anyway, followed by her disciples. When they reached Sarnath the train suddenly developed some kind of mechanical problem and pulled to a halt. After Ma and her devotees jumped off, the engine started up again and the train rumbled off.

Ma strode purposefully into town. "Where are you headed?" the disciples asked. "The hotel," she answered. Neither she nor they had any idea where the local hotel was, yet Anandamayi Ma walked directly to it. Inside the hotel they heard a woman crying. It turned out she had gotten stranded in Sarnath without any money. She was terribly frightened and started mentally calling out to Anandamayi Ma, her guru. In those days there were no telephones or telegraphs in the area, but Ma had obviously received the message!

FYI   *At the Eleventh Hour* by Pandit Rajmani Tigunait relates the true story of Bengali Baba, one of the most famous miracle workers of twentieth-century India. The extraordinary powers of this sage were thoroughly documented by investigators and verified in court proceedings. The book is a mind-expanding account of the potentials of human consciousness.

Anandamayi Ma was a meditation master of the first caliber who naturally remained in the highest states of consciousness at all times. She had no interest in psychic powers whatsoever, yet often spontaneously displayed them. Yet she made no claims to special powers. According to her, she simply listened to her inner guidance, which effortlessly led her to serve and inspire others.

My meditation teacher had a secluded ashram in Nepal. There were no phones on the grounds so it was always a mystery how the ashram attendant invariably knew when to drive to the Katmandu airport to pick up his guru when he returned from India. "Oh it's easy," the attendant explained. "The night before he arrives he appears in my dreams and gives me the flight arrival time."

Westerners can scarcely comprehend that powers like these actually exist. Yet many people in traditional Eastern cultures take them completely for granted. These types of events are so common it doesn't occur to people there to question them. Like the yogis, they recognize that the powers of the mind are virtually limitless, once they're harnessed through meditation and self-discipline.

YOGIC SLEEP

One of the advanced abilities adepts develop is yoga nidra, or yogic sleep. Advanced yogis are constantly doing their inner work, even while they're asleep. For the yogis whose goal is nothing less than enlightenment in this lifetime, embodied life is all too short and there isn't a moment to spare. Therefore the dream and deep sleep states are also used for spiritual practice.

FYI *Yoga Nidra* by Swami Satyasanganananda Saraswati is an excellent introduction to the yogic discipline of sleep. Tongue-in-cheek, the swami renames the hypnagogic state between waking and sleep the "hypnayogic" state. The founder of the Yoga Research Foundation goes on more seriously to explain in detail how to enter yogic sleep and the results to expect from your experience.

That yogis could be meditating even while asleep seems incredible, yet it's a scientifically proven fact. In 1970, Swami Rama of the Himalayas was hooked up to an EEG (electroencephalograph, a machine that monitors brain function) at the Menninger Foundation Voluntary Controls Program in Topeka, Kansas. Eventually the swami fell asleep, the EEG confirming that he was no longer awake. Yet when researchers awoke him, he was able to report everything that had occurred in the room while he was physically unconscious. The scientists were staggered but to the swami, the ability to remain completely lucid during sleep was just a basic yogic skill.

"All of the body is in the mind, but not all of the mind is in the body," Swami Rama explained. Yogis believe that there is much more to human consciousness than the gray matter of our brains. The body may be sound asleep, but the Higher Self is always awake according to yoga science. If we identify our entire reality with the waking state, we quickly forget most of our dreams when we wake up, and don't remember having been in the deep sleep state at all, even though we know we *must* have been sleeping soundly.

The technique of yogic sleep, or lucid sleep, is different from lucid dreaming, in which you become aware that you're dreaming while the dream is still going on. In lucid sleep, you will not experience dream imagery, but will be intensely mentally alert even though your body is technically asleep. The full yogic sleep technique can be performed by advanced yogis only and involves a demanding level of breath control. But beginners can enter a light state of yogic sleep by performing the following practice taught by Swami Rama.

PREPARE FOR LUCID SLEEP

To complete the following exercise, you will need to have mastered the Corpse Posture and the 61 Points exercise taught in Hour 3. Go back to that hour to make sure you can remember all 61 points in the correct order. This concentration technique will help you deeply relax your body while sharply focusing your mind, so that you can remain alert in the sleep state. You will also need to be familiar with the chakras you learned about in Hour 18.

There are five important prerequisites for the practice of lucid sleep:

- Do not try this practice when you are tired. The first few times in particular, you should be fully awake and well rested to avoid slipping into unconsciousness.

- Do the practice in a dark, quiet room. Cover your eyes with a light blanket if you need to shut out the distraction of light.

- Do not do the practice on a soft mattress! A firm mattress or cot is better, or the floor if it is well cushioned. You might start to nap if you're too comfortable. Use a thin pillow, not a very thick one. Your head should be lightly supported but not lifted so high it's out of alignment with your spine.

- You should not have eaten for at least two hours before beginning your session. Otherwise, the activity of your digestive system will prevent your brain from operating optimally during the session. You need to be as clearheaded and focused as possible.

- Do the practice every day at the same time. Be prepared to practice daily for some time before seeing full results. Most beginners take a few days to a few weeks to get the knack of the technique.

JUST A MINUTE

You will be in full control throughout the process of yoga nidra or lucid sleep. This is not a passive state. This is one yoga practice in which it is not helpful to have someone else guide you through the routine. You need to be fully in command, exercising your will and concentrating sharply in order to avoid napping rather than doing yoga! Remember, your body falls asleep but you, as a conscious observer, remain awake.

PRACTICE LUCID SLEEP

The following technique is fairly demanding. It will require your intensive focus for 10 to 15 minutes. Memorize the steps in advance so you can lead yourself through the exercise without having to stop midway to check the instructions. This might seem like a daunting task, but avoid the temptation to speak the steps into a tape recorder and play it back for yourself. It is essential that you *not* place yourself into a state of auto-hypnosis, as you may if you passively listen to a tape. Your active will must be fully engaged during this exercise! Otherwise, you are likely to fall asleep or drift into reverie. The steps are complex for the very purpose of creating intense meditative focus.

During the practice of lucid sleep, you are required to breathe down to each of your chakras from the top of your skull and inhale back up. Yoga texts specify that you skip the center associated with the sex organs during this practice, going directly from the root chakra to the navel center. This helps prevent the tendency to slip off into romantic fantasies.

1. Lie down in the Corpse Posture. Close your eyes.

2. Bring your full awareness to the chakra behind your eyebrows. Breathe diaphragmatically. Do not entertain any thoughts, even the sound of your mantra. Just focus on the chakra behind your eyebrows as if you were breathing in and out from the center of your brain.

3. Bring your full awareness to the chakra at the pit of your throat. Breathe diaphragmatically as if you're breathing from your throat center. Relax but stay focused.

4. Bring your full awareness to the chakra between your breasts. Breathe diaphragmatically from your heart center. Allow yourself to relax deeply but don't lose consciousness. Stay with the feeling of the breath at your heart. As you relax, your breath will become slower and very refined.

5. Return your focus to your eyebrow center and begin the 61 Points concentration exercise you learned in Hour 3. Stay focused! Move your mind through your body, systematically relaxing each part. By the time you complete the 61 Points you should be very deeply relaxed but your mind should be intensely focused from tracing a path through your body.

6. At this point you begin to breathe much more deeply but not forcefully. Slowly exhale as though you're breathing out from the top of your skull down to the tips of your toes. As you exhale, feel any residual tension, inner blocks, and physical or mental toxins being expelled

down out of your body. As you inhale, feel revitalizing energy surging up through your body from the bottom of your feet to the top of your head. Do this 10 times. Your body will remain deeply relaxed but the extra oxygen will enhance your mental alertness.

7. Exhale tensions from the top of your head to your ankles 10 times. Inhale fresh energy from your ankles to the top of your skull.

8. Exhale tensions from the top of your head to your knees 10 times. Inhale revitalizing energy from your knees to the top of your skull.

9. Exhale from the top of your head to the bottom of your spine. Breathe out bad energy, breathe in good energy. This time repeat the exhalation and inhalation only five times.

10. Exhale from the top of your head to the chakra at your navel, releasing tensions. Inhale fresh energy back up. Do this five times.

11. Exhale from the top of your head to the center between your breasts, releasing tensions. Inhale fresh energy back up. Do this five times.

12. Exhale from the top of your head to your throat chakra, releasing tensions. Inhale revitalizing energy back up to the top of your skull. Do this five times.

13. Exhale from the top of your head to your nasal septum, the bridge between your two nostrils. Sense whether both nostrils are open so that you are breathing equally through your right and left nostrils at the same time. If one nostril is more open than the other, focus on the other until it, too, opens and you can breathe freely through both. Expel tense or blocked energy as you exhale. Then inhale fresh energy up to the top of your skull five times.

14. Exhale from the top of your head to the center behind your eyebrows. Exhale used energy, inhale fresh energy. Repeat this five times. By now your breathing process is very soft and subtle. You're getting enough air to sustain you in your present deeply relaxed state, but a person watching you would barely be able to see you breathe, your respiratory cycle has become so refined.

15. Now repeat the process, breathing five more times each down from the top of your head to the eyebrow center, then to the nostrils, then to the throat center, next the heart center, then the navel center, then the root center at the bottom of the spine. With each exhalation you are expelling used gas and toxins. With each inhalation you are taking in fresh energy.

16. Continue the process breathing 10 times each from the top of your head to your knees, then to your ankles, and finally down to your toes. Breathe out used energy, breathe in fresh energy.

17. Turn over and lie on your left side. Breathe as if your entire right side is breathing. Take 10 full breaths through the right side of your body.

18. Now turn over onto your right side. Take 10 full breaths through the left side of your body.

19. Turn onto your back. Breathe 10 times as if your entire body is expelling used air from the top of your head to your toes, and taking in fresh air from toes to top. Your body and mind are relaxed but filled with vitality.

20. Bring your full attention to the center behind your eyebrows. Focus there for a moment as you breathe naturally.

21. Shift your full attention to the center in the pit of your throat. Breathe naturally for a moment.

22. Now focus fully at your heart center, breathing naturally. Don't think about anything. Just be conscious of yourself as a breathing being, observing the flow of your breath at your heart chakra.

23. Sit up and experience the present moment fully. You will feel very clear and alert, and rested yet energized.

This is the preliminary exercise yogis do to begin mastering the state of deep sleep.

REDUCE YOUR NEED FOR SLEEP

The name Buddha literally means "the awakened one." Being awake, living consciously, is the goal of yoga practice.

Advanced yogis spend very little time sleeping, rarely more than 2 hours in 24. They do, however, spend a great deal of time in meditation, often eight hours or more per day. Ordinary people have to sleep in order to clear their brain circuitry in a process known as dreaming, and to replenish depleted biochemicals during deep sleep. Yogis discharge their excess mental energy during meditation rather than dreams, and recharge their physical bodies through Hatha Yoga and relaxation exercises rather than in deep sleep.

PROCEED WITH CAUTION

Yogic adepts can often go for long periods with little or no sleep. Beginning yoga students, however, should not artificially force themselves to cut short their natural sleep cycles in an effort to appear more "yogic." As you deepen your yoga practice, your need for sleep will lessen at a natural pace. Listen to your body. It will let you know how much sleep it needs.

Through your practice of Hatha Yoga postures, breathing exercises, and meditation, you will find yourself remaining much more relaxed and stress-free throughout the day. Before long, you'll find yourself needing less sleep at night, and resting more deeply when you do sleep. Special techniques like Yogic Sleep can also revitalize your body and release tensions from your mind, gradually reducing your need for sleep.

HIGHER STATES OF CONSCIOUSNESS

Advanced yogis shift the focus of their attention from the physical body to the Higher Self, and remain fully conscious in an illumined state that is called *turiya* in Sanskrit. This "fourth state" is accessible to all meditators and, with a little concentrated effort, is not actually that difficult to experience. Yogic sleep leads you to turiya. So do the states of mental absorption you experience in deep meditation.

STRICTLY DEFINED

Turiya, which literally means "the fourth state," is the superconscious state beyond the three conditions of waking, dreaming, and deep sleep.

Patanjali's *Yoga Sutras* lists several levels of absorption that you may encounter as your meditative practice deepens. Here is what to watch for:

- **Unbroken meditation on an external object.** You are meditating with your eyes open on an object outside yourself, such as a picture of a saint or guru, or a symbol of God, your breath, or a glowing light. You are not distracted but remain completely focused for three minutes or more at a time.

- **Unbroken meditation on an internal object.** You are meditating with your eyes closed on an object you are picturing or hearing in your mind, such as an image of God or the Goddess, or the sound of your mantra. Your attention doesn't waver.

- **Unbroken meditation on the bliss within.** Sitting with your eyes closed, you don't see or hear any object. You simply feel incredible joy or profound peace or deep contentment. It suffuses your entire awareness for three minutes or more at a time.

- **Unbroken meditation on your own existence.** Sitting with your eyes closed, you experience nothing but the sense of your own existence. You remain completely focused on the reality of your own inner being without becoming distracted.

This condition of unbroken meditation, where you remain completely focused for three minutes or more, is called samadhi in Sanskrit. (You might remember this state of total meditative absorption from Hour 15.)

THE EXPERIENCE OF SAMADHI

There are three types of samadhi. In the first you still have an experience of yourself as the individual who is sitting in meditation.

In the second type of samadhi, however, you're so focused that your very identity vanishes. Perhaps you've noticed that when you're deeply mentally absorbed, you may actually forget you exist. This occurs, for example, when you're watching a really good movie. Only the characters in the film exist in your consciousness—you actually forget you're a separate person sitting in a theater looking at projected images on a screen. Likewise, in the second kind of samadhi you forget that you're chanting your mantra and, for all practical purposes, *become* the sound of the mantra reverberating in the sky of your consciousness. You forget that you're blissful and simply become bliss itself. You forget that you exist and become pure existence itself. You become one with the object of your meditation.

In the third and highest type of samadhi you're not meditating on any object or image or feeling at all. There is nothing you're focused on. Your own innermost being is simply shining of its own accord. Your attention is no longer fixed on any object in the external environment or in your mind. You are pure awareness itself. Now you are in turiya, the fourth state of consciousness beyond waking, dreaming, and deep sleep.

According to the yoga tradition, everyone has experienced turiya, but most of the time they don't recognize it for what it is: a portal into their innermost being. You have experienced this state if any of the following events have happened to you:

- You've received sudden, terrible news, such as that a friend or loved one has just died. Your mind is stunned into a deep silence and sober clarity.

- You're abruptly thrust into great danger, such as when you lose control of your car. Suddenly, your mind becomes extremely calm and clear, as if you're simply witnessing the car going off the road.

- You suddenly experience an unexpected shock of pleasure, such as learning you've just been hired for a coveted job or won an award, or someone you're in love with walks in the door unexpectedly. It's as if you're thrown out of space and time into a place of total lucidity. You're suddenly totally focused in the present moment.

 FYI What would it be like to live with a person who is constantly in the highest state of consciousness? In the nine volumes of *Awaken Children!* by Swami Amritswarupananda, a swami from southwestern India relates his experiences with Ammachi, one of the great women yogis of modern India.

RECOGNIZE YOUR OWN PRESENCE

Gurus often advise their students to carefully watch the train of their thoughts. In the split second between one thought and the next, turiya occurs. For a moment, your mind becomes still. Thoughts stop their incessant chatter and you are simply intensely aware. This experience of pure awareness is greatly valued in yoga. In some Buddhist traditions it's called *satori*. Zen masters play shocking tricks on their students in order to stun them into this state, such as slapping them very suddenly on the back while they sit meditating.

Yogis work to stay in this state of intense, living awareness at all times. To be in *sahaja samadhi* means to naturally remain fully present and lucid in every moment. In this state, full yoga or union with the Higher Self has been attained. There is no longer a lower self—one's day-to-day personality—in addition to a Higher Self hidden within. Instead the Higher Self is now fully manifest in the personality. You have become the best you can be. The greatest saints and yogis live in continual sahaja samadhi. The wisdom, creativity, and healing power of the divine within constantly pours through them for the benefit of others.

STRICTLY DEFINED

Sahaja samadhi means to naturally remain in a state of meditation at all times, whether you are awake, dreaming or sleeping, sitting with your eyes closed, or actively engaged in any activity. *Sahaja* literally means "natural."

EVALUATING YOUR PROGRESS

Some students have an unstoppable inner drive to explore the deepest states of meditation. Whether they're searching for answers to life's ultimate questions or just curious about the amazing phenomena of consciousness, they focus inward with innate talent or intense motivation and quickly find their way into higher states.

The majority of people who take up meditation, however, don't want or expect to become enlightened in this lifetime. They just want some relief from the stress of their jobs and relationships, want to bring more balance into their lives, or simply want a little mental peace and quiet knowing how much it can contribute to their emotional well-being.

Whatever your goal is in taking up a meditation practice, here are a few questions to help you assess whether you are making progress in your meditation. Wait till you've been meditating for about a month before giving yourself this evaluation. Rate yourself on a scale of 1 to 3, with 1 meaning "not at all," 2 meaning "a little," and 3 meaning "a lot." You may want to make copies of the blank table, so you can repeat this evaluation every month or two to keep track of the benefits meditation is adding to your life.

	Not at All (1)	A Little (2)	A Lot (3)
Since I started meditating …			
My emotions are more stable (less dramatic ups and downs).			
I feel more cheerful.			
Minor irritations in life don't bother me as much.			
I have more perspective on my life.			
My relationships have been improving.			
I feel physically healthier.			
I can think more clearly.			
I sleep better.			

You have now been introduced to the three most practical components of the yoga tradition: the Hatha Yoga postures, breathing exercises, and meditation. In Part 5, you'll go on to learn about the yogic lifestyle, with its cuisine, cleansing techniques, and ethical vision. You'll also learn about the different types of yoga that are suitable for various personality types. The last hour will map out avenues of further study should you be interested in traveling further along the path of yogic self-transformation.

HOUR'S UP!

Here is your quiz for Hour 19. Answer true or false to the following statements:

1. According to yoga, there is no state of consciousness beyond waking, dreaming, and deep sleep.

2. Yogis have demonstrated in scientific experiments that they can remain alert while their bodies are sleeping.

3. Psychic powers are the main goal of yoga practice.

4. Meditation is one of several ways to gain access to the hidden potentials of the human mind.

5. It's a basic yogic truism that the mind is totally contained in the body.

6. It's best to practice the yogic sleep technique when you're just about to fall asleep anyway.

7. Yogis often need very little sleep.

8. Very high states of consciousness can be attained when the chatter in the mind becomes still.

9. In some yogic states, the meditator and the object she's meditating on become unified.

10. Trying to live in the present moment defeats the whole purpose of yoga.

Part V

Live Your Yoga

Hour 20   The Yoga Lifestyle

Hour 21   Yoga Psychology

Hour 22   Yoga Ethics

Hour 23   Types of Yoga

Hour 24   The Yoga Universe

HOUR 20

The Yoga Lifestyle

CHAPTER SUMMARY

LESSON PLAN:

In this hour you will learn …

- The traditional yogic diet is vegetarian, using bean and grain combinations to supply vital protein.

- Yoga stresses the importance of cleanliness, including the cleanliness of your internal organs.

- Regularly cleansing the nasal cavity is as important as brushing your teeth.

- The traditional Ayurvedic medical system of India is rooted in yogic principles of health and well-being.

For avid yoga students, yoga is much more than a series of physical exercises. It's a lifestyle. The yoga way of life is strongly oriented toward physical, mental, and spiritual health. It works with every level of your being, including your relationships with other people and with the cosmos as a whole.

If you're interested in taking advantage of the numerous health-promoting aspects of yoga science, you'll want to learn about the yogic diet, special cleansing techniques to wash not only the outside but the inside of your body, and how yogic principles are applied medically.

YOGA AND NUTRITION

Traditionally, yogis are vegetarian. There are two reasons for this. The first is ethical. Yogis believe that unnecessarily taking life is bad karma. All living beings are conscious entities and the life force in each of them should be respected. The second reason is physiological. As numerous studies have demonstrated, a balanced vegetarian diet is much better for you than meat-based meals. In general, vegetarians are healthier and live longer.

Yogis noted that unlike carnivorous animals who were designed by nature to eat meat, humans have a comparatively long digestive tract. Your teeth and gut are designed to process grains, fruit, vegetables, beans and legumes, nuts, and to a certain extent, dairy products. Unlike carnivorous animals, you don't have teeth or claws designed for killing prey. As in the case of other primates such as chimpanzees and gorillas, meat was meant to be an insignificant part of the human diet.

If the yogic contention that humans are inherently vegetarian seems unlikely to you, try the following thought experiment:

1. Imagine it's a beautiful spring day. You're very hungry. You pass an apple tree and see hundreds of fresh, ripe apples hanging from its branches. You pluck one off the tree and sink your teeth into its juicy flesh.

2. Imagine it's a beautiful spring day. You're very hungry. You pass an apple tree and see a large bird sitting in one of its branches. You leap upward, catch the bird with your hands, and sink your teeth into its juicy flesh.

Creatures designed by nature to eat meat will find the second visualization far more appealing. Yet few humans do. Yogis take this as a signal that people are meant to live in harmony with the animal creation, avoiding killing whenever possible. Even in traditional societies where animals are killed for food, most aboriginal people make reparations to the soul of the slain animal. Modern Western society may be one of the first cultures in human history that slaughters animals for food on a massive scale without any thought of the suffering of these creatures.

 FYI If you'd like to learn more about a healthy vegetarian diet, two books by Rudolph M. Ballentine, M.D., are essential reading. *Diet and Nutrition: A Holistic Approach* examines the largely vegetarian diets of the world's healthiest cultures, and *Transition to Vegetarianism* can help make your switch to a meat-free diet as painless as possible.

EAT LIKE A YOGI

The traditional yogic diet excludes meat, fish, poultry, eggs, and alcohol. Dairy is used however. You may ask why eggs aren't eaten while milk products are included. The reason is that if you leave eggs out, they'll quickly rot just like meat. If you leave milk out, however, it turns into useful products like yogurt and paneer, which is strained milk curd. Paneer makes an excellent cheese, and I'll show you how to make it in the next section.

Supper for yogis usually includes whole-grain or parboiled rice or an unleavened whole-grain bread combined with a curry called dahl (sometimes spelled dal or dahlbhat), which is a spiced Indian dish made of beans, peas, or lentils. I'll show you how to make it a little later in this hour. There'd be a vegetable dish on the side or combined with the dahl, and a small helping of dairy such as a yogurt-cucumber salad called raita. The dahl and grain together with the serving of milk would provide more than enough protein and vitamins to make up for the lack of meat in the meal. Dessert might consist of a piece of seasonal fruit.

All six basic flavors are included in a traditional Indian dinner: salty, sweet, sour, astringent, bitter, and pungent. Chutneys, which are usually very spicy fruit preserves, are served with the meal in order to provide the flavors the main entrees may not contain. Yogis believe that when all six flavors are present, the taste buds will be satisfied even if the amount of food in the meal is meager.

PROCEED WITH CAUTION

Don't adopt a vegetarian diet unless you understand the principles of healthy meatless eating! Simply giving up meat can cause serious health problems if you don't know how to substitute vegetable protein for the protein you were previously getting from animal products. Take a vegetarian cooking class or consult a good-quality vegetarian cookbook for entrees that are well balanced, tasty, and cruelty-free.

EASY YOGA RECIPES

Here are a few yoga recipes adapted from Indian cuisine. You might want to experiment with these to see if you care for the flavors, which are typical of North India. Fortunately, there are many dozens of excellent vegetarian cookbooks available now which also offer recipes from other cultures like the rice and bean dishes of Mexico, pasta-based dishes from southern Europe, hummus and falafel recipes from the Mediterranean, tofu stir fries from Japan, bean cakes from China, garden burgers from North America, and so on.

Start by making ghee (sometimes spelled ghi), the favored cooking oil of traditional India. Known as clarified butter in the West, ghee is so highly regarded in the yoga tradition that it's incorporated in many Indian medicines. It can be stored for weeks at a time at room temperature, and doesn't burn when you fry it. Instead it coats the vegetables you fry in it, adding a delicious flavor.

Ghee

Ingredients: 1 lb. fresh, unsalted butter

1. Cut the butter into small slices. Put it in a frying pan or shallow pot. Place the pan over low heat.

2. When the butter starts melting, skim the white milk solids that form on the top with a large spoon. Keep skimming until no more solids form over the yellow oil. Then discard the white solids and remove the melted oil from the stove. When it cools a bit, pour it into a glass jar for storage.

You now have a jar full of the finest-quality cooking oil in the world! Note that it turns semi-solid at room temperature.

Ghee takes only a few minutes to make, but is now available in many better-stocked grocery stores and in all Indian groceries, if you prefer to purchase it pre-made. It's high in calories and fat, so always use it in moderation. You'll quickly discover that a little ghee goes a long way.

FYI Want to try cooking like a yogi? Probably the best yoga cookbook in English is *Himalayan Mountain Cookery* by Martha Ballentine. It introduces you to the vegetarian cuisine of North India's yogis, thankfully substituting ingredients that are easy to find in virtually any supermarket in America in place of some obscure Indian ingredients.

You might also want to experiment with making paneer at home. This is also a quick recipe. Paneer is more similar to cottage cheese than the harder cheeses you're familiar with, except that it's incredibly tasty.

Only whole milk will do in this recipe. Low-fat milk will yield far less cheese. You will also need a cheesecloth, which you can purchase at most supermarkets. A clean, thin dish towel will do if you can't find cheesecloth.

Paneer

Ingredients: 1 gallon fresh whole milk

2 medium-size lemons

1. Slowly bring the milk to a rolling boil. (If you heat the milk too fast it will burn.) While the milk is heating, juice the two lemons.

2. The moment the milk begins to boil, pour the freshly squeezed lemon juice into it. Remove the milk from the stove immediately.

3. Stir the milk. The lemon juice will make the milk curdle instantly. When no more milk solids separate out from the fluid, the paneer is ready for straining.

4. Pour the curdled milk through the cheesecloth. The cloth will catch the fresh cheese. Use the cloth to squeeze out fluid from the cheese until the paneer reaches the consistency you desire.

Paneer that's still a little soggy can be eaten like cottage cheese or whipped like whipped cream with a touch of honey. You won't believe how good it tastes. If you squeeze all the fluid out, the cheese will become quite thick. You can slice it into cubes and keep it in the refrigerator. Stir it into your subzi, the vegetable dish you'll learn to make in a moment.

The milk fluid out of which the paneer has condensed is called whey in English. Whey was traditionally used to cleanse the urinary system and treat urinary tract infections. But be forewarned: Most people agree it tastes awful! It's least obnoxious tasting while it's still warm.

Now let's make a dahl, a spicy Indian curry that's an important source of protein in a vegetarian diet. There are two processes involved in making a curry. First you cook the beans, then you prepare a masala, a combination of tasty Indian spices, to mix in with the bean dish.

TIME SAVER

If you own a pressure cooker (stainless steel is best), you're ahead of the game because it will save cooking time. In traditional societies, people place heavy stones on top of the lids of their pots to produce a pressure cooker–like effect.

You can substitute virtually any kind of bean, lentil, or hard pea (such as yellow peas) for the mung beans in this recipe. Each creates a completely unique flavor, though harder beans take longer to cook.

Dahl

Ingredients: 1 cup whole mung beans

1 quart water

3 TB. ghee

2 tsp. ground coriander

2 tsp. ground cumin

2 tsp. ground turmeric

1 tsp. salt

1. If you are preparing the dish well in advance, soak the mung beans in water for a few hours or overnight. If you don't have a pressure cooker, soaking the beans will help reduce cooking time. Throw out the water, which now contains compounds from the beans that cause flatulence.

2. Place the mung beans and water in a pressure cooker or covered pot. Cook until the beans are mushy. This will take about 15 minutes in a pressure cooker. You can reduce cooking time by using split mung beans instead of whole mung. However, split mung should not be cooked in a pressure cooker since they will clog the vent.

3. When the beans are almost done cooking, heat the ghee in a frying pan. Add the coriander, cumin, and turmeric, frying them over low heat until they are brown and fragrant.

4. When the beans are done they'll be a little soupy. Pour the spice mixture over the beans and add the salt. Stir.

You now have a classic Indian dahl. Pour the dahl over rice or serve it with another cooked grain or whole grain bread. North Indians eat dahl with a thin, fried bread called chapati.

Subzi is Hindi for any spiced Indian vegetable dish. Just about any fresh vegetables that lend themselves to frying will do, though some (like sliced carrots or fresh green beans) will take longer to fry than others. Adding cubes of paneer to the vegetables just as they're finished cooking will make the dish even more appealing.

Subzi

Ingredients: 3 TB. ghee (see previous recipe)

2 tsp. ground coriander

2 tsp. ground cumin

2 tsp. ground turmeric

1 diced onion

1 cup sliced mushrooms

1 sliced zucchini

1 cup sliced broccoli florets

1 cup cut spinach

¼ tsp. salt

1. Heat the ghee in a large frying pan. Add the coriander, cumin, and turmeric, stirring the spices over low heat until they are brown.

2. Stir in the vegetables. Fry them for a few minutes until they're lightly cooked. If the vegetables get too dry, add a few tablespoons water and cover the pan. Sprinkle the vegetables with salt just before serving them.

You're now ready to enjoy a delicious, well-balanced vegetarian meal. The food you've just prepared is similar to the meals served to the yogis and swamis at ashrams and pilgrimage places throughout India. Yogis value this kind of dinner because it's both appetizing and extremely nutritious, yet it's easy to digest.

CLEANING OUT YOUR BODY

"Cleanliness is next to godliness" is a phrase you sometimes hear in the West. The yoga tradition agrees. If you've ever visited India you may have seen yogis who have smeared their entire bodies with ash. You might think they're about as dirty as anyone can get. In fact the sacred ash is from ritual fires and is completely sterile. It protects them from sunburn and insect bites. Most yogis, however, bathe before Hatha Yoga practice and meditation.

Yogis are not only concerned with external cleanliness but internal cleanliness as well. Optimal health requires a well-tuned digestive and respiratory system that moves waste products out efficiently. Let's look at a few of the methods yogis use to keep the insides of their bodies clean.

NASAL WASH

The nasal wash, called *Jala Neti* in Sanskrit (*jala* is Sanskrit for "water" and *neti* means "cleansing the nose"), is the single most important yogic cleansing technique you can learn. The technique is very simple, takes just a minute, and can make a dramatic difference in the way you feel, particularly if you suffer from respiratory allergies, frequent upper respiratory infections, or sinus problems. Yogis value this technique highly because it clears their nasal passages, making breathing exercises more effective and easier to do. You'll be amazed at how much more freely you can breathe after the nasal wash becomes part of your daily routine.

To do the nasal wash you need three things:

- A neti pot
- Lukewarm water
- Up to a teaspoon or so of salt

You can purchase a porcelain neti pot from the Himalayan Institute by calling 1-800-822-4547 or logging on to www.himalayaninstitute.org. Or check your local yoga center, which may sell nasal wash kits in its bookshop. If you

GO TO ▶
Success with relaxation and meditation techniques depends in part on being able to breathe freely. This can be problematic for people with allergies or who tend to catch colds frequently. Doing the nasal wash will help with this. See Hour 3 for a refresher on the breathing exercises that form the core of yoga practice.

don't have a neti pot, you can use any clean vessel that has a spout that fits comfortably into the entrance of your nostril.

1. Fill the neti pot with lukewarm water. (If you're using another type of vessel, fill it with a cup or so of water.) Add a bit of salt. You'll be able to tell you've found the right amount of salt when the saline solution tastes like tears.

2. Bend over a sink and tilt your head to the left. Insert the spout of the neti pot just inside your right nostril and lift the pot till the water runs in your right nostril and out your left nostril. You may have to adjust the angle of your head to facilitate the flow of water. If you hold your head too far upright, the water will flow in your right nostril, down the back of your nasal cavity, and into your mouth. This is also a good cleaning practice. Simply spit out the water.

3. After you've poured all the water through your nostrils, refill the pot with tepid water and a little salt. Bend over the sink, tilt your head to the right, and insert the spout just barely inside your left nostril. Pour the lightly salted water into your left nostril, allowing it to flow out the right nostril.

4. It's important that you get all the water out of your nasal cavity after the nasal wash. From a standing position, bend forward, allowing your head to dangle nearly upside down. Tilt your head to various angles to allow any extra water to drain out of your sinuses. Because the angles of the passages into the sinuses vary from one person to the next, you'll have to experiment to find which angles work for you.

Add the nasal wash to your morning routine after brushing your teeth. If you have upper respiratory tract problems like hay fever, it's a good idea to do the nasal wash two or three times a day.

Beginning yoga students are sometimes horrified at the prospect of pouring water into their nose. However, the technique is easier and far less unpleasant than you might think, provided you've got the temperature of the water right and have added the proper amount of salt. Remember that your nasal passages are constantly being bathed with mucus, the temperature and salinity of which you're trying to imitate with your solution. If the water in your nose stings or feels uncomfortable, it's either too hot or too cold, or you've dissolved too much or not enough salt into the fluid. It's worth experimenting to get it right.

Yogis also do *Sutra Neti,* which means "string cleaning." In this technique a specially designed, sterilized cotton cord is passed in one nostril and out the other, and in one nostril and out the mouth. This very effectively cleans the nasal passages. Don't try this at home without having first been taught by an experienced teacher!

What you can do, however, is pick up a tongue scraper. These used to only be available at well-stocked yoga centers and Indian grocery shops, but are now widely available in drug stores. Yogis not only clean their nasal passages and teeth, they also lightly scrape their tongues to remove germs and excess mucus. If you check your tongue in the bathroom mirror you may find it's covered with a white or yellowish coating and could definitely use a good cleaning.

Stomach Wash

The Stomach Wash or Upper Wash is called *Gajakarani* in Sanskrit. It cleans out the stomach, esophagus, and bronchial tubes. You'll feel mentally clearer and less lethargic afterward. Do this practice only occasionally, perhaps once a month. This is another technique that you shouldn't try at home without first learning it from an experienced teacher.

PROCEED WITH CAUTION

Don't confuse the Stomach Wash with bulimic practices in which a person vomits after eating. Forcibly induced vomiting following a meal is considered an extremely unhealthy practice in yoga. Bulimia is a serious eating disorder that must be treated by a professional.

1. Start with an empty stomach! The best time to do the Stomach Wash is in the morning, a couple of hours before breakfast.

2. Mix a little salt into two to four quarts of lukewarm water. Smaller individuals may use less water; big males should use more. The mixture should taste like tears.

3. In a squatting position, rapidly drink as much of the water as you can without stopping.

4. Drinking this much salt water this fast will probably make you throw up. If it doesn't, bend over a basin or toilet and insert your fingers into the back of your throat, activating your gag reflex and making yourself vomit.

5. Vomit all the water back out of your system. You may be amazed at how much mucus comes up with the water.

6. Don't eat for a couple hours, though you may take light fluids.

In addition to learning it from an experienced yoga teacher, there are two cautions you need to be aware of if you attempt the Stomach Wash. First, be careful not to vomit so violently that you start to choke. Second, stop immediately if you notice the bitter taste of bile in your mouth.

The biggest hurdle to mastering the yoga washes (there are many more body washes not mentioned here) is psychological. Westerners are often obsessed with the external appearance of their bodies but disgusted by the inner contents of their bodies. However, after a teacher takes you through the process once, it's really surprising how easy the washes turn out to be. Vegetarians usually have an easier time with the Stomach Wash because they don't need to contend with the flavor of partially digested flesh.

Remember that the simplest and best cleansing technique of all is to drink plenty of fresh, clean water throughout the day. This bathes all the cells in your body and keeps your body well hydrated.

Ayurveda: Yoga Therapy

According to legend, the Indian medical tradition (called Ayurveda) was created by yogis. This shouldn't be surprising because in ancient times very few people had a better understanding of the body and mind, and the energy dynamics that run them, than the yogis.

The *Charaka Samhita*, the bible of Ayurveda, relates that in vast antiquity as people's lives grew more and more out of sync with nature, physical and mental ailments became increasingly common. Yoga masters convened to find a solution to the problem. The great adepts sat down together, and collectively went into samadhi, the deepest state of meditation. Connecting with the inner genius that emanates from the Higher Self, they saw into the very root of disease and intuitively understood how to treat it. Returning to ordinary waking consciousness, they taught humanity the new science of Ayurveda, the yogic medical system.

Ayu means "life" or "longevity." *Veda* means "knowledge" or "science." So Ayurveda is "the knowledge of life" or "the science of longevity." It is a brilliant system that has been used for thousands of years to treat every kind of disorder imaginable, often quite successfully.

FYI There has been a surge of interest in traditional yogic medicine in the West in recent years. For more information about Ayurveda, see *Ayurveda: The Science of Self-Healing* by Dr. Vasant Lad; *Prakruti: Your Ayurvedic Constitution* by Dr. Robert Svoboda; and *Yoga for Your Type: An Ayurvedic Approach to Your Asana Practice* by Dr. David Frawley.

WHAT'S YOUR AYURVEDIC TYPE?

Ayurvedic physicians divide people into three fundamental types:

- *Vata* people are nervous, quick, alert, restless, and wear out quickly. They're easily agitated and scattered. Vata is associated with the elements air and ether. Its qualities are dry, cold, rough, lightweight, fast, and insubstantial.

- *Pitta* people are hot-tempered, fiery, and emotional. They are aggressive and have strong appetites. Pitta is associated with the element fire. Qualities connected with it include hot, intense, mobile, and irritable.

- *Kapha* people are stable, slow starters, reliable, and placid. Kapha is associated with both the elements earth and water. Its qualities are cold, heavy, wet, oily, smooth, and dense.

In Western terms, these are basically people with different metabolic rates. Vata or air people have a high metabolism and burn a lot of energy. Kapha or earth people have a low metabolism and move more slowly to conserve energy. Pitta or fire people are somewhere in between, sometimes simmering and other times boiling over.

Air people especially benefit from yoga because it teaches them to sit still and to focus their minds. Fire types benefit because they learn to calm down and get a handle on their feelings. Earth types gain because yoga energizes their body and mind so they can get up and get moving.

Most people are a combination of these elemental types. Some people might have an earth body but an air mind, or fiery digestion but airy hair and skin. Ayurvedic doctors take all these factors into account when they prescribe diets, medications, treatment modalities, or exercises for their patients, knowing that the three different types tend to respond differently to the same stimuli.

If you're familiar with medieval European history, you're aware that until comparatively recently, doctors in the West analyzed patients in a remarkably

GO TO ▶
Refer to Hour 9 for the Ayurvedic perspective on the stomach, small intestine, and colon. When they are not functioning properly, these three organs can be the root of many disease processes. Yoga postures and several of the yoga washes work very specifically with these areas to restore excellent health.

similar way. Fire types were called choleric, earth types phlegmatic, and air types pneumatic. In addition, European doctors recognized a bilious, ill-tempered type.

FINDING BALANCE

The *Charaka Samhita* says that one of the main causes of disease is imbalance. The secret to good health is to stay in balance with nature, with other people, and with yourself. Ayurveda, like yoga, is about finding the point of equilibrium. From ancient times, Ayurvedic doctors were as concerned with mental health as physical well-being because they recognized that many physical ailments originate in our thoughts and attitudes. In the next hour, you'll be introduced to the fascinating subject of yoga psychology.

HOUR'S UP!

QUIZ

Take this short quiz to see how much of the material in Hour 20 you absorbed. Answer true or false to the following statements:

1. While switching to a vegetarian diet is a way to express nonviolence toward animals, meat eating is actually healthier.
2. Yoga teaches that you should keep not only the outside of your body clean, but the inside as well.
3. The nasal wash requires you to pour a soapy solution through your nostrils.
4. The Ayurvedic medical system of India and the yoga tradition are totally unrelated.
5. It's best to do the Stomach Wash immediately after a meal.
6. Ayurveda recognizes three basic constitutional types.
7. Dairy and eggs are not included in the yogic vegetarian diet.
8. Clarified butter is the cooking oil favored by traditional yogis.
9. Ayurveda recognizes the psychological root of some health problems.
10. A yogic diet includes six distinct flavors: salty, sweet, sour, astringent, bitter, and pungent.

HOUR 21
Yoga Psychology

CHAPTER SUMMARY

LESSON PLAN:
In this hour you will learn …

- Yoga sees the mind as a living energy field operating through the physical brain.

- The mind has four major functions: sensory awareness, judgment, memory, and self-identity.

- Traditional yoga psychology accepts the existence of karma and reincarnation.

- Karma directs the flow of your destiny, but you direct your karma.

When you watch a program on television, you know perfectly well that the people you're watching don't actually live inside your television. The events you're watching are being enacted somewhere else and broadcast into your television set. The yoga tradition claims that much the same is true about your brain.

According to yoga psychology, your experience of consciousness is *not* produced by your physical brain. Your brain is just a receiver that registers the broadcasts of your mind, and relays back to the mind information it's picked up from your eyes, ears, and senses of taste, touch, and smell. The mind itself is a living energy field that acts through your brain but also has access to other channels your brain can't pick up. When you tune in to those other channels you have extrasensory or psychic experiences. Advanced yogis claim that, with practice, minds can even travel outside their physical bodies.

Deeper even than the mind field is consciousness itself, the Higher Self that, according to yoga, is immortal. This Inner Self changes bodies at birth and death the way you change your clothes at the beginning and end of the day. The Self doesn't change but carries the experiences, desires, talents, and liabilities of its past incarnations from one life to the next like luggage.

In your meditation practice you will directly experience the different parts of the mind field already explored by millions of meditators before you. You will also gradually get to know your Higher Self, that immortal entity Western religions call the soul or spirit.

UNDERSTAND YOURSELF

Understanding your thinking process, how intuition works, how habits are formed and how they can be broken, and how you create your self-identity is necessary for any genuine self-knowledge. To do this, yoga psychology breaks down the mind into four essential functions:

- **Manas.** The sensory processing part of your mind, the work-a-day part of your awareness that's operating when you're mentally "on automatic"

- **Buddhi.** The higher functions of your mind, your rational and intuitive faculties, your willpower, judgment, and conscience

- **Chitta.** The storehouse of your memories and habit patterns, your subconscious mind

- **Ahankara.** Your sense of self, how you identify what is distinctly you and yours

ANALYZE YOUR MIND

It's extremely important to understand manas, because that's the level of awareness most people experience most of the time. It's your ordinary state of consciousness when you're merely noting what's going on in your environment and responding as usual. The Sanskrit word *manas*, which literally means "the thinking faculty," is related to the English words *man*, *woman*, and *human*. Manas is almost always in motion, continually activating the physical brain. Even when you're not interfacing with the world around you, there is usually a continual stream of mental chatter going on inside your head. Even while you're asleep the fluctuations of your manas produce dreams.

Only in deep sleep and in deep meditation does the manas become still. However, in deep sleep you become unconscious while in meditative absorption you're fully awake. In deep meditation all thought, all sensory input and all motor output (except that necessary to sustain life) come to a halt.

That's why when scientists at the Menninger Foundation checked Swami Rama's brain waves and heart rate during deep meditation, they could barely detect a thing.

The experience of remaining fully conscious when the manas stops acting is truly astonishing. You have never felt more alive, clearer, more balanced, or more at peace. Learning to remain in this state, called turiya, even as you go about your business in the world is what enlightenment is all about.

ANALYZE YOUR INTELLECT

The *buddhi* is the most subtle part of the human mind, and the part yogis say is closest to the Inner Self. Buddhi is sometimes translated "intellect" and other times "intuition," but actually represents a range of higher mental functions. At the lower end of the spectrum it includes your ability to think rationally and to exercise your will to make decisions, whether they're rational or not.

Most of the time the manas responds for you. You see a person who was rude to you in the past and instantly feel dislike and try to avoid that individual. But buddhi gives you the ability to respond in a noninstinctual way. You can make the conscious choice to go out of your way to be nice to that person. Yogis say that the capacity to act out of free will is a function few animals are able to exercise but that all healthy humans can use if they want to. The ability to consciously direct your actions comes from the buddhi.

At its higher end the buddhi grants full-fledged intuition. This is real intuitive power rooted in superconsciousness, as opposed to instinctual responses that come straight out of the circuitry of the physical body.

Working with the intuition is a large part of a yogi's inner work. Genuine intuition operates at three levels of your buddhi:

- *Dhi.* The field of knowledge that flashes in your mind as intuitive insight or a flash of genius following the process of rational thought
- *Pratibha.* The field of knowledge that's instantly accessible to your mind through the simple movement of your will or desire
- *Prajna.* The field of knowledge that continually pours forth into your mind as spiritual wisdom

You might concentrate deeply on a problem for hours without finding a solution. Later, the answer spontaneously occurs to you. Your rational mind had grappled with the problem but your reasoning powers alone were insufficient to identify the correct answer. However, when you finally gave up reasoning and relaxed your mind, the information in your dhi simply presented itself to your conscious awareness. There are many famous examples of researchers who wrestled with scientific questions to no avail. Later, while they were relaxing or even dreaming, the right answer appeared in their minds.

What about pratibha? You may wonder about some topic about which you know very little, and immediately—even though you have no possible access to this knowledge in your ordinary awareness—you simply *know* the information you need. In the case of dhi, you had to reason through the problem first before the answer came to you. With pratibha you just reach out with your mind, and almost effortlessly you catch a glimpse of the answer. It flashes in your mind in a sudden burst of illumination like a meteor flashing across the night sky. Savants are good examples of pratibha. You ask them an impossibly difficult mathematical question and see the solution faster than you can key it into a calculator.

GO TO ▶
Yogis specifically use the Gayatri mantra to purify their minds and gain access to the field of their intuition. Turn back to Hour 16 for more information about this important mantra.

Prajna is an even higher form of intuitive knowledge. You don't have to stop and reason through a problem, or even stop for a moment to ponder it. You simply already know the answer. Someone asks you a question you've never thought about before in your life, yet out of your mouth pops a perfect, deeply insightful reply. You don't *have* knowledge—in a sense you simply *are* the knowledge. Spiritual masters illustrate prajna in their lives. Whatever you ask them, they are able to answer immediately with stunning insight without having to think about it or even without knowing a thing about the subject. In the yoga tradition, continual access to prajna is a commonly recognized symptom of yogic mastery.

ANALYZE YOUR MEMORY

In the West, Sigmund Freud is given a lot of credit for discovering the subconscious mind. However, the subconscious had been recognized and thoroughly explored in yoga psychology thousands of years earlier. In Sanskrit it's called *chitta*.

Chitta is the vast inner storehouse of all your experiences. It's the basement of your mind, filled with both treasures and trash. If you're not a particularly conscious person, it can actually control your life. Here's how.

If you think a thought only once or twice, it will probably disappear into the wastebasket of your memory and never be recalled again. However, if you keep thinking about some experience, fear or desire, or if you have an experience that moves you deeply, this memory trace forms what's called a *vasana* or a "groove" in your chitta—a thought pattern that has constellated in the subconscious. It keeps calling attention to itself because of the emotional charge or mental force it generates. You keep returning to that thought whether you want to or not. As the groove keeps getting deeper the *vasana* becomes a *samskara*, a living force in your subconscious that begins to run your life for you, affecting the way you think and behave. The groove is now a ditch, or even a canyon! This is how habits, phobias, and obsessions become rooted in your personality.

JUST A MINUTE

Meditators quickly become acquainted with the vasanas or thought complexes "stuck" in their mind field. These will continually rise into your awareness as you sit for meditation. Do not mentally engage with these thought forms. Calmly watch them pass by, allowing them to dissolve of their own accord, without feeding them any more energy. According to yoga they're just constellations of energy, which dissipate when not fed with the fuel of your attention.

According to yoga psychology, samskaras can become so powerful that you carry them with you into the after-death state and even into your future lives. Note that many samskaras can be quite positive. If you devote a lot of energy to mastering a musical instrument, for example, according to yoga in your next life that samskara may be so strong that from childhood you'll show an amazing aptitude for music.

Yoga is about awakening and living consciously. One of the reasons advanced yogis spend so much time in meditation is to become fully aware of the thought grooves hidden in the subconscious. They discharge the energy associated with negative grooves by dispassionately watching them arise in their awareness during meditation and calmly releasing them. Then they replace unhealthy thought patterns that may dominate their chitta with the purifying vibrations of their mantra. In this way they bring everything dark in their minds into the light of consciousness, and begin to live freely rather than at the mercy of unconscious compulsions.

ANALYZE YOUR SELF-IDENTITY

The term ahankara is a combination of two Sanskrit words: *aham*, which means "I," and *kara*, which means "make." So ahankara is the "I-maker" or self-identity in humans and animals. Westerners are often surprised to learn that yogis believe that various natural phenomena such as planets, weather patterns, or diseases are fields of intelligence, not just blind, lifeless energies. However, unlike humans, these fields may not have an overriding organizing principle called ahankara that allows them to recognize themselves as conscious entities. To translate this into Western terms, imagine a robot programmed to act like a human. Without ahankara, no matter how realistically the robot simulates human behavior, it wouldn't actually be self-conscious.

Ahankara allows you to identify your fingers and toes, as well as your thoughts, as essentially yours. Extending it outward, you also start to identify certain objects, like a toothbrush or a house, as yours also. Certain forms of mental illness or some head injuries may interfere with the brain's ability to register self-identity. Physicians have reported cases of people who no longer recognized their arms or legs as part of their own bodies. Some psychotics believe the thoughts passing through their minds are not really theirs but belong to some other entity. The damage to the brain prevents the ahankara from manifesting properly. The brain has become like a broken television set, unreceptive to signals from the ahankara.

FYI *From Death to Birth: Understanding Karma and Reincarnation* by Pandit Rajmani Tigunait, Ph.D., offers one of the clearest explanations of the karmic process available in English, and is filled with real-life examples. *Aghora III: The Law of Karma* by Robert E. Svoboda is another excellent introduction to this fascinating topic, drawn from the teachings of the twentieth-century Aghora adept Vimalananda.

Ahankara is sometimes translated "ego," though it should not be confused with egotism. Every human being needs ahankara in order to function in the world and think in a sane fashion. However, yoga ultimately leads you—in a safe and gentle way—beyond the ego. It takes you to a transcendent mind field that unites all individual mind fields in one vast, interconnected whole.

FROM LIFE TO LIFE: REINCARNATION

If there's one thing most people notice in life, it's that there doesn't seem to be any justice in this world. The innocent are often victimized while the guilty commonly get away with their crimes. Yogis claim this apparent lack of justice in the universe is an illusion caused by most people's inability to remember their past lives or foresee their future births. They say memory traces of your activities in past lives are recorded in a part of your subtle body called the *karmashaya*. The karmashaya or "collection of karma" travels with you from life to life. It is the depository of memory traces in the subtle body where your karmic balance sheet is preserved. The subtle forces it emanates ensure that your good actions in past lives lead to good consequences in this life, and that your selfish actions lead to less pleasant results.

Some children remember details from their past lives, but most people forget these by the time they're four or five years old. In deep states of meditation, memories from past lives can come back. If you'd like to try connecting with a past life, try the following exercise.

1. Sit down at a table with a pen and pad of paper in front of you. Focus on the bridge between your nostrils and breathe diaphragmatically for a minute or two. When you feel relaxed and your mind is clear, go on to step 2.

2. Think back to your early childhood. Were there certain talents or interests that you displayed early on? Perhaps your parents were even amazed at certain skills you seemed to display as a child with very little or no training. Jot down a few notes about these interests. These memories are important clues to talents you may have developed in past lives.

3. Are there certain things that frighten you horribly, even though you've never actually had a bad experience with them? These might include deep, irrational fear of insects, the sight of blood, deep water, explosive sounds, contracting a particular disease? Write this down. This material could provide valuable clues about how you may have died in a past life.

4. Are there certain people in your life who from the very first moment you met them, perhaps even before you had spoken to them or knew their names, very powerfully attracted or repelled you? Were there friends you were completely comfortable with from the first moment or other relatives or acquaintances who, despite knowing them for years, you still mistrust? Note down their names. The yoga tradition suggests you probably had dealings with these people in previous incarnations.

Surprisingly, scholarly studies of the history of religions show that belief in reincarnation was a significant part of early Christianity and appeared in the early Jewish tradition as well. By the fifth century, when Christianity had become more politicized, Christian clergy started discouraging belief in reincarnation. This was in spite of the fact that several times in the New Testament, Jesus explicitly says that John the Baptist was the reincarnation of the prophet Elijah.

UNDERSTAND THE KARMIC PROCESS

According to yoga psychology, every time you think, speak, or act, you are producing *karma*. Because the ability to choose your own course sets human beings off from most animals and plants, you are responsible for your actions. If a tiger kills a man, it's not morally responsible because its instincts controlled its behavior. But if a human being kills a man, the killer is accountable. The action was his conscious choice. He has generated karma and nature will hold him liable for his action, according to yoga. Here or in a life to come, humans experience the consequences of their actions.

STRICTLY DEFINED

Karma simply means an action and its effect. It is the law of cause and effect in the moral sphere.

ACTION AND ITS CONSEQUENCES

Yogis catalog four types of karma:

- *Sanchita.* All the karma you have created in all your previous incarnations

- *Prarabdha.* All the karma from past lives that's destined to play out during your current life

- *Kriyamana.* The karma you are creating in your present life through your speech and actions

- *Agama.* The karma you are creating in your present life through your thoughts, plans, and desires

Within the confines of time and space, only a small part of the mass of karma you may have accumulated over many lives can play out in your current incarnation. This prarabdha karma—which shaped the personality you were born with and governs the events that are "destined" to occur in your present life—comes in three strengths, depending on how much energy you put into certain actions, positive or negative, in past births:

- **Mild.** These are karmas that can easily be changed if you make a bit of effort.

- **Medium.** These karmas can be changed only if you make a lot of effort.

- **Fixed.** These karmas are unalterable; you will have to undergo these experiences sometime in this life.

Yogis say only God has the power to alter fixed karma. You may at various times undergo experiences that have a distinctly "fated" quality to them, such as a bad marriage or an incredibly inspiring meeting with a spiritual teacher. It's possible these events *had* to happen as part of your "course curriculum" for this life. In yoga the universe is seen as a vast university in which we are evolving toward greater spiritual awareness. Many of the events in life, even difficult ones like a serious accident or terminal disease, may represent lessons your soul needs to learn or tests it must repeat until it passes.

But you do have the ability to redirect mild and medium-strength karma. For example, if you worked in the medical profession in several previous lives, your family may pressure you to become a doctor in this life. However, if you really want to be an artist or painter instead this time around, you can use the force of kriyamana karma, the karma you're creating now, to reshape your future even if this causes serious conflict with your family.

WATCH WHAT YOU THINK

Bear in mind that not only do people generate karma, but organizations and communities do, too. Don't assume that when something tragic happens to a person, it was that person's karma. Many of the really awful things that happen in life are due to group karma. Sometimes innocent individuals suffer because of the negative karma of the community or nation they belong to.

Karma takes effect wherever one or more people generate conscious intention. Sometimes innocent victims are caught up in a vortex of very painful group karma, such as a war, a crime, or a terrorist act. Another example of collective karma is the rising crime rate that may accompany increasingly horrible images of violence in the entertainment industry. As millions of people focus on violent imagery in movies or computer games, they may unconsciously invoke greater violence in their society through the sheer force of their collective imagination.

This is because yogis believe that people are responsible not only for what they do but for what they think. This is called agama karma. The effects of agama karma are obvious. People who tend to think positive, generous, cheerful thoughts are most often cheerful people who generally attract favorable outcomes to themselves. People whose thoughts tend to be sour, cynical, or malevolent often find events in their lives confirming their worst fears.

One of the best exercises you can do to help purify your own mind field as well as the psychic atmosphere of the world around you is to deliberately

GO TO ▶
The importance of thinking positively and behaving ethically are strongly emphasized in yoga psychology. Hour 22 will explain the role good thoughts and actions play in yoga. Yogis are not self-righteous about their morality, but they do recognize the role ethics plays in purifying the mind and correcting karmic imbalances.

generate positive mental energy, radiating it out to the world as blessing power. This is what the great saints and advanced yogis do continually. You might want to incorporate the following yogic meditation into your daily routine.

1. Sit in your meditation posture with your head, neck, and trunk straight. Close your eyes.

2. Check to ensure that you're breathing diaphragmatically. Then focus on the bridge between your nostrils, breathing slowly, smoothly, and evenly until your breath starts flowing equally in both your nostrils.

3. Remember a scene or event in your life that made you very happy. That memory is connecting you with your anandamaya kosha or innermost level of bliss (which you learned about in Hour 1). Turn your focus from the memory to the feeling of joy within yourself.

4. Vividly imagine the joy you feel emanating outward from your heart chakra to the people you love. Imagine it flowing into their heart chakras. Visualize their faces lighting up as they sense the love and joy pouring out of your soul.

5. Vividly imagine the joy you feel radiating out from you to the people you ordinary dislike. Imagine it flowing into their heart centers. Visualize their faces lighting up as they feel love and joy entering their spirits.

6. Vividly imagine your inner joy emanating outward to all the people in the world. Visualize them sensing their own inner happiness and peace. Imagine that all over the world hostility and distrust are dissolving away. Imagine people everywhere feeling joyous, content, and loving. Imagine even the bitterest enemies recognizing the goodness in each other and embracing each other warmly.

7. Clear your mind of any visual images and simply sit still enjoying the inner sensation of warmth and peace for a moment. Then open your eyes.

Erase Bad Karma

Karma is a completely impartial force. Whether it's "good" or "bad" karma depends on how you feel about it. For example, a person may be born with unalterable karma that in this life they won't have children. For some this is an unbearable tragedy. For others it's a huge relief.

Generally speaking, though, no one wants to be sick, to get in an accident, to be so poor they can't support their families, or to fail in their career. The vast majority of karma is of mild or medium strength, however, which means you can completely avoid some difficult karma headed your way, or at least lessen its effect in your life. Gurus who see the challenging karma coming will often prescribe *upayas*, spiritual practices you can do to alleviate the effects of bad karma.

Here are a few of the numerous upayas recommended in yoga texts.

- **Charitable donations.** Making a generous donation can help repay karmic debts from previous lives. For example, if ill health is a problem, money should be donated to support medical research, hospitals and hospices, and indigent patients. If infertility is the problem, donate to orphanages and child welfare programs. Giving freely of your money, or of your time if you have no financial resources, develops generosity of spirit and helps correct the karmic imbalance causing the difficulty.

- **Hatha Yoga and breathing exercises.** Yoga postures improve and prevent many medical conditions. Breathing exercises are superb for releasing the tension supporting stress-related symptoms.

- **Prayer.** Praying, singing hymns, and reading holy scriptures helps you connect with divine guidance during troubled times. The sense of grace and peace that flows from these spiritual practices can greatly lessen the negative emotional impact of difficult experiences.

- **Meditation and honest self-examination.** Meditation can release the karmic complexes causing problems in your life, while self-analysis can help you understand how in some cases your own attitudes or behavior may be subtly contributing to your difficulties.

JUST A MINUTE

According to the ancient sage Manu, one of the best ways to discharge bad karma involves three steps. First, repent sincerely. Second, take action to correct any problems your mistake may have caused. Third, don't repeat the mistake.

BANISH NEGATIVITY

Difficulties can't always be avoided. Sometimes they're absolutely essential for your growth. There an old Hindu proverb, "He who walks through fire won't fade in the sun." By putting you in touch with your Higher Self, yoga and meditation provide the strength and inner resources you need to deal with the troubles that life sends your way.

According to Patanjali, author of the *Yoga Sutras*, in very deep states of meditation the seeds of karma are "fried" in the heat of self-awareness. Bad karmas can no longer germinate when the full force of consciousness is brought to bear on action and its consequences.

The yogic view is that karma shapes your destiny but you shape your karma. Everyone has the power to reshape their lives when they choose to live consciously. Doing yoga and meditation is good karma—it's positive action with positive effects that will help you move through life with greater self-awareness and understanding.

CALCULATE YOUR KARMA: YOGA ASTROLOGY

Very advanced yoga masters are said to have full knowledge of their past lives. According to legend, when he became enlightened the Buddha remembered numerous previous incarnations, including some in animal form. Most people don't have that advantage.

To help people who can't remember their past lives understand their karma, great sages of antiquity like Parashara, Jaimini, and Bhrigu developed the science of yoga astrology. In the West, astrology is often considered a "flaky" subject and is frowned upon by both scientists and clergy. In India, however, astrology is a respectable profession and is taught at leading universities.

 FYI   For more information about yoga and astrology contact the American College of Vedic Astrology at 1-800-900-6595 or ACVA108@aol.com. Astrology is called *Jyotir Vidya* in the yoga tradition, which means "the science of light."

Yoga astrology uses 12 Sun signs (which are calculated differently from the 12 signs in Western astrology) and 27 Moon signs. Depending on where in the horoscope the seven classical planets (Sun, Moon, Mercury, Venus, Mars, Jupiter, Saturn) were in the sky at the time of a person's birth, a yogic astrologer can determine whether a client will be getting good or bad results in areas such as health, finances, relationships, progeny, career, education, or spiritual practices. Areas in a birth chart where the planets are strong and well configured show good karma from past lives. Areas where the planets are weak or poorly configured reveal bad karma. Carefully calculated planetary cycles are said to show when a certain destined karmic event is most likely to occur.

A sample yoga horoscope.

(SkyClock software)

RASI PLANET POSITIONS		Ramakrishna Paramahansa	MAHA DASA	START DATE
LG 02♒49 Dhanishtha		Feb 18, 1836	♃ Jupiter	02/18/1836 AD
☽ 22♒01 Purva Bhadra		06:22:25 ST TZ:-05:54	♄ Saturn	09/16/1849 AD
☉ 06♒52 Shatabhistak		Kamarpukur, India	☿ Mercury	09/16/1868 AD
☿ 15♒04℞	☊ 02♉36	088E24 22N54	☋ Ketu	09/16/1885 AD
♀ 09♓04	☋ 02♏36		♀ Venus	09/18/1892 AD
♂ 22♑15	♅ 09♒44	Event Chart	☉ Sun	02/17/1912 AD
♃ 14♊05℞	♆ 12♑04	Lahiri Ayanamsa	☽ Moon	09/17/1918 AD
♄ 14♎34℞	♇ 21♓51	21 D 35 M	♂ Mars	09/17/1928 AD
		Harmonic 1	☊ Rahu	09/18/1935 AD

In India almost every Hindu has their horoscope read so they have some idea what their karma from past incarnations is and how to manage their karma in this life. In fact, most children in India are given a name that corresponds to their Moon sign.

Interestingly, K. N. Rao, one of the best-known Indian astrologers of the late twentieth and early twenty-first centuries, made the following remark in a recent interview. "If you are practicing yoga, you don't need to have your horoscope done." He explained that your spiritual practice will help nullify the effect of your bad karma and amplify the effect of your good karma. If you are interested in reshaping your karma to create as positive a future as possible, then by doing yoga and sitting for meditation, you're already on the right track.

GET OFF THE KARMIC WHEEL

Ultimately, the point of spiritual practice is not to stop creating bad karma and only create good karma. The final goal is not to be subject to karma at all. *Moksha*, the ultimate goal of yoga practice, literally means "freedom from karma." A *jivanmukta* is a completely conscious person, a liberated master who has achieved moksha. (*Mukta* means "free," and *jiva* means "soul.") This person acts totally freely because he or she is not driven by compulsions, complexes, and needs hidden in the subconscious mind. Through the process of meditation, this person has made the entire contents of their mind, including the memories hidden in the chitta, transparent to consciousness. They know themselves completely and act as they choose to act, rather than simply reacting to the circumstances of life, as most people do.

When a person has illuminated his or her entire mind through the practice of yoga, and moved into an unshakable center of tranquility, then the light of the Higher Self can shine through unimpeded. According to the tradition, the focus of identity has shifted from the lower personality into the immortal inner awareness that is not subject to karma. This is what the yoga tradition means when it speaks of jivanmuktas or liberated masters.

HOUR'S UP!

Test your comprehension of the information in this hour with this quiz. Answer true or false to the following statements:

1. According to yoga, consciousness is a biochemical process generated by the brain.

2. Yoga assigned four functions to the mind: memory, ego, intellect, and sensory awareness.

3. Thought waves are stilled in deep sleep and very deep states of meditation.

4. Meditation helps activate the part of the mind that grasps knowledge intuitively.

5. Sigmund Freud was the first person in world history to understand that humans have a subconscious mind.

6. Meditation releases the emotional charge associated with thought complexes stored in the memory.

7. According to yoga, all events in your life are predestined and you can't change that.

8. Feeling strongly attracted to or repelled by a person you've just met may mean you knew that person in a past life, according to yoga psychology.

9. Actions produce karma but thoughts on which you don't take action do not produce karmic effects.

10. Astrology is considered a legitimate part of the yoga tradition.

HOUR 22
Yoga Ethics

CHAPTER SUMMARY

LESSON PLAN:
In this hour you will learn ...

- The four basic goals of life are meaningful work, prosperity, enjoyment, and enlightenment.

- The *Yoga Sutras* lists 10 commitments that every serious yoga student is asked to make.

- Gurus are highly venerated in the yoga tradition, but the human side of the guru needs to be recognized, too.

- Living consciously in the present moment is the key to successful yoga practice.

Yoga is not only a collection of physical postures or a set of meditation exercises. Practiced fully, it's an inner attitude and an outer way of life. Yoga teaches you to travel through life consciously, fearlessly, and respectfully.

Centuries before the dawn of the Christian era, the great yogic adept Patanjali drew up a code of life that included 10 commitments that traditional yoga teachers expected every sincere student to make. These commitments affect every department of your life, challenging you to direct all your actions, all your words, and even all your thoughts to becoming the very best you can be.

THE TEN COMMITMENTS

The high ethical standards Patanjali sets for you are called *dharma* in Sanskrit. To live according to dharma means to do the right thing for its own sake. It is to live in harmony with the laws of nature, and to give expression to spirit in the most elegant manner possible. It calls you to moral action and to purposeful work not only for your own benefit, but for the good of all beings.

Dharma is the first of the four goals of life sanctified by the yoga tradition. These goals are as follows:

- **Dharma.** To live meaningfully, virtuously, and respectfully

- **Artha.** To acquire enough money and worldly goods so that you and your family can live comfortably

- **Kama.** To enjoy the pleasures life has to offer

- **Moksha.** Be become enlightened here and now

Westerners think of yogis as ascetics living in caves, but the vast majority are householders living normal family lives. They deal with financial and sexual issues just like everyone else. However, artha, which means wealth, and kama, which means sensual pleasure, are always seen within the context of dharma and moksha in the yogic lifestyle. That means the acquisition of material goods and the acting out of sensual desires are always done in the moral, mutually respectful way defined by dharma. Yoga students are asked to avoid earning money in a manner that causes harm to others (such as drug dealing). They are also asked to treat sensual pleasures such as sexuality with respect, in a way that honors others rather than exploiting them.

Moksha literally means freedom, and refers specifically to spiritual liberation. Money and sexual relationships are not viewed as ultimate values, but are seen as adjunct parts of your life as you evolve toward the final goal of enlightenment.

Patanjali's 10 commitments are seen within this fourfold framework except by monks and renunciates, who choose to bypass marriage and material prosperity and devote themselves full-time to the pursuit of spiritual liberation.

GO TO ▶
The 10 commitments of Patanjali are the foundation of Raja Yoga or "the royal path of yoga." They are described in Chapter 2, verses 29 through 45 of his *Yoga Sutras.* You'll learn more about Raja Yoga in Hour 23.

YOGA'S DO'S AND DON'TS

Patanjali's code is divided into two equal halves. The first five rules are called yamas, which regulate what a yogi should avoid doing. The second five rules are called *niyamas*, and define what a yogi should definitely be doing.

These are the 10 ethical precepts that are central to yoga practice:

- *Ahimsa.* Don't harm anyone.
- *Satya.* Don't lie.
- *Asteya.* Don't steal.
- *Brahmacharya.* Don't overindulge.
- *Aparigraha.* Don't be greedy.
- *Saucha.* Keep clean.
- *Santosha.* Stay content.
- *Tapas.* Be self-disciplined.
- *Svadhyaya.* Study yourself.
- *Ishvara Pranidhana.* Surrender to a Higher Force.

Let's look at each precept more closely.

Don't Harm Anyone

The first of the 10 commitments is ahimsa, nonviolence. This means never hurting others or oneself.

This is a huge commitment that asks students to overhaul their whole way of thinking. It requires you to consider carefully whether your words and actions, even your thoughts, are causing damage. Malicious gossip, for example, might be a pleasurable indulgence, but it's a form of violence. Needlessly using products that contribute to the destruction of the environment is another often-overlooked way of causing damage.

Patanjali says that when nonviolence truly becomes part of your nature to the extent that ill will toward others no longer exists in your psychic makeup, then no violent act can occur in your presence. Even wild animals will become tame near you. Your perfect inner peace creates an aura around you that draws other creatures into your tranquil state.

PROCEED WITH CAUTION

The yoga tradition teaches nonviolence but recognizes your need to protect yourself in dangerous situations. In ancient times, yogis relied on the warrior caste to keep their neighborhoods safe so they could perform their spiritual practices unmolested. Advanced yogis were said to become so psychically powerful that no violence could occur in their presence.

Don't Lie

Patanjali emphasized the need for satya or truthfulness in your speech and all your dealings. Yogis in ancient times took this precept so seriously that they would literally rather die than tell an untruth. However, nonlying comes second after nonharming, which Patanjali's followers took to mean that although speech should always be honest, it should not be callous or hurtful.

The classic *Yoga Sutras* associates a special psychic power with yogis who never deviate from truthfulness. It is said that whatever these yogis utter, however unlikely it may sound, will come true. At first your speech always conforms to reality. Ultimately, however, reality conforms to your speech. You gain the power to alter reality through the power of your unbroken connection with truth. In India to this day people go to advanced yogis hoping the adept will heal their diseases or grant them prosperity simply by uttering a blessing. It's believed that the words of a truly great master *must* come true.

Don't Steal

Asteya, taking what rightfully belongs to others or hoarding more than you need, especially if someone else could really use it, has always been considered wrong in the yoga tradition.

It's said that if a person masters this precept, going through life without ever stealing, then wealth will automatically find its way to him or her. In India you can actually watch this occur. Some of India's saints and yogis own next to nothing. They ask for nothing and would never dream of taking anything from anyone else. Instead, they constantly look for ways they can offer whatever they do have to others. Though they don't try to acquire anything, lavish gifts and enormous donations are continually showered on them. In most cases the yogi redirects these goods toward humanitarian projects.

Don't Overindulge

Brahmacharya literally means "walking in God consciousness." The implication is that you make spiritual life, not sensual overindulgence, your top priority. Brahmacharya is often translated "celibacy," although in the yoga tradition a couple in a committed relationship is considered to be practicing brahmacharya because they are disciplining their sex drive through their faithfulness to each other.

Brahmacharya doesn't refer exclusively to sex, however. Sensual overindulgence of any kind, as per the Ayurvedic medical tradition, can lead to ill health. A balanced or moderate lifestyle is preferred in yoga. Having a sweet after dinner would not be considered bad; in fact, you'll often find trays full of sweets served at ashrams. But yogis feel that helping yourself to one dessert after another reveals a mind that is out of balance.

Patanjali says that when you lead a life free from overindulgence, you gain immense power to influence others. Perhaps this is because resisting temptation requires a lot of self-awareness and willpower. Anyone with these traits strongly established in their personality will begin to develop some charisma. People usually believe that a person who has control over his own nature can be trusted to manage others.

FYI *The Divine Romance* by the late Paramahansa Yogananda is filled with practical advice for facing the everyday dilemmas of life in a yogic manner. Yogananda was one of the greatest yoga masters of the twentieth century. He was one of the first yogis to settle in America. The organization he founded, Self Realization Fellowship, is based in Los Angeles and still has a large membership today.

Don't Be Greedy

Greed is the mainstay of the national economies of the entire Western world. These cultures are geared toward fostering more and more desires. Things that were considered luxuries only a few years ago, like a telephone answering machine or a computer, seem like necessities now. There is always something else people are encouraged to go out and buy.

Aparigraha, or greed, is considered a serious problem in yoga. Continual craving prevents peace of mind. It also keeps you so busy earning money to pay for your new purchases that there's less time for inexpensive pastimes like meditation!

Curiously, Patanjali says that if you stop running after things and can even stop accepting gifts, then you'll acquire the ability to know your past and future lives. This may be because the nongreedy mind can finally become still, allowing the light of higher awareness to shine through with all the knowledge it contains of the past and future.

FYI Pandit Rajmani Tigunait is a columnist for *Yoga International* magazine. In *Inner Quest: The Path of Spiritual Unfoldment* he answers more than 100 questions sent in by readers about a range of topics yoga students often wonder about. His sound advice helps new students take their first steps on the inner path, and helps more advanced students expand and invigorate their spiritual practices.

Keep Clean

The first of the five niyamas or yogic observances is saucha or cleanliness. Advanced yoga students strive for three levels of purity:

- **Cleanliness of the body, inside and out.** Bathing keeps the outside of the body clean. Regular elimination and the body washes you learned about in Hour 20 keep the inside of the body clean.

- **Cleanliness of the emotions.** This means purifying the mental field of hatred, anger, and jealousy. Hatred and envy block the emotional nature, while anger makes it erupt in an unhealthy way. Positive emotions like joy and compassion keep emotional energy light and flowing. The mind remains cheerful and relaxed.

- **Cleanliness of the intellect.** This means thinking in a constructive way rather than dwelling on thoughts that are selfish, delusional, or destructive. A positive frame of mind facilitates meditation. A negative mental state only creates more internal garbage that has to be cleaned out during the meditative process.

Patanjali says that as you become increasingly purified, you become less overly attached to your body. This makes the flight into spirit during meditation easier and quicker. He also promises an abiding sense of happiness, the ability to concentrate, and an increased aptitude for self-realization.

STAY CONTENT

In yoga, santosha or contentment is considered the greatest form of wealth. Although conditions in India are changing rapidly today, you can still find communities where people don't realize that because they own very little, according to modern thought they're not supposed to be happy.

Yoga encourages contentment but discourages complacency. It's good to be happy with what you have, but not good to be smug, lazy, or self-satisfied. In yoga you are continually working on self-development, growing in spirit even as you're letting go of frivolous desires that only make you anxious and avaricious.

The result of practicing contentment, according to Patanjali's *Yoga Sutras*, is "unsurpassed happiness."

BE SELF-DISCIPLINED

Discipline is a word a lot of Westerners don't like to hear, yet very few people get anywhere without it. Athletes need discipline to win competitions, politicians need discipline to win elections, business people need discipline to run their businesses effectively. In yoga also, there's no achievement of excellent physical and mental health without some tapas or self-discipline. This doesn't mean you completely ignore your desires. It does mean you control your desires; your desires don't control you.

Practicing self-discipline, even a little austerity, grants "perfection of the body" according to Patanjali. Abiding health and a mind and senses that stay sharp into old age are the outcome of this practice, he says.

JUST A MINUTE

Some advanced yogis practice very rigorous forms of self-discipline. These are not appropriate for beginning level students. Go easy on yourself but don't stop challenging yourself. If you're new to yoga, just adding a hatha routine to your schedule four or five times a week may be as much additional discipline as you need right now!

STUDY YOURSELF

Svadhyaya or self-study is another important component of a yogic lifestyle. It entails honest examination of your mind and emotions, as well as awareness of your physical condition and energy state. If you buy a fancy new car, you need to understand how to operate it and get a feel for how it rides. Likewise, your body and mind are your vehicles, according to yoga. Watching what kinds of foods make you feel clearer and more energetic, and which foods make you irritable or lethargic, helps you operate your body more effectively, for example.

Reading books about yoga and other spiritually inspirational texts is part of self-study because they can help point you toward greater self-awareness. Mantra meditation is also an important component of svadhyaya, says Patanjali, because it leads to dispassionate examination of the contents of your mind and helps free you from mental and emotional complexes.

The *Yoga Sutras* state that through self-study you will gain communion with your Higher Self. Its guidance, healing power, and creative energy will become readily accessible to you once you truly know yourself.

SURRENDER TO A HIGHER FORCE

Most people know about surrender. They surrender to their television sets, to a good novel, to a great meal, to a lively conversation. Patanjali advises to once in a while surrender your attention to the Higher Self within you. Ishvara pranidhana can also be translated "surrender to God."

Patanjali uses the word *surrender* because you have to release the concerns and preoccupations, interests and desires of your lower mind in order to connect fully with the higher part of yourself. The more you surrender to your innermost being, the more its power and radiant peace can become part of your daily consciousness.

The *Yoga Sutras* say that perfect self-surrender leads to samadhi, the deepest states of consciousness in which you connect with a part of yourself that transcends time and space, that even—according to yoga—transcends death.

These 10 commitments are the guidelines to a yogic lifestyle, whether you're a recluse living in a Himalayan cave or a busy executive living in New York or Chicago.

GO TO ▶

Hour 17 lists obstacles that meditators often encounter when they first begin a spiritual practice. These issues were raised by Patanjali, author of the *Yoga Sutras,* who also codified the 10 commitments presented in this hour. In Hour 17, you'll find advice on such concerns as laziness, poor health, and self-delusion, explaining how these obstacles can be overcome.

TAKE STOCK OF THE DAY

Many yoga teachers recommend that before you go to sleep each night, you take stock of the day in a candid self-review.

1. Before bed at the end of the day, sit up straight and close your eyes. Breathe diaphragmatically.

2. Quickly review the events of the day. Were there times when you lost your center, getting caught up in negative reactions or behavior? Don't judge yourself! Simply dispassionately note areas in your day where they may have been room for improvement. Don't mull over grievances or failures. Just note them and pass on to the next event of the day.

3. Were there things you did, said, or thought today that reveal an improvement in your attitude or behavior over previous days? Don't congratulate yourself! Just honestly note what happened and pass on to the next event of the day.

4. Quickly note your plans for tomorrow. What can you do tomorrow as well or even better than you did today? Don't worry or spend time planning events in detail. Just quickly decide how you can best put your commitment to yoga to work tomorrow.

5. Now release all thoughts of the past and future. Shift your awareness into the present moment. Bring your full awareness to the bridge between your nostrils or to your heart center, and breathe diaphragmatically for a moment or two. Open your eyes.

JUST A MINUTE

You have enough problems in life without further burdening yourself with guilt. If you do the self-review exercise at the end of the day, merely note areas where perhaps you could have done better. Don't scold yourself! This is an exercise to help increase your awareness of your behavioral and emotional patterns. It should lead to greater clarity, not shame!

THE GURU-DISCIPLE RELATIONSHIP

Traditionally, yoga students always worked with a guru, someone far more experienced on the yoga path who could teach them how to do yoga exercises and meditation properly, formally initiate them in a mantra, guide them around the obstacles they may encounter in their practice, and ultimately lead them to vastly expanded self-awareness.

In the ageless tradition of yoga, the guru is honored because he or she has achieved genuine spiritual greatness through the self-mastery that comes from years of concerted yoga practice. The guru has the wisdom born of personal experience to introduce you to your Higher Self. This makes the guru more valuable and venerable than a king.

There is no comparable status in Western culture where a mentor takes so such responsibility for a student's spiritual development, or where a student surrenders so completely to a teacher. Western students' confusion about the guru-disciple relationship has led to misunderstandings, scandals, lawsuits, and disillusionment in recent decades.

PROCEED WITH CAUTION

Not everyone who claims to be God-realized or an enlightened master is what he or she pretends to be. Most truly enlightened saints don't make any such claims at all! Be very cautious in selecting a guru. Real gurus won't try to manipulate you or extort money from you. Genuine saints live to serve, not to be served.

RECOGNIZE THE GURU

The yoga tradition distinguishes between the guru and guru shakti. Shakti means energy, specifically the living energy directed by a conscious will. The guru is just a human being but guru shakti, or the enlightening energy of the guru tradition, was generated in antiquity and has been transmitted across time to the present generation of spiritual aspirants by illumined, self-sacrificing individuals called gurus. The human guru can transmit guru shakti in an initiation called *shaktipat*, which literally means "the descent of grace." It refers to the transmission of the energy of enlightenment from teacher to disciple.

But the human guru is not the guru shakti itself. In fact, if the guru falls off the path he or she can lose the ability to transport students into higher states of consciousness. When people honor the guru, they're really expressing their reverence for the grace that pours through their teacher. True gurus are often extraordinarily humble people, because they feel a tremendous sense of responsibility and humility in the face of the guru shakti their spiritual lineage has empowered them to transmit.

The human guru deserves your respect, but you should not lose sight of the fact that the guru is, after all, human, and may still be subject to some of the same foibles that ordinary folk are.

THE LEVELS OF ENLIGHTENMENT

According to the tradition, there are three levels of enlightenment. The experience of enlightenment is the same in all three, but the person's capacity to remain continually in that state differs.

The first and by far most common level is the yogi who has not yet learned to stabilize his attention in the superconscious state. He moves in and out of that state like a child learning to ride a bicycle, who loses and then regains his balance. Many very great gurus are at this level. They are really enlightened, but not all the time.

The second level, which is commonly seen in the East but rarely witnessed in the West, is the yogi who is totally established in the superconscious state, to the extent that she has to a large extent lost contact with the physical world. She remains in states of extraordinary bliss most of the time, and might even have difficulty leaving meditation to relate to other human beings on the physical plane. This person is not crazy, though she may appear catatonic or disoriented to the uninitiated. Really crazy people are often frightened and make others feel uncomfortable. Saints at this level of consciousness may not be functioning normally, but everyone who enters their presence feels an extraordinary sense of peace and joy.

The third and rarest level of all is the sat guru or true master who is fully established in the superconscious state, yet fully capable of continuing to speak and act in the external world. These exceptional souls have conquered both the inner and outer worlds.

Fully realized masters are rare. Most spiritual teachers can be in a very high state while lecturing or counseling, but then slip out of that state when they go about their own affairs. Remember the guru is human. Take advantage of the guru shakti that pours through him while he is in the superconscious state, but don't be thrown off when you see him return to his ordinary level of awareness. Chances are this person is only a first-level master.

CRAZY WISDOM

One of the most abused concepts in the Western world of yoga is "crazy wisdom." Students hear inspiring stories about great disciples like the Tibetan yogi Milarepa who was severely tested by his guru Marpa. Marpa forced Milarepa to do countless hours of agonizing physical labor building stone towers, and then commanded him to tear the towers down again. At the time Milarepa didn't understand why his teacher was so cruel, but Marpa saw that his student would never progress spiritually till he atoned for several murders he had committed earlier in life, and used the ego-grinding experience of hard labor in the guru's service to help Milarepa burn away vast amounts of terrible karma.

Some yoga students understand tales like these to mean they must obey whatever the guru commands, whether it seems right to them or not. And some would-be gurus take these stories as permission to freely abuse their students.

Don't be naive. The greatest teacher is the teacher within. If your spiritual mentor tells you to do something you feel is wrong, trust your conscience. A sat guru or true guru will respect you for it.

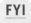 **FYI** *The Play of Consciousness* by the Siddha Yoga master Swami Muktananda describes his experiences in India with a number of avadhuts or crazy-seeming yogis, who were in fact highly advanced masters. These great adepts were at the second and third stages of spiritual realization described in this hour.

TEST THE TEACHER

If you have found a spiritual mentor whom you think may be your guru, examine that person's words and actions very carefully. Ask yourself the following questions:

- Does this teacher seem more interested in serving others or in being served?

- Does this teacher charge exorbitant amounts of money for her teaching, beyond what she needs to take care of her basic needs and support genuine charitable projects?

- Does this teacher behave in a principled, ethical manner, as outlined by Patanjali in his list of 10 commitments, or does he manipulate students for his own gain?

- When you are in the presence of this teacher, do you feel tranquil and centered, or anxious and on edge?

A genuine teacher will test your spiritual mettle, but before you allow him to do that, test him first. You need to determine two things. Is this teacher authentically enlightened? And even if she is, is she the right teacher for you?

Be advised that in a very few Indian lineages such as some Pashupati Shaivites, yogis are actually instructed by their gurus to behave in bizarre, hostile, or sexual ways during part of their spiritual training. But if any would-be yoga teacher approaches you in these ways, you are generally well advised to be on your guard.

Maybe you're attracted to yoga philosophy or you've met a guru who inspires you, but hatha postures and meditation just don't appeal to you. You can still practice yoga! The yoga tradition is extremely broad and includes practices for every personality type imaginable. In the next hour, you'll be introduced to whole new sets of yoga techniques designed to expand your awareness and enhance your life. Whether you're interested in hatha and meditation or not, you're likely to find a form of yoga that works for you.

HOUR'S UP!

Take this quiz to help you review the contents of Hour 22. Answer true or false to the following statements:

1. In the *Yoga Sutras*, Patanjali offers yoga students a code of 10 commitments to guide their actions.

2. Not causing harm is the first commitment a yoga student is asked to make.

3. Making money and having fun are not considered worthy pursuits for students on the path of yoga.

4. Yogic purity includes cleanliness of the body but also of the mind.

5. Yogis do not believe in the presence of a higher spiritual power.

6. The *Yoga Sutras* teach that the words of a person who never lies have special power.

7. Everyone who achieves enlightenment remains in the enlightened state forever after.

8. If your meditation teacher tries to take advantage of you, you should always accept this as valuable crazy wisdom training.

9. Mantra meditation is a valuable adjunct to yogic self-study.

10. Evaluating your thoughts and actions for the previous 24 hours is a good way to increase your self-awareness.

QUIZ

HOUR 23

Types of Yoga

CHAPTER SUMMARY

LESSON PLAN:

In this hour you will learn …

- Raja Yoga is the eightfold path of yoga defined by Patanjali in his *Yoga Sutras*.
- Karma Yoga is the path of active service.
- Bhakti Yoga involves loving devotion to a higher power.
- Jnana Yoga is the path of spiritual discernment.

The yoga tradition is both ancient and vast. It includes hundreds of thousands of techniques directed toward achieving physical and mental health, longevity, and enlightenment. There are numerous different branches of yoga, designed to accommodate every personality type imaginable. Yoga is an all-encompassing methodology that has something to offer everyone.

While yoga philosophy and psychology are fascinating topics, the living essence of yoga is *sadhana*, or spiritual practice. You can read a dozen books about swimming pools, swimming styles, and champion swimmers, but until you get in the water you don't really know much about swimming. It's the same with yoga. A university professor may have studied hundreds of Sanskrit yoga texts, but until she's actually tried the practices herself she doesn't really understand what yoga is about.

RAJA YOGA

Raja Yoga is by far the best-known type of yoga in the West. *Raja* means "king" in Sanskrit, so Raja Yoga is often called "the Royal Path." This is the system taught by Patanjali in the *Yoga Sutras*. It has eight components so you'll sometimes hear it called *Ashtanga Yoga*, which means "the branch of yoga with eight limbs." The first four limbs deal primarily with your body and behavior, the things of the physical world. The second four deal with your inner reality. The eight limbs are as follows:

- **Yama.** These are the first five of the ethical precepts you learned in Hour 22, the "don'ts" of yoga. Don't cause harm, lie, steal, over-indulge, or insist on having more than you need.

- **Niyama.** These are the second five of the ethical principles described in Hour 22, the "do's" of yoga. Be clean, content, self-disciplined, self-aware, and surrendered.

- **Asana.** These are the famous Hatha Yoga postures. Patanjali especially meant the meditation postures you learned in Hour 14. He defined an asana as a posture in which you can sit up straight steadily and comfortably for the length of your meditation practice.

- **Pranayama.** These are yogic breathing exercises. You learned some of the most important of these in Hour 4. They include diaphragmatic breathing, alternate nostril breathing, and so on.

- **Pratyahara.** This means turning your attention away from the outside world and focusing inward on your own awareness and its contents. The 61 Points exercise from Hour 3 is an excellent beginning-level sense withdrawal practice. It redirects your sensory apparatus to your inner world.

- **Dharana.** This is yogic contemplation, as you learned in Hour 15. You zero in on one topic, thinking of only one thing.

- **Dhyana.** This means yogic meditation. Now you hold only one image, sound, or feeling continuously in your mind.

- **Samadhi.** This is the deepest state of meditation, in which your mental focus remains absolutely one-pointed and unbroken. You and the object you're focusing on seem to merge into a seamless unity.

STRICTLY DEFINED

Ashtanga Yoga is the eightfold path described in the *Yoga Sutras*. *Ashta* means "eight," and *anga* means "limb."

Patanjali's school of yoga is wonderfully systematic and highly scientific. Its techniques have been tested and re-tested by advanced practitioners from many different cultures over thousands of years. It requires concentration and self-discipline, but is amazingly effective and mind-expanding when practiced diligently.

KARMA YOGA

Raja Yoga requires you to sit still and focus your mind. But some people just can't sit still! They're too dynamic; it's their nature to always be doing something. Trying to meditate bores or frustrates them. The outer world is the only reality they relate to. Diving into higher states of consciousness is too abstract and intangible a process for them.

Karma Yoga or the path of action is more appropriate for these types of individuals. (You might recall from Hour 21 that karma means "action and its consequences.") In Karma Yoga, the yogi performs all his actions without expecting any reward. Every act is directed solely toward experiencing a higher reality. Most people tie themselves up in knots doing things to get something back. But yogis perform all their acts simply as worship of God. They're not concerned with what the outcome of their activities may be, or whether they benefit personally.

Karma Yoga teachers advise that you should always fulfill your duties and obligations to the best of your ability. But don't be anxious about the future. Don't bind yourself with expectations about what's supposed to happen as a result of your deeds. Surrender every act and its consequences to God. Then you'll be free from worry and free also from the bondage of karma.

Remember, it is willful intention that creates karma. Most animals and young children don't generate karma because they're acting instinctually. Nature is responsible for their behavior. But when you consciously choose to perform an action, you are responsible for the results. Whenever you perform an action, repercussions from it return to you sooner or later, positive or negative.

However, when you sincerely perform your actions as service to a higher power, two things automatically happen. First, your words and deeds will be noble because only good actions are worthy offerings. Second, when you hand these actions over to God, the karmic results go with them. For the karma yogi, all actions become *seva* or selfless service to God and the world.

GO TO ▶
Go back to Hour 21 to review the mechanics of the karmic process. Karma Yoga frees you from bondage to *kriyamana karma* or the consequences of actions you're performing now. Deep states of meditation are still necessary to free you from *sanchita karma*, or the mass of karma you accumulated during previous lives.

WORK WITHOUT WORRY

Approaching all your activities as Karma Yoga has a profound effect on the way you experience life. Try the following experiment.

1. Choose one workweek in the near future as your "Karma Yoga Week."
2. When you go to work, perform your job to the best of your ability, as if it were your gift to God himself.

3. Don't worry about whether anyone else appreciates your work. Don't be concerned if anyone else criticizes it, either. Simply do your job as selfless service to the higher power that placed you on this planet.

4. Accept any results that accrue to you, whether that's praise or blame from your boss, good or bad relations with your fellow employees, public success or lack of recognition, and even your paycheck, as the grace of God, all provided for your benefit.

5. At the end of the week, look back and see if living without expecting a reward didn't make your life far less stressful.

You simply did your work as well as you possibly could, and relaxed and left the consequences to God. The work was still there but the emotional burden connected with it was gone. The emotional ups and downs that come with worrying about other people's reactions or about your own worth or about what the future holds just don't occur.

A tremendous sense of freedom comes with letting go. Karma yogis feel they are responsible for doing the best they can in the moment, but the future is God's responsibility.

 Which of the different types of yoga is most appropriate for you? *Choosing a Path* by Swami Rama helps you find the brand of yoga that best suits your inclinations and talents. You may also find four short books by Swami Vivekananda especially helpful: *Raja Yoga*, *Jnana Yoga*, *Karma Yoga*, and *Bhakti Yoga*. Vivekananda was the first yogi to teach in America.

SERVE SELFLESSLY

Students often hear the word *seva* at their yoga centers or ashrams. Seva or selfless service lies at the root of yoga. Until very recently in Eastern cultures, students would work for their gurus free for years on end out of love and respect. To this day many of the leading yogis of India sponsor enormous humanitarian projects. Feeding, clothing, and housing pilgrims and the poor is still common at many ashrams. Yoga centers in India fund and staff free medical camps, hospitals, orphanages, and schools.

Whether or not there's any payment involved is not an issue for the yoga students who spend part of their lives working in these institutions. Many students report that even if they're completely penniless, in the most miraculous ways life arranges to provide for all their needs while they do their charitable work.

It's easy to think of meditation as a mind-expanding exercise. But freely serving others also helps to expand the perimeter of your self-identity and unfold your inner potentials. Helping others is yoga in action.

PROCEED WITH CAUTION

Working selflessly does not mean opening yourself to economic exploitation, ignoring your family's financial needs, or becoming a doormat. Whether or not she's being paid, the karma yogi surrenders her work as an offering to the higher power within herself. This disconnects her from the cycle of karma while solidifying her connection with her own inner power.

BHAKTI YOGA

Some people are innately oriented to inner life. Raja Yoga is ideal for them. Others are action-oriented. Karma Yoga was meant for them. But there's another personality type the yoga tradition also accommodates. Some people are predominantly emotional. It's hard for them to get excited about any sort of activity, whether it's meditation or selfless service, unless their feelings are fully engaged. Bhakti Yoga is specially designed for these students.

Bhakti means "loving devotion." Traditionally, bhakti was directed at God or the Goddess, or the guru. Most yoga centers in the West downplay this aspect of the yoga tradition out of respect for Western religious sensibilities. Almost every yoga teacher you'll meet is careful to avoid imposing Eastern religious norms on his or her Western students. Some people in the West don't believe in God or are uncomfortable with the image of a Goddess. Nevertheless, in its original cultural setting, devotion to a higher power has always been an important part of yogic practice. Bhakti Yoga works within the context of all religions, whatever your conception of the higher power may be.

FYI The nineteenth-century Bengali saint Ramakrishna Paramahansa is a premier example of a bhakti yogi. *The Gospel of Sri Ramakrishna* by his disciple Mahendranath Gupta is one of the greatest spiritual classics of all time. It records what it was actually like to sit in the presence of this love-intoxicated master.

EMPOWER YOUR PRACTICE

To begin a program of Hatha Yoga and meditation is like putting up sails on the boat of your spiritual life. But love is like a strong wind that fills the sails and sends the boat racing across the sea. Bhakti Yoga is designed to work with the energizing power of positive emotions.

In the yoga tradition the Supreme Being, called *Ishvara*, is conceived as a limitless immaterial consciousness from which grace and inspiration flow. It doesn't have a body, form, or gender. Nevertheless, for the sake of devotional practice, the Supreme Being is pictured in some shape. In India this could be a pillar of white light, an oval shaped stone, the divine incarnation Krishna, the fierce but loving goddess Kali, the elephant-headed deity Ganesh, or any of thousands of other images. In the West it could take the form of Jesus Christ, his mother Mary, or an aged white male with a white beard in a white robe. The yoga tradition accepts all of these as valid images of the Divine Being, provided that students keep in mind these are just images, but that the actual reality they point to lies beyond the reach of the human imagination.

In yoga, the form in which you visualize the Supreme Being is called your *Ishta Devata* or "personal God." Bhakti yogis place more emphasis on worship than on formal meditation. They strive to develop and deepen their relationship with their Ishta Devata rather than struggling with challenging yogic techniques. They feel this makes spiritual life a pleasure, rather than a chore.

Bhakti Yoga texts recommend a number of techniques for worship. If soul-stirring emotion comes easily to you and you feel particularly close to God, the Goddess, or a saint or divine incarnation like Jesus or Krishna, you might enjoy the following techniques recommended in the bhakti tradition.

- Pray, whether spontaneously from the heart or formally with prayers you've memorized such as the Lord's Prayer.
- Sing hymns to your personal God.
- Prostrate before an image of your deity.
- Perform rituals honoring the deity.
- Read inspiring stories about your deity.
- Constantly repeat the mantra or an affirmation associated with your deity.

In early Christianity, Jesus' devotees used to repeat the formula *Maranatha*, which in Aramaic means "Come, lord." Astonishingly, *maranatha* means "lord of love" in Sanskrit. The Indians have preserved an ancient tradition that Jesus lived for some time in Kashmir at a site called Amaranatha. Many Indian yogis believe Jesus studied yoga there!

Orthodox Judeo-Christian-Islamic practitioners are adamant that their deity is the only Supreme Being, and everyone else is worshiping a false God. The yoga tradition has a radically different perspective. Yoga texts say, "There is one God though people call him by different names." Yogis believe that no matter what religion you practice, you are ultimately worshiping the same God as everyone else in the entire universe.

Express Your Emotions

Bhakti Yoga techniques, performed wholeheartedly, produce a tremendous sense of euphoria. Some bhakti yogis weep with emotion. There is an extensive Indian tradition of great yogis who cried for God night and day, until they were finally blessed with a mystical vision. "Five minutes of sincerely crying to God is worth more than hours of unfocused meditation," says Amritanandamayi Ma, a contemporary saint from South India.

Emotional catharsis is not the same as enlightenment. Nevertheless, raja yogis respect Bhakti Yoga's ability to blast open the anahata chakra or heart center. This can lead to intensely concentrated mental states in which deep states of meditation spontaneously occur. The yogi experiences a profound and loving connection with the entire cosmos and a deep sense of peace. Yogis claim it's not unusual for miraculous healings and life-transforming visions to occur in this state.

Whether you understand God as a separate entity that exists outside yourself, or simply as the center of love and light within yourself, there are ample historical examples of bhakti yogis who went on to become beloved saints and enlightened masters.

Jnana Yoga

Jnana Yoga is usually translated "the path of the intellect" but to some extent this creates the wrong impression. *Jnana* (pronounced *gyah-na*) actually means "spiritual intelligence." Jnana Yoga is not primarily about mastering a subject intellectually, though many jnana yogis are in fact brilliant men or women renowned for their scholarship. But scholarship in and of itself doesn't make you enlightened. There are many references in yoga literature, some going back thousands of years, to intellectuals who believe they know all about yoga but have never actually practiced it. They're "like the blind leading the blind," the texts say.

Jnana yogis use their incisive intelligence to discriminate between the things in life that have lasting value and the things that don't. Having a lot of money or being famous can be fun and flattering, but you can't take these things with you when you die. However, the strength of character you develop by doing good deeds and the insights you gain from meditation *can* be transported with you into your next life. But the highest value is Self-Realization, a prize you can keep forever. Jnana yogis evaluate all their experiences in time and space in terms of their value in eternity.

Jnana is not knowledge about the ultimate reality. It's the living experience of the ultimate reality. Try the following Jnana Yoga practice to see if this yogic methodology appeals to you.

 FYI The most profound books on Jnana Yoga or the path of the intellect ever written are the *Upanishads*. These extremely ancient classics are among the oldest yoga books in existence. There are many translations, but one of the clearest is *The Upanishads* by Swami Nikhilananda.

STUDY, CONTEMPLATE, REALIZE

There are three steps to enlightenment, according to the most famous jnana yogi of all time. His name was Shankaracharya and he was born in South India at least 800 years ago. The three steps are as follows:

1. *Shravana.* Study.
2. *Manana.* Contemplate.
3. *Nididhyasana.* Experience for yourself.

Here's how it works. The first step is to select a spiritual affirmation you feel is true, such as "We are all one" or "God is love" or "At the center of my soul lies perfect peace." Then pick up a biography of a saint or an inspiring spiritual book (a number of them are listed in Appendix D) that illustrates this principle. Read as much as you can about it. For example, read a collection of writings by mystics from different spiritual traditions who actually experienced the unity of all being or who tasted the love of God or perfect inner peace. Study the concept you have chosen as fully as you can.

Once you've taken in as much information as you can find about your affirmation, you're ready for the second step. Put aside your research materials and sit down and really think about the words you chose. Look at them closely from every angle. What does it really mean to say there is perfect peace at the center of your being? Does everyone feel the same thing? Why don't you feel it now? When have you felt it? Where does it come from?

Is this your peace or God's? Really mull it over. As you contemplate, you're no longer concerned what other people think about the subject. Now you want to determine what *you* think about it.

The third step requires you to sit in your meditation posture. Breathe diaphragmatically. If you have mastered the process of opening your central channel, focus on the bridge between your two nostrils until your breath flows equally through both. Now that your body is relaxed and your physical energy is settled, turn your full attention to your affirmation. Dive deep within yourself till you experience the actual reality of what you have been contemplating.

Go inward until you find the peace that passes all understanding, divine love, or a sense of oneness with all things. This might well require a series of meditation sessions. You are looking for a level within yourself where you're not simply emotionally attracted to an idea or intellectually convinced of it, but where you actually experience its reality in a living way.

PROCEED WITH CAUTION

Ancient texts warn that of all the yogic paths, Jnana Yoga may be the most dangerous. Treading this path is said to be like "walking the razor's edge." That's because while the intellect has the ability to generate profound spiritual insight, it also has the power to inflate the ego and delude the mind. Jnana Yoga should be practiced under the supervision of a qualified teacher.

EXPERIENCE TRUTH

Jnana yogis contemplate the four great statements you encountered in Hour 16, such as "My Inner Self is one with the Self of all beings." Their goal is to know these truths experientially. Studying is building a rocket. Contemplating is filling its tanks with rocket fuel. Realizing is blasting off the surface of the earth into orbit. Jnana yogis are using words and concepts as fuel to propel themselves toward Self-Realization.

Karma Yoga, Bhakti Yoga, and Jnana Yoga, the paths of action, devotion, and intellect, sound like separate and distinct avenues to enlightenment. But most yogis counsel that working with all three at once is the best method of all. It's often said that spiritual practice is like a soaring bird. The bhakta path of the heart is one wing. The karma path of the hand is the other wing. The bird can't fly unless it uses both wings. Loving without giving makes you a stagnant pond rather than a running stream. Giving without love exhausts you.

But Jnana Yoga, the path of the head, is the bird's tail. The bird uses its tail feathers to navigate its way through rising and falling currents in the atmosphere. Action without wisdom can be self-defeating. Love without wisdom can curdle into fanaticism. When knowledge, love, and service blend together in your spiritual practice, your yoga takes flight.

FYI The best-known exponent of Jnana Yoga or the path of the intellect in recent centuries was the great South Indian sage Ramana Maharshi. *A Search in Secret India* by Dr. Paul Brunton is the best-selling account of Brunton's meeting with this extraordinary master. This book has sold more than a quarter of a million copies.

In Hour 24, you'll learn about one more type of yoga, the ancient tradition of Tantra.

Hour's Up!

Ready for your quiz? Answer true or false to the following statements:

1. Serving others is considered a distraction on the path of meditation.
2. Raja Yoga or "the royal path" refers to Patanjali's system of spiritual practice defined in the *Yoga Sutras*.
3. Jnana Yoga or the yoga of the intellect uses a three-step process to proceed from study to realization.
4. The karmic process is short-circuited by selflessly performing actions, without expecting any rewards.
5. Withdrawal of the senses means turning your attention away from the flood of data entering through your senses and focusing inward instead.
6. Praying, singing hymns, and reading inspiring spiritual stories are part of the yoga of devotional love.
7. Combining yogic paths, such as the path of love and the path of action, is a mistake that can only lead to confusion.
8. Raja Yoga is the ideal path for people who find it difficult to sit still.
9. People who practice Jnana Yoga are like the blind leading the blind.
10. Bhakti yogis cultivate a loving personal relationship with the Supreme Being.

HOUR 24

The Yoga Universe

- The yoga tradition challenges you to become healthier and more self-aware at every level of your being: physical, emotional, mental, and spiritual.

- Tantra Yoga uses ritual work and the manipulation of the body's subtle energies to reach for enlightenment.

- Classic yoga texts invite you into the inner world of the yoga masters.

- Being fully present in the moment is the essence of yoga practice.

In the previous 23 hours, you've learned a full range of Hatha Yoga practices, from the simplest to some exceptionally challenging postures. You've learned breathing exercises and internal cleansing techniques yogis use to keep themselves healthy and energized.

You have also learned how to meditate. Meditation is the practice at the very heart of yoga, the inward journey for which the Hatha Yoga poses and breathing techniques prepare you.

In addition, you've learned a great deal about yoga psychology: the four components of the mind, the five "bodies" in which consciousness is encased, and higher states of consciousness you're likely to encounter as you progress in your meditation practice. You've been introduced to the ethical standards by which yogis measure their lives, and various schools of yoga designed to help every personality type achieve a state of harmony and illumination.

You've studied the view of karma and reincarnation held in the yoga tradition, and the attitudes and actions yogis strive to maintain in order to live an enlightened life. You deserve a lot of credit for your enthusiasm and persistence in mastering this material! Much of the information in these 24 hours is radically new to individuals raised in Western culture. Yet incorporating the insights of the East into the lifestyle of the West is one of the best gifts you can give yourself.

In this, your final hour, your vision will expand to include the integral vision and techniques of Tantra Yoga. You will also be offered more avenues to travel if you wish to tread farther along the path of yoga practice to ever-increasing self-awareness. And you'll be given one final exercise to try, as you're challenged to live like a yogi, centered, tranquil, and fully present in the moment.

TANTRA YOGA

Tantra Yoga is the technical science of mysticism. It employs all kinds of ritual objects, such as mantras and the yantras you learned about in Hour 16, to expand consciousness and galvanize the kundalini into rising through the central canal of the subtle body to the top of the head, spiritually enlivening every aspect of your personality.

People in the West are very conscious of the distinction between inner and outer realities. That distinction breaks down almost completely in Tantra. Tantrics see the external universe as infinite interlocking energy patterns that are replicated inside every living being. Learning to control those living energies, called *devatas*, inside yourself is said to bring control of those same energy patterns in the external universe.

JUST A MINUTE

Sexual practices are described in significantly less than 1 percent of tantric texts. Yet during the Victorian era, puritanical European scholars obsessed about this minor aspect of the tantric tradition, magnifying its significance in their books and lectures until Western students got the impression Tantra was all about sex. When students go to India they're often shocked (and disappointed!) to find how little Tantra has to do with sexuality.

For example, you may recall from Hour 18 that the manipura chakra or navel center is associated with fire. By meditating deeply in the manner prescribed by the guru on this energy center, the tantric yogi gains control of the element fire. If you travel in India in winter you will see yogis sitting stark naked in sub-zero weather, as comfortable as if they were lazing on a beach in Hawaii. By igniting their inner fire at the navel center, they can regulate their internal temperature under just about any conditions. (It might be this mechanism that's involuntarily activated in women's bodies during menopause, causing hot flashes.)

Full mastery is believed to bring not only inner control, but a conscious connection with the fire element throughout the cosmos. Patanjali says that activating the navel center gives knowledge of astronomy. This is because the sun and stars represent the fire principle as it manifests in the sky. That "contemplating your navel" could unlock the secrets of the universe may sound ludicrous to people raised in Western culture. But very ancient astronomy texts composed by yogis show a phenomenally advanced knowledge of the Earth's geography and other world systems. It's easy to laugh at yogis who said they could use this chakra to gain knowledge of the stars. It's harder to explain where, in an age before telescopes, their advanced knowledge actually did come from.

MENTAL MECHANICS

To the tantrics, the whole universe is alive. If you stub your toe, your entire body reacts. Likewise, tantrics say, what happens in one part of the universe affects every other part. The whole cosmos is a vast, interconnected organism that operates according to a series of different sets of laws. There is one set of laws for the physical world. For example, you can't see a thing unless light illuminates the space in front of you. And if you drop your candle and set your house on fire, it burns to the ground.

But there's another set of laws for the mental universe. If you burn down your house in your imagination, a split second later it reappears in perfect shape if you will it to. Note that although flames were burning in your mind, not only did your head not catch on fire, but your temperature didn't even go up. Also, you can squeeze your eyes shut, closing out all the light in the universe, yet if you mentally command it, your mind's eye will be flooded with light.

In the West, physical laws of nature are taken seriously. The laws of the mental world, however, aren't given a moment's thought. Yet by carefully mapping these inner realities, the tantric yogis came to a profound understanding of the mechanics of consciousness. They learned how to work with the subtle energies of the inner universe, and how these living fields of energy interact with the energy of the outer world.

Remember that yogis do not accept that the mind and the brain are the same thing. To them, the brain is an organism the mind can act through the way broadcast wave bands can act through a television set if your antenna is hooked up. The brain allows the human mind to interact with the material world. But when the brain dies, the mind remains in the mental or astral world, and lives exclusively according to the laws of that plane of reality.

FYI The fascinating subject of Tantra is often misrepresented in the West. Two of the best introductions to Tantra as it is practiced authentically in Eastern lineages are *Tantra Unveiled* by Pandit Rajmani Tigunait, Ph.D., and *Tantra: The Path of Ecstasy* by Georg Feuerstein, Ph.D.

THE VALUE OF SYMBOLS

In the material world, cause and effect operate through the mechanism of physical laws. In the mental universe, cause and effect act through symbolism. In the physical world, you might feel intensely frustrated that your job is going nowhere. But when you go to sleep, instead of dreaming about work you may dream that you're trapped in an elevator or unable to get the elevator to stop at the floor you want. Your mind is processing your thoughts and emotions in a symbolic way, following the laws of the inner realm.

This understanding is critical to tantrics who believe that the material world was originally projected out of an underlying matrix of intelligence, a sort of cosmic mind. Therefore, objects and events in the outer world can be controlled through the manipulation of the symbols from which they materialized.

There are three broad approaches to Tantra Yoga. The first uses ritual objects in the external world, such as honoring the statue of a deity that symbolizes a particular blessing power, to achieve a result. The second uses no external objects at all, but works only in the mental universe. The third uses both methods, depending on what's most appropriate at the time.

If a yogi's progress in meditation is being blocked by huge amounts of repressed anger, he may make an offering to an image of the fierce goddess Kali, who controls anger. She likes red flowers so he may offer some of these, along with incense and red cloth and other objects symbolically connected with Kali. This is an example of the first type of Tantra. Another yogi might simply visualize all the things that disturb his peace, and then offer them into a fire he imagines burning in his Jnana Chakra between his eyebrow center and the top of his head. He does all his work mentally. A third yogi might opt to work with both sets of techniques. Either way, the yogi is using symbols to help release hostilities that have taken root in his subconscious mind.

INVOKE BLESSING FORCE

Here are two easy sample tantric rituals you can try—one outer, the other inner—to see if the tantric path is right for you. The purpose of these rituals is to invoke blessings and success for your yoga practice, excellent physical health and emotional well-being, and spiritual growth.

For the first ritual, you will need to collect several ritual implements:

- A photo or other image of a deity, saint, or a spiritual teacher you especially esteem
- A fresh, ripe piece of fruit
- A metal or porcelain bowl filled with pure water or fresh milk
- A candle and matches (the candle should be a light color such as white, yellow, or a pastel shade)
- A handheld fan
- A pleasant fragrance (incense, an aromatic oil, or a bottle of perfume will do)

If there is no deity or saint you especially relate to, then substitute a symbol that in your mind stands for a higher reality, such as a cross, a Star of David, a copy of the *Koran,* or the symbol "Om."

1. Wash your hands and face and put on fresh, clean clothes before beginning this ritual.

2. Sit down in your meditation posture with the photo or image representing spiritual awareness in front of you. Place the other articles within easy reach.

3. Close your eyes and breathe diaphragmatically. Relax your body but keep your spine straight. Focus on the bridge between your nostrils until the air flows equally through both your nostrils. Open your eyes.

4. Place your hands in the namaste position (palms pressed together, fingers pointing upward) in front of your heart center. Bow to the image before you.

5. Mentally speak to the image, humbly requesting the grace of a higher power to help you be healthy and happy, and to bless your yoga and meditation practice. Let the words pour out from your heart center. Try to really feel the words deeply and to connect with the living reality that the image in front of you represents.

6. Offer the fruit, leaving it right in front of the image. This represents offering everything made of the element earth within your being to a higher reality.

7. Offer the water or milk to the image. This represents offering everything in you connected with the element water.

JUST A MINUTE

Your bones and flesh are made of the element earth, according to the yoga tradition. Your blood is made of the watery element, the oxygen in your lungs of the air element. The fire in you corresponds to the digestive power in your abdominal organs and the heat that keeps your temperature around 98.6 degrees. The empty spaces in your body, such as in your nasal and oral cavities, represent ether.

8. Light the candle and wave it several times in a circle, clockwise, before the image. You are now offering the fire in yourself to a higher reality.

9. Fan the image for a moment or two. You are now offering the element air.

10. Release the fragrance by opening the bottle of perfume or scented oil, or by lighting the stick of incense. Offer it to the image. This signifies offering the element ether.

11. Sit up straight in your meditation posture and close your eyes. Breathe diaphragmatically. Feel peace, trust, and contentment in your heart center.

12. When you're ready, open your eyes and rise.

MEDITATE ON BLESSINGS

Now try the ritual again, this time performing it only mentally.

1. Begin by washing your hands and face. Your clothes should be clean and fresh.

2. Sit down in your meditation posture. Close your eyes and breathe diaphragmatically. Relax your body but keep your spine straight. Focus on your nasal septum until the air flows equally through both your nostrils.

3. Bring your full awareness to the center behind your eyebrows. Adjust your attention upward about halfway between the eyebrow center and the top of your skull. This is the Guru Chakra, from which blessings for your yoga practice continually flow.

4. Sit absolutely silent for a moment or so, focusing in a relaxed but attentive manner on the Guru Chakra. Simply be aware of your awareness focused there. Anchor yourself in the present moment, dismissing all extraneous thoughts about the past and future.

5. Mentally speak to your Higher Self, humbly requesting its grace in granting you health and happiness, and success in your yoga and meditation practice. Try to connect with the living reality of the inner guru. Feel the living presence of its blessing power.

6. Inhale upward from your root chakra to your Guru Chakra. This represents offering everything made of the element earth within your being to this higher reality.

7. Exhale back down to your sex center. Then inhale from this center back up to your Guru Chakra. This represents offering everything in you connected with the element water.

8. Exhale back down to your navel center. Then inhale from this center back up to your Guru Chakra. You are now offering the fire in yourself to the highest part of your being.

9. Exhale back down to your heart center. Then inhale from this center back up to your Guru Chakra. You are offering the element air.

10. Exhale back down to your throat center. Then inhale from this center back up to your Guru Chakra. This signifies offering the element ether.

11. Exhale back down to your eyebrow center. Then inhale from this center back up to your Guru Chakra. You are now offering the essence of yourself as a thinking, conscious entity to the very source of thought.

12. Remain focused in the Guru Chakra for a few moments. Breathe diaphragmatically. You will experience a profound sense of clarity, peace, and illumination.

13. When you're ready, open your eyes and get up.

READ THE CLASSICS

Want to learn more about yoga? There are dozens of excellent books on the market that will teach you the basic Hatha Yoga postures and guide you through the beginning stages of meditation. If you're a particularly enthusiastic student, you might eventually want to learn more than the fundamentals, and move on to a more complete understanding of yoga. In that case, it's time to turn to the classics, the great books of the yoga tradition.

PROCEED WITH CAUTION

Some advanced yogic texts describe unusual practices such as gradually severing the tongue muscle from the bottom of the mouth so that the tongue can be turned backward into the throat. These bizarre-sounding techniques often have symbolic rather than literal meaning. Don't attempt any extreme technique unless a qualified teacher has explained to you what it actually means!

Yoga has been around for thousands of years and the literature on every aspect of the subject is voluminous. You could literally spend lifetimes reading yoga texts and still barely make a dent in all the texts available. Be aware that some classic yoga texts encourage the reader to adopt a lifestyle of extreme asceticism. It's important to distinguish texts that were specifically composed for monks from those written for householders. Generally, the yoga tradition encourages moderation, not extreme behavior, as a more balanced approach to the enlightened life.

Most yoga texts are written in Indian languages like Sanskrit and Tamil. As of the beginning of the twenty-first century, only a fraction of yoga texts have been translated into English.

Here are a few of the most important texts available in English. You might want to start your in-depth study with these great works. Refer to Appendix D for other excellent books on the yoga tradition.

THE *YOGA SUTRAS*

The first of the two most essential texts on yoga is one you've encountered numerous times in these 24 hours, the *Yoga Sutras* by the North Indian adept Patanjali. This great yoga master, who lived more than 22 centuries ago, composed a series of 195 aphorisms (*sutras* in Sanskrit) in which he summarized the doctrines and techniques of Raja Yoga. The text is divided into four sections:

 FYI *The Heart of Yoga: Developing a Personal Practice* is by T.K.V. Desikachar, one of the most respected yoga teachers of the last half-century. In addition to offering invaluable advice on how to customize your yoga session, Desikachar includes a highly readable translation of Patanjali's classic *Yoga Sutras.*

- **Meditation.** These sutras explain the nature of the mind and delineate the stages of consciousness you pass through as your concentration becomes deeper.
- **Practice.** This section deals with the problems you may encounter as you begin your meditation practice, and the benefits that accrue from specific techniques.
- **Psychic abilities.** This series of sutras describes the hidden powers of the mind that you may uncover as your meditation practice matures.
- **Spiritual liberation.** The last portion of the text is about very advanced states of consciousness that occur when your awareness merges permanently in your Higher Self.

Many translations of the *Yoga Sutras* are available. There are excellent ones by Georg Feuerstein, Ph.D., and by Swami Satchidananda. *Meditation and Mantras* by Swami Vishnu Devananda also contains a very clear translation of Patanjali's master work, as well as the swami's reader-friendly introduction to the inner world of yoga practice.

THE *BHAGAVAD GITA*

The second of the two most important texts on yoga is the *Bhagavad Gita* by Veda Vyasa. There is no information about Hatha Yoga in this work, but the advice the *Bhagavad Gita* offers about how to live a yogic life has made this the single most popular book on the yoga tradition ever written.

With simplicity and brilliance, the *Bhagavad Gita* spells out the paths of Karma Yoga, Jnana Yoga, and Bhakti Yoga, which you studied in Hour 23. Perhaps the most inspired translation is the best-selling *The Song of God* by Swami Prabhavananda and Christopher Isherwood.

HATHA YOGA TEXTS

The *Hatha Pradipika* by Svatmarama is especially valuable for students working with Hatha Yoga. (The title means "Light on Hatha Yoga.") Svatmarama describes the action of the hatha postures both on the physical level and on the subtle body. He treats the breathing exercises at length, confirming their immense value in any Hatha Yoga routine. A number of fine translations are available, including one edited by Swami Digambarji and Pandit Raghunathashastri Kokaje.

GO TO ▶
Hour 21 expands on the system of psychology Patanjali developed in his *Yoga Sutras.* Hour 22 lays out the code of behavior Patanjali also described. Hour 23 explains the three types of yoga—Karma Yoga, Bhakti Yoga, and Jnana Yoga—advocated in the *Bhagavad Gita.*

In the *Hatha Pradipika* Svatmarama says "Success in yoga is attained by those who actually do the practices. It is not achieved just by reading books." He goes on to promise, "Those who practice yoga regularly will achieve results even if they are old, sick, or weak." He had seen for himself the immense benefits of consistent yoga practice, and particularly noted how much yoga helps the people need it most: those who are out of shape, aged, or unwell.

TEXTS ON INNER AWARENESS

The amount of literature on higher states of consciousness in the Sanskrit language is immense. Because much of it deals with levels of awareness far beyond the experience of most Westerners, you might find it nearly impossible to understand even if it was available in English. However, there are a number of translations that are more accessible to Western readers because they couch their teachings about alternate states of consciousness within the framework of entertaining stories about great yoga masters.

The *Yoga Vasishtha* is the story of a teenage boy's attempt to understand why there is so much suffering and injustice in the world. A yoga adept named Vasishtha sits down with him and explains the nature of human experience from an advanced yogi's point of view. Vasishtha's yoga powers have enabled him to visit other dimensions of reality and to move backward and forward in time, giving him a comprehensive view of human life. This is one of the greatest spiritual classics ever written, a truly unforgettable book. The complete text by the sage Valmiki, which is four volumes long, has been translated by Vihari Lala Mitra. An abridged version, *The Concise Yoga Vasistha*, was prepared by Swami Venkatesananda.

The *Tripura Rahasya* is another mind-expanding odyssey in yoga. It describes the cosmos from the point of view of enlightened men and women who experience the universe as an ocean of consciousness and energy. It includes stories of yoga adepts who live in a state of full enlightenment while fully engaged in the world, raising families and doing their jobs. *Sakti Sadhana: Steps to Samadhi* by Pandit Rajmani Tigunait, Ph.D., is the latest translation of this classic.

JUST A MINUTE

You might remember from Hour 22 that one of the 10 commitments suggested by Patanjali was self-study. This includes studying books that help you understand yourself better. Yoga classics like the *Yoga Vasishtha* and *Tripura Rahasya* make yoga philosophy and psychology more comprehensible by illustrating metaphysical principles in the form of entertaining stories.

REACH FOR ENLIGHTENMENT

You have now been exposed to a wide spectrum of yoga techniques. At one end of the range are the Hatha Yoga postures, designed to keep you healthy, young looking, and energized. At the other end are meditation techniques that begin by keeping you calm and centered and end by leading to the highest states of consciousness any human being can attain. Yoga starts by inviting you to embrace well-being and ends by showing you how to embrace your own inner being, your innermost self.

Yoga challenges you to live consciously and to maximize your full potentials. Many people sleepwalk through life. Yoga encourages you to become a *buddha,* that is, an "awakened" person. The yogis say that the difference in the level of consciousness between an enlightened master and an average human being is like that between a person who's awake and another who's still dreaming. An awakened person lives in the light of inner spirit. This light provides continual illumination in the form of inner guidance, healing, and creative power.

STRICTLY DEFINED

A **buddha** is a person who's spiritually awake, who travels through life consciously. A buddha is literally someone whose *buddhi* or higher mental faculties are fully functional, making the person spiritually illumined.

LIVE CONSCIOUSLY

Try the following experiment to test what it feels like to live consciously.

1. Select a half-hour period during the day when you're active—working, preparing food, visiting with friends, or otherwise engaged in some activity that occupies you both physically and mentally.

2. When your chosen time begins, make a firm mental resolution, "For the next 30 minutes I will be fully awake and self-aware. I will complete my tasks but still keep fully focused in the light of my Higher Self as if I were sitting in deep meditation."

3. Now bring your full awareness to the bridge between your nostrils (your nasal septum). Make sure you're breathing diaphragmatically. Breathe smoothly, evenly, and deeply without any jerks or pauses in your breath.

4. Breathe diaphragmatically until you feel centered and clear. Then begin your activities. For the next half-hour, every minute or two return your attention to your breath. Focus momentarily on the bridge between your nostrils and re-center yourself. Try to check in on your breath without interrupting the task you're working on.

5. After 30 minutes, evaluate how this exercise affected you.

Continual breath awareness is a trick yogis and kung fu adepts use to keep their attention focused in the present moment and to remain alert and self-aware. They stay with their breath, riding it like they might ride a horse.

Martial arts masters report that when they stay with their breath as they go into battle, they are not distracted by fear or anxiety. This is because fear is concern about what's going to happen in the future, and breath awareness keeps their attention squarely in the present. Because they are living in the moment, they are able to respond to any attacks more rapidly and effectively. There is no longer that split-second delay necessary to call the mind back from the past or future or from some fantasy or internal chatter. These masters respond instantaneously to whatever comes at them because they never leave the present moment.

Like the great martial arts adepts, yogis live consciously, fully awake in every activity whether they are meditating, speaking, cooking dinner, standing in line at the supermarket, or working on the job. Not only are their head, neck, and trunk aligned, but their work-a-day consciousness is also fully aligned with the center of awareness within. This alignment of body, mind, and spirit is what yoga is all about. Remember, yoga is a Sanskrit word that means "union." When you are united with the center of consciousness in yourself, you have become a yogi.

Hour's Up!

Here is your last quiz to test your understanding of the material in Hour 24. Answer true or false to the following statements:

1. Tantrics use rituals to help expand their awareness and control both inner and outer energies.

2. The primary focus of Tantra Yoga is spiritualized sex.

3. According to Tantra, the laws of the inner world work symbolically.

4. Tantrics believe that the images in our minds have no value, unlike the real objects in the external world.

5. One school of Tantra uses meditation and visualization rather than external rituals to center the mind.

6. The *Bhagavad Gita* is primarily a manual on ritual practices to help you raise your kundalini.

7. The *Yoga Sutras* describe what happens when your awareness merges permanently in your Higher Self.

8. Studying books on yoga is the single best way you can master yoga science.

9. Yoga masters do not recommend practicing breath awareness while you go about your daily activities.

10. Living consciously in the present moment is the essence of yoga practice.

APPENDIX A
Twenty-Minute Recap

HOUR 1

Hour 1 introduces you to the history and worldview of the yoga tradition. It describes the five levels of the human personality, all of which yoga aims to make healthy and balanced. You learn about the three basic energy states, active, passive, and perfectly poised. You also read about the ultimate goal of yoga, enlightenment, and what that really means.

HOUR 2

Before you begin a program of Hatha Yoga postures, you need to know a few preliminary stretches and some general precautions to ensure that you avoid injuring yourself as you exercise. You discover why yoga places so much importance on working with the spine. In yoga, you'll be conditioning not only your body, but your mind. The vital role of self-awareness in Hatha Yoga is explained.

HOUR 3

The relaxation postures are the body positions in which you begin and end your Hatha Yoga program. Because it's important to relieve residual tension in your muscles so normal blood flow can be restored after each pose, you'll pause to relax frequently during your yoga routine. Because working with your mind is part and parcel of Hatha Yoga, you learn two new exercises that require you to balance both your body and your mental state. You also learn two concentration exercises that help you attune to every part of your body.

Hour 4

Breathing exercises are one of the most valuable components of your yoga practice. Hour 4 explains how regulating your breath provides a shortcut to gaining mastery over your autonomic nervous system. The concept of *prana* or vital energy, analogous to *chi* in the martial arts, is clarified for you. Then you begin practicing several of the most important breathing techniques, including diaphragmatic breathing, alternate nostril breathing, and the complete breath.

Hour 5

In this hour, you start practicing the classic Hatha Yoga postures. You begin with the back bending poses you hold while lying on the floor. You learn the Cobra, Locust, and Boat, which are done lying on your stomach, and the Arch, Bridge, and Fish, in which you begin by lying on your back.

Hour 6

Hour 6 introduces more of the beginning level poses all yoga students need to know. Five of these begin on the floor: the Staff, Shoulder Stand, Plow, Pigeon, and Down Facing Dog. Then you get up to begin work with two standing postures: the Warrior Pose and the Horse Riding Posture. You learn that although aerobic exercises work your cardiovascular system, Hatha Yoga poses focus on toning your internal organs and glands.

Hour 7

The bending exercises of the Hatha Yoga tradition provide a massage for your internal organs. You learn three standing bends, the Side, Forward, and Backward bends. Then you bend from a sitting position on the floor, forming the Churn, Butterfly, Symbol of Yoga, and Sitting Forward bends. For the first time you'll practice a yoga position in which you're in constant motion, rather than simply holding still in the posture.

Hour 8

In Hour 8, you go on to master beginning-level twisting postures. You discover how their action on the spine and your internal organs differs from simple bends. You do the Angle and Triangle Poses, the Revolving Triangle, Torso Twist, Half Spinal Twist, and Reclining Twist. You also practice the Rocking Chair, which releases tension and strain in the spinal column.

HOUR 9

In this hour, you practice a series of postures that firm and tone your abdominal muscles while enhancing the vitality of your visceral organs. These postures are great for improving your vitality and daily elimination. You incorporate into your daily routine the Stomach Lift, Leg Lift, and Balance Pose.

HOUR 10

In Hour 10, you go on to learn some more challenging Hatha Yoga postures. These include the Eagle and King Dancer, which demand balance and concentration. You practice the Back Bending Monkey, Archer, Camel, and Inclined Plane Pose. You will learn how to expand beyond your previous physical limitations without straining yourself.

HOUR 11

Hour 11 teaches you the most famous of the difficult Hatha Yoga postures. You will learn the Dolphin, Headstand, Crow, Full Spinal Twist, Peacock, Wheel, and Scorpion. These challenging poses are harder to do than any posture you've learned before. However, they're not necessarily better for you than the easier postures, so if they are beyond your capacity, you're encouraged to continue practicing the Beginning and Intermediate exercises.

HOUR 12

Many traditional yogis begin their day with the Sun Salutation, a flowing series of 12 yoga poses you'll learn in this hour. This exercise is designed to help you start your day with an attitude of inner composure and connectedness with nature. It also energizes your body and helps get you moving in the morning. Because it gently stretches your muscles it provides a perfect warm-up for your daily Hatha Yoga program.

Hour 13

Hour 13 shows you how to customize your own Hatha Yoga routine. You are also offered four sample routines, based on your level of strength and flexibility. You learn how to create an atmosphere conducive to yoga practice and what items you can purchase that will simplify and enrich your experience of Hatha Yoga.

Hour 14

Traditionally, Hatha Yoga postures were taught to help create the physical health and mental steadiness necessary for meditation practice. In Hour 14 you learn the physiological and psychological benefits of adding meditation to your routine. You are also encouraged to experiment with the five basic meditation postures until you find a pose you can sit in comfortably, without moving, for the length of your meditation.

Hour 15

In Hour 15, you are given the two most important tools you need for a successful meditation practice. The first is a breathing exercise that allows you to breathe equally through both nostrils at the same time, a technique that places the two halves of the brain in a state of equilibrium. The second is a mantra, a special sound on which you will focus in order to concentrate your mind. You also learn how meditation calmly and safely helps you release painful emotions and memories.

Hour 16

During Hour 16, you have the opportunity to set up a daily meditation routine. You are given several more tools to help deepen your meditation practice, including images for visualization, inspiring affirmations, and mantras to help you connect with your inner guidance. You are also cautioned about pitfalls on the path of meditation you need to watch out for.

Hour 17

More than 2,000 years ago, the yoga master Patanjali frankly addressed the problems beginning-level meditators are likely to face. He also offered invaluable advice about how to deal with these difficulties. You learn what Patanjali had to say, as well as what to do about challenges that are unique to modern Western civilization, which Patanjali could hardly have imagined so many centuries ago.

Hour 18

Yoga students are often curious about kundalini and the chakras. Kundalini is the energy of consciousness that travels through your nervous system, up and down your spine, and into your brain. The chakras are way stations along the spine and brain where this energy manifests through particular personality traits. You learn the qualities and powers associated with each chakra, and what happens when the kundalini reaches the highest center in the brain.

Hour 19

As you progress in your meditation, you may begin to encounter higher states of consciousness delineated in the yoga texts. Hour 19 lets you know what to expect, and describes the highest states of awareness attained by advanced yogic adepts. You will learn about the fourth level of consciousness beyond waking, dreaming, and sleep, and about the extrasensory abilities traditional yogis say may begin to appear as meditation deepens.

Hour 20

It's not necessary to be a vegetarian to practice yoga, but yoga masters have found that a balanced meatless diet can be more healthful for the body and more helpful for meditation. You learn some easy vegetarian recipes. Yoga addresses not only what goes into your body but what comes out, so you also learn some basic cleansing techniques to keep not just the outside, but also the inside, of your body clean. You are also introduced to Ayurveda, the yogic medical system.

Hour 21

Thousands of years before Sigmund Freud, the yoga masters explored the depths of the subconscious mind. Unlike Western psychologists, who focus mostly on the subconscious, yoga adepts also work with the superconscious.

The yoga view of how the mind operates is explained, along with how the concepts of karma and reincarnation are incorporated in the yogic understanding of the inner dynamics of the psyche.

HOUR 22

Although this book began by teaching you the Hatha Yoga postures, in the traditional yoga system, personal ethics, not physical exercises, are considered the foundation of all yogic practice. In Hour 22, you are introduced to the yogic perspective on right action, and the powers the adepts say you develop when you live in harmony with the basic moral laws of the universe. You are also advised on what qualities to look for in a guru, should you decide to look for a meditation mentor.

HOUR 23

Not everyone is interested in Hatha Yoga postures or meditation, but everyone can practice yoga! Other branches of yoga are introduced which may be more appealing to different personality types. You discover Bhakti Yoga, which is helpful for deeply emotional people; Karma Yoga, which works for active, dynamic personalities; and Jnana Yoga, which is oriented toward intellectually focused people. You'll also learn how these three modalities are integrated in the holistic system of yoga.

HOUR 24

The final hour introduces you to Tantra Yoga as it's actually practiced in the Eastern world. You will also be directed to resources that can help you deepen your knowledge of the amazing insights and techniques of the yoga tradition.

APPENDIX B
Glossary

This yoga glossary is a compendium of Sanskrit terms students are likely to run into in their Hatha Yoga and meditation classes. Many are Sanskrit words that describe a particular yoga posture. For example, when the Sanskrit word *dhanu*, which means "bow," is combined with the word *asana*, which means "posture," you have *dhanurasana*, the name for the Bow Pose.

Ahankara   Your sense of yourself as a distinct entity.

Ahimsa   Nonviolence.

Agama Karma   The karma created by thoughts, plans, and desires.

Agni   Fire or the state of burning.

Ajna Chakra   The center of consciousness behind the eyebrows.

Akarna Dhanurasana   The Archer Posture.

Akasha   The subtle element of space, from which the material elements emerge.

Anahata Chakra   The center of consciousness at the heart.

Ananda Maya Kosha   The subtle body made of inner joy (*ananda*).

Anna Maya Kosha   The physical body, composed of food (*anna*).

Ap   Water or the state of being liquid.

Apana   The downward moving energy in the body responsible for eliminating waste products.

Apanasana   The Knees-to-Chest Posture.

Aparigraha   Nongreediness.

Ardha Matsyendrasana   The Half Spinal Twist.

Artha   Wealth.

Asana   A yoga posture. Also, the cushion one sits on for meditation.

Ashram   A spiritual community.

Ashtanga Yoga   The eightfold path described in the *Yoga Sutras*.

Asteya   Nonstealing.

Avadhut   An enlightened adept who may appear crazy.

Ayu   Life or longevity.

Ayurveda   The traditional medical system of India.

Baddha Konasana   The Butterfly Posture.

Balasana   The Child's Posture.

Banarasana   The Monkey Posture.

Bhajan   A devotional song.

Bhakti   Loving devotion.

Bhastrika   The Bellows breathing exercise.

Bhujangasana   The Cobra Posture.

Bindu   A point of origin from which energy or consciousness emerge.

Brahmacharya   Celibacy; not overindulging in sensuality.

Buddha   A person who's spiritually awake, who travels through life consciously.

Buddhi   The rational and intuitive faculties including the will, judgment, and conscience.

Chakra   An energy center in the subtle body.

Chakrasana   The Wheel Pose.

Chakshu The ability to see.

Chalan The Churning yoga exercise.

Chitta The storehouse of memories.

Dahl A spiced Indian dish made of beans, peas, or lentils.

Danda A wooden staff.

Devata A living field of intelligent energy.

Dhanurasana The Bow Posture (as in bow and arrow).

Dharana Contemplation.

Dharma Virtue. Righteousness.

Dhauti A yogic cleansing technique involving swallowing a thin strip of cotton.

Dhi The field of knowledge accessible to the human intuition.

Dhyana Meditation.

Diksha Mantra initiation.

Dvipada Pitham The Arch Posture.

Gajakarani The Stomach Wash.

Gandha The experience of smelling.

Garudasana The Eagle Posture.

Ghee Clarified butter.

Ghrana The ability to smell.

Guru Mentor or spiritual teacher.

Guru Chakra A center of consciousness in the brain associated with intuitive guidance.

Halasana The Plow Posture.

Ida The primary left energy channel of the subtle body.

Ishta Devata Your personal image of God.

Ishvara The yogi's name for God.

Ishvara Pranidhana   To surrender to a higher force.

Jala Neti   The Nasal Wash.

Jalandhara Bandha   The Chin Lock.

Japa   The continuous repetition of a mantra.

Jathara Parivartanasana   The Reclining Twist.

Jihva   The ability to taste.

Jivanmukta   A liberated soul.

Jnana   Spiritual intelligence.

Jnana Chakra   A center of consciousness in the brain associated with spiritual discernment.

Jnani   A sage.

Jyotir Vidya   The "science of light," meaning yoga astrology.

Jyotish   Yoga astrology.

Kakasana   The Crow Pose.

Kama   Sensual pleasure, especially sex.

Kapha   The earthy quality in a person's body and personality.

Kapalabhati   The Glowing Face breathing exercise.

Kapotasana   The Pigeon Posture.

Karma   Willful action and its consequences.

Karmashaya   The depository of karma in the subtle body.

Khichari   A mixture of cooked beans, rice, and Indian spices.

Kirtan   Singing devotional songs.

Konasana   The Angle Posture.

Kriyamana Karma   The karma you create in your present life through your speech and actions.

Kundalini   The energy of consciousness as it operates within the subtle body.

Mahat   The network of cosmic consciousness connecting all things.

Maha vakya The four "great sayings" used in Jnana Yoga.

Maitri Asana The Chair Posture.

Makarasana The Crocodile Posture.

Mala A yoga rosary that usually has 108 beads.

Manana To deeply contemplate a truth.

Manas The part of the mind that deals with sensory data.

Manipura Chakra The center of consciousness at the navel.

Mano Maya Kosha The subtle body made of thought (*manas*).

Mantra A sound used in the yoga tradition to deepen meditation.

Maranatha Lord of love.

Masala A combination of Indian spices.

Matsyabhedasana The Dolphin Posture.

Matsyasana The Fish Posture.

Mayurasana The Peacock Posture.

Moksha Freedom from karma and rebirth.

Mudra Special hand positions which create specific energetic effects in the subtle body.

Muladhara Chakra The center of consciousness at the bottom of the spine.

Nadi Any one of 72,000 energy channels in the subtle body which conduct prana or vital energy.

Nadi Shodhana The Alternate Nostril breathing exercise.

Namaste Greeting meaning "I bow to the divinity in you."

Natarajasana The King Dancer Pose.

Naukasana The Boat Posture.

Nauli The Stomach Roll.

Navasana The Balance Posture.

Neti Cleansing or washing the nasal cavity.

Nididhyasana   To assimilate knowledge into your being until it becomes your living experience.

Niyama   Five moral principles guiding what you should do.

Pada   The act of moving, locomoting.

Padahastasana   The Standing Forward Bend.

Padmasana   The Lotus Posture.

Paneer   Strained milk curd.

Pani   The ability to handle objects.

Parivritta Trikonasana   The Revolving Twist.

Parshvottanasana   The Angle Posture.

Paschimottanasana   The Sitting Forward Bend.

Paya   The act of excreting.

Pingala   The primary right energy channel of the subtle body.

Pitta   The fiery element in the body.

Prajna   Spiritual wisdom.

Prakriti   The energy and matter of which the universe is composed.

Prana   Life force or breath.

Prana Maya Kosha   The subtle body made of life force (*prana*).

Pranam   To bow in respect.

Pranayama   Breathing techniques used to control prana.

Pranidhana   Self-surrender.

Prarabdha Karma   The karma from past lives destined to play out during the present life.

Prasad   Food that has been blessed.

Pratibha   Intuitive insight or genius.

Pratyahara   Sensory withdrawal leading to inward focus.

Prithivi   Earth or the state of being solid.

Purana Yoga's ancient chronicles, outlining yoga cosmology.

Purascharana The vow to chant a mantra a certain number of times within a certain period.

Purusha The immortal soul.

Purvottanasana The Inclined Plane Posture.

Raja Yoga Patanjali's eightfold yoga path.

Rajas An active, dynamic energy state.

Rasa The experience of flavor.

Rishi A sage.

Rupa The experience of sight.

Sadhana Spiritual practice.

Sahaja "Natural" as in sahaja samadhi, to naturally remain in meditative absorption.

Sahasrara Chakra The thousand-petaled center of consciousness at the top of the brain.

Samadhi Full mental absorption experienced in very deep states of meditation.

Samskara A deep thought groove in the subconscious that affects the way a person behaves.

Sanchita Karma The karma you created in your previous incarnations.

Sankhya The philosophical system on which yoga is based.

Santosha Contentment.

Sarvangasana The Shoulder Stand.

Sat Guru A genuine spiritual master.

Satsang Spiritual fellowship.

Sattva A balanced, harmonious energy state.

Satya Truthfulness.

Saucha Cleanliness.

Setu Bandhasana   The Bridge Posture.

Seva   Selfless service.

Shabda   The experience of sound.

Shakti   The energy of consciousness.

Shaktipat   The transmission of the energy of enlightenment.

Shalabha   The Locust Posture.

Shanti   Peace.

Shavasana   The Corpse Posture.

Shirshasana   The Headstand.

Shravana   To listen to a teacher or to study.

Siddha   A yoga adept.

Siddhasana   The Accomplished Pose.

Siddhi   A supernatural or psychic power.

So Hum   A mantra meaning "I am one with higher consciousness."

Soma Chakra   A center of consciousness in the brain associated with bliss.

Sparsha   The experience of feeling.

Stotra   The ability to hear.

Subzi   Hindi for any spiced Indian vegetable dish.

Sukhasana   The Easy Posture.

Surya Namaskar   The Sun Salutation.

Sushumna   The primary central energy channel of the subtle body.

Sutra   Any Sanskrit text composed of a string of short aphorisms.

Sutra Neti   A yogic cleansing technique in which the nasal passages are cleaned with a cotton cord.

Svadhisthana Chakra   The center of consciousness near the genital organs.

Svadhyaya   Self-study.

Svarodaya   The yogic science of breath.

Swastikasana   The Auspicious Pose.

Tadasana   The Mountain Posture.

Tadasana Parshvabhangi   The Torso Twist.

Tamas   An inert, dull energy state.

Tanmatra   The five subtle elements.

Tantra   A yogic path using rituals and the control of internal energy states.

Tapas   Self-discipline; austerity.

Tattva   The essential constituents of reality, the evolutes of matter and energy.

Trataka   Yogic gazing exercise.

Trikonasana   The Triangle Posture.

Turiya   The fourth state of consciousness beyond waking, dreaming, and deep sleep; superconsciousness.

Tvak   The ability to touch.

Uddiyana Bandha   The Stomach Lift.

Ujjayi   The Humming Breath exercise.

Upastha   The ability to procreate.

Upaya   A spiritual practice undertaken to offset the effects of bad karma.

Ustrasana   The Camel Pose.

Utkatasana   The Horse Riding Posture.

Utthita Dvipadasana   The Double Leg Lift.

Utthita Ekapadasana   The Single Leg Lift.

Utthita Hastapadasana   The Balance Pose.

Vak   Speech.

Vasana   A groove of thought in the subconscious.

Vata   The air element in a person's physical constitution.

Vayu   Air or the gaseous state.

Veda   Knowledge or science. This is also the name of the basic scripture of Hinduism.

Vijnana Maya Kosha   The subtle body composed of intelligence.

Vimana   Legendary ancient flying vehicles.

Virabhadrasana   The Warrior Posture.

Vishuddha Chakra   The center of consciousness at the throat.

Viveka   Spiritual discrimination.

Vrata   The vow to perform some type of spiritual practice for a certain length of time.

Vrishchikasana   The Scorpion Pose.

Vriskshasana   The Tree Posture.

Yama   Five moral principles suggesting what you should avoid doing.

Yantra   A geometric design used in meditation.

Yoga   The physical and mental exercises developed in India that "yoke" the mortal mind and immortal spirit together.

Yoga Mudra   The Symbol of Yoga Posture.

Yoga Nidra   Yogic sleep.

APPENDIX C
Resources

If you want to sign up for a yoga class, learn to meditate, take a course in vegetarian cooking, pick up a yoga outfit or meditation cushion, or learn more about the fascinating philosophy and worldview of yoga, here are some places to begin your search for more information.

GENERAL

Ananda Yoga Retreat
1618 Tyler Foote Road
Nevada City, CA 95959
1-800-346-5350
www.ExpandingLight.org

B.K.S. Iyengar Yoga Association
PO Box 941
Lemont, PA 16851
1-800-889-9642
www.Iyengar-Yoga.com

Himalayan International Institute
RR#1 Box 400
Honesdale, PA 18451
1-800-822-4547
www.HimalayanInstitute.org

Jivamukti Yoga Center
404 Lafayette Street
New York, NY 10003
1-800-295-6814
www.JivamuktiYoga.com

Institute of the Himalayan Tradition
1317 Summit Avenue
St. Paul, MN 55105
651-645-6808
www.IHTyoga.org

Kripalu Center
PO Box 793
Lenox, MA 01240
1-800-741-SELF
www.kripalu.org

Midwest Yoga and Wellness Conference
1-800-599-9642
www.CenterForYoga.net

Mount Madonna Center
445 Summit Road
Watsonville, CA 95076
408-847-0406
www.MountMadonna.org

Omega Institute
150 Lake Drive
Rhinebeck, NY 12572
1-800-944-1001
www.eomega.org

Satchidananda Ashram
Yogaville
Buckingham, VA 23921
804-858-YOGA
www.Yogaville.org

Shoshoni Yoga Retreat
PO Box 410
Rollingsville, CO 80474
303-642-0116
www.Shoshoni.org

Sivananda Yoga Vedanta Center
243 W. 24th Street
New York, NY 10011
1-800-783-YOGA
www.Sivananda.org

Southeast Yoga Conference
1-800-599-YOGA
www.SouthEastYoga.com

AYURVEDA

For more information about Ayurveda, the system of medicine developed by yoga masters, contact:

The Ayurvedic Institute
PO Box 23445
Albuquerque, NM 87192
505-291-9698
www.Ayurveda.com

JYOTISH

For more information about Jyotish, the system of astrology created by yoga adepts, contact:

The American College of Vedic Astrology
PO Box 2149
Sedona, AZ 86339
1-800-900-6595
www.VedicAstrology.org

Remember, you can always log on to www.YogaFinder.com for worldwide access to teachers, classes, and events related to yoga. Or stop by your local bookshop and ask for copies of *Yoga Journal* and *Yoga International* magazines.

YOGA MODELS

Delia Quigley, the Dynamic Yoga instructor who posed for most of the pictures in this book, is Director of StillPoint Schoolhouse and is host of a weekly radio program called "Food for Thought." In 1999, she developed the Body Rejuvenation Cleanse Program. For information about Delia's work, log on to www.DeliaQuigley.com.

Ramaiah Collins, who also posed for photos in this book, is a popular Ashtanga Yoga instructor teaching at the Yoga Company in Sonoma, California. Log on to www.SonomaYoga.com for details about his classes.

APPENDIX D
Further Reading

HATHA YOGA

Anatomy of Hatha Yoga: A Manual for Students, Teachers and Practitioners by H. David Coulter, Ph.D.

Asana Pranayama Mudra Bandha by Swami Satyananda Saraswati

Back Care Basics: A Doctor's Gentle Yoga Program for Back and Neck Pain Relief by Mary Pullig Schatz, M.D.

The Complete Idiot's Guide to Power Yoga by Geo Takoma and Eve Adamson

The Complete Illustrated Book of Yoga by Swami Vishnu-Devananda

Hatha Pradipika by Svatmarama

The Heart of Yoga: Developing a Personal Practice by T.K.V. Desikachar

Integral Yoga Hatha by Swami Satchidananda

Joints and Glands Exercises by Rudolph Ballentine, M.D.

The Muscle Book by Paul Blakey

Relax and Renew: Restful Yoga for Stressful Times by Judith Lasater

The Sivananda Companion to Yoga by Swami Vishnu-Devananda

Structural Yoga Therapy: Adapting to the Individual by Mukunda Stiles

Yoga Journal's Yoga Basics by Mara Carrico

Yoga: Mastering the Basics by Sandra Anderson and Rolf Sovik, Psy.D.

Yoga Mind and Body by Sivananda Yoga Vedanta Center

Yoga Mind, Body and Spirit: A Return to Wholeness by Donna Farhi

Yoga: The Path to Holistic Health by B.K.S. Iyengar

PRANAYAMA

Breath, Mind, and Consciousness by Harish Johari

The Breathing Book by Donna Farhi

Path of Fire and Light by Swami Rama (two volumes)

Science of Breath: A Practical Guide by Swami Rama, Rudolph Ballentine, M.D., and Alan Hymes, M.D.

Swara Yoga by Swami Muktibodhananda

MEDITATION

How to Know God by Swami Prabhavananda and Christopher Isherwood

How to Meditate: A Practical Guide by Kathleen McDonald

How to Meditate Using Chakras, Mantras and Breath by Dennis Chernin, M.D.

Mantra and Meditation by Pandit Usharbudh Arya, D.Litt.

Meditation and Its Practice by Swami Rama

Meditation and Mantras by Swami Vishnu Devananda

Meditation in Christianity by Swami Rama, et al.

Meditation Is Boring? Putting Life in Your Spiritual Practice by Linda Johnsen

The Power of Mantra and the Mystery of Initiation by Pandit Rajmani Tigunait, Ph.D.

Yoga Philosophy of Patanjali by Swami Hariharananda Aranya

Yoga and Health

Ayurveda: The Science of Self-Healing by Dr. Vasant Lad

The Ayurvedic Encyclopedia: Natural Secrets to Healing, Prevention, and Longevity by Swami Sada Shiva Tirtha

The Charaka Samhita translated by P. V. Sharma

Diet and Nutrition: A Holistic Approach by Rudolph M. Ballentine, M.D.

Freedom from Stress by Phil Nuernberger, Ph.D.

Himalayan Mountain Cookery by Martha Ballentine

A Practical Guide to Holistic Health by Swami Rama

Prakruti: Your Ayurvedic Constitution by Dr. Robert Svoboda

Psychotherapy East and West: A Unifying Paradigm by Swami Ajaya, Ph.D.

The Quiet Mind edited by John Harvey, Ph.D.

Transition to Vegetarianism by Rudolph M. Ballentine, M.D.

The Wellness Tree by Justin O'Brien, Ph.D.

Yoga and Ayurveda: Self-Healing and Self-Realization by David Frawley

Yoga and Psychotherapy by Swami Rama, Rudolph Ballentine, M.D., and Swami Ajaya, Ph.D.

Yoga for Your Type: An Ayurvedic Approach to Your Asana Practice by Dr. David Frawley

Yoga Psychology: A Practical Guide to Meditation by Swami Ajaya, Ph.D.

Yoga Lifestyle

The Art of Joyful Living by Swami Rama

Bhakti Yoga by Swami Vivekananda

Choosing a Path by Swami Rama

Creative Use of Emotion by Swami Rama and Swami Ajaya, Ph.D.

The Divine Romance by Paramahansa Yogananda

First Lessons in Sanskrit Grammar and Reading by Judith M. Tyberg

Freedom from the Bondage of Karma by Swami Rama

Inner Quest: The Path of Spiritual Unfoldment by Pandit Rajmani Tigunait

Jnana Yoga by Swami Vivekananda

Love and Family Life by Swami Rama

The Power of Now: A Guide to Spiritual Enlightenment by Eckhart Tolle

Raja Yoga by Swami Vivekananda

Yoga Gems: A Treasury of Practical and Spiritual Wisdom from Ancient and Modern Masters by Georg Feuerstein, Ph.D.

YOGA SCIENCE

Aghora III: The Law of Karma by Robert E. Svoboda

Chakras: Energy Centers of Transformation by Harish Johari

From Death to Birth: Understanding Karma and Reincarnation by Pandit Rajmani Tigunait, Ph.D.

I Have Lived Before: The True Story of the Reincarnation of Shanti Devi by Sture Lonnerstrand

Kundalini: The Arousal of the Inner Energy by Adjit Mookerjee

Layayoga: An Advanced Method of Concentration by Shyam Sundar Goswami

The Royal Path: Practical Lessons on Yoga by Swami Rama

The Serpent Power by Sir John Woodroffe

Tantra: The Path of Ecstasy by Georg Feuerstein, Ph.D.

Tantra Unveiled by Pandit Rajmani Tigunait, Ph.D.

Tattva Shuddhi by Swami Satyasangananda Saraswati

Tools for Tantra by Harish Johari

The Upanishads translated by Swami Nikhilananda

The World as Power by Sir John Woodroffe

Yantra: The Tantric Symbol of Cosmic Unity by Madhu Khanna

Yoga Nidra by Swami Satyasangananda Saraswati

The Yoga Sutras of Patanjali translated by Swami Satchidananda

YOGIS AND YOGA HISTORY

Aghora: At the Left Hand of God by Robert Svoboda

At the Eleventh Hour by Pandit Rajmani Tigunait

Autobiography of a Yogi by Paramahansa Yogananda

Awaken Children! by Swami Amritswarupananda

Be Here Now by Baba Ram Dass

The Complete Idiot's Guide to Hinduism by Linda Johnsen

The Concise Yoga Vasistha translated by Swami Venkatesananda

Daughters of the Goddess: The Women Saints of India by Linda Johnsen

The Gospel of Sri Ramakrishna by Mahendranath Gupta

The Living Goddess: Reclaiming the Tradition of the Mother of the Universe by
    Linda Johnsen

Living with the Himalayan Masters by Swami Rama

The Play of Consciousness by Swami Muktananda

Radha: Diary of a Woman's Search by Swami Sivananda Radha

Sakti Sadhana: Steps to Samadhi by Pandit Rajmani Tigunait, Ph.D.

A Search in Secret India by Dr. Paul Brunton

The Tradition of the Himalayan Masters by Pandit Rajmani Tigunait, Ph.D.

Walking with a Himalayan Master by Justin O'Brien

The Yoga Tradition: Its History, Literature, Philosophy and Practice by Georg
    Feuerstein, Ph.D.

The Yoga Vasishtha Maharamayana of Valmiki translated by Vihari Lala Mitra

APPENDIX E
Quiz Answers

HOUR 1

1. True
2. True
3. False
4. False
5. True
6. True
7. False
8. True
9. True
10. True

HOUR 2

1. True
2. False
3. False
4. True
5. True
6. False
7. True
8. True
9. True
10. False

HOUR 3

1. True
2. True
3. False
4. False
5. True
6. False
7. False
8. True
9. True
10. True

HOUR 4

1. False
2. True
3. True
4. False
5. True
6. False
7. True
8. False
9. True
10. True

Hour 5

1. False
2. False
3. True
4. False
5. True
6. True
7. False
8. True
9. True
10. False

Hour 6

1. True
2. True
3. True
4. False
5. True
6. False
7. False
8. False
9. True
10. True

Hour 7

1. True
2. True
3. True
4. False
5. False
6. False
7. False
8. False
9. True
10. True

Hour 8

1. True
2. True
3. False
4. False
5. False
6. True
7. True
8. True
9. False
10. True

Hour 9

1. True
2. True
3. False
4. False
5. False
6. True
7. False
8. False
9. True
10. True

Hour 10

1. True
2. False
3. True
4. False
5. True
6. False
7. True
8. False
9. False
10. True

Hour 11

1. False
2. True
3. False
4. True
5. False
6. False
7. False
8. True
9. False
10. True

Hour 12

1. True
2. False
3. False
4. True
5. True
6. True
7. True
8. True
9. True
10. False

Hour 13

1. True
2. False
3. False
4. False
5. True
6. True
7. True
8. False
9. True
10. True

Hour 14

1. True
2. False
3. True
4. False
5. True
6. True
7. False
8. False
9. True
10. True

Hour 15

1. False
2. False
3. True
4. True
5. True
6. False
7. True
8. False
9. True
10. True

Hour 16

1. False
2. False
3. True
4. True
5. True
6. False
7. True
8. False
9. False
10. True

Hour 17

1. False
2. True
3. False
4. True
5. False
6. False
7. False
8. True
9. True
10. False

Hour 18

1. True
2. False
3. False
4. False
5. True
6. True
7. True
8. True
9. False
10. False

Hour 19

1. False
2. True
3. False
4. True
5. False
6. False
7. True
8. True
9. True
10. False

Hour 20

1. False
2. True
3. False
4. False
5. False
6. True
7. False
8. True
9. True
10. True

Hour 21

1. False
2. True
3. True
4. True
5. False
6. True
7. False
8. True
9. False
10. True

Hour 22

1. True
2. True
3. False
4. True
5. False
6. True
7. False
8. False
9. True
10. True

Hour 23

1. False
2. True
3. True
4. True
5. True
6. True
7. False
8. False
9. False
10. True

Hour 24

1. True
2. False
3. True
4. False
5. True
6. False
7. True
8. False
9. False
10. True

Index

Symbols

31 and 61 Points: A Technique for Health and Relaxation, 41

31 Points exercise, 38, 40-41

61 Points exercise, 38, 41-42

A

abdominal poses, 120-121
  Balance Pose, 125-127
  Leg Lift, 124-125
  safety, 120-121
  Stomach Lift, 121-122
  Stomach Roll, 123

Accomplished Posture (Siddhasana), 197-198

ACVA (American College of Vedic Astrology), 292

Adho Mukha Svanasana (Down Facing Dog Posture), 85-86

Advanced routine, designing your session, 182-183

advanced yoga postures, 143-144
  Crow Posture, 150-152
  Dolphin Posture, 144-146
  Full Spinal Twist, 153-154
  Headstand, 146-150
  Peacock Pose, 152
  Scorpion Posture, 156-157
  Wheel Posture, 155-156

agama karma, 288-289

Aghora III: The Law of Karma, 286

Aham Brahmasmi, 224

ahankara, as function of the mind, 282-286

ahimsa (do not harm anyone), 297

ajna chakra (eyebrow center), 250

Akarna Dhanurasana (Arch Posture), 138-140

All Limbs Posture. *See* Shoulder Stand

Alternate Nostril Breathing, Channel Purification, 52-56

American College of Vedic Astrology. *See* ACVA

anahata chakra (heart center), 248

Ananda Maya Kosha, 8

Anandamayi Ma, 256

Anatomy of Hatha Yoga: A Manual for Students, Teachers and Practitioners, 71

Anderson, Sandra, 79

Angle Pose (Parshvottanasana/ Konasana), 106-107

ankle roll, 22-23

Anusara Yoga, 7

apana, 59

Apanasana (Knees-to-Chest Posture), 34

aparigraha (do not be greedy), 299

apnea, 48

Apollonius of Tyana, 4

approval by a physician, 16

Arch Posture (Akarna Dhanurasana), 138-140

Ardha Matsyasana (Half Fish Posture), 71

Ardha Matsyendrasana (Half Spinal Twist), 112-113

Arousal of the Inner Energy, The, 242

artha (wealth), 295-296

asana (posture/pose), 30

Asana (Raja Yoga limb), 308

ashrams, 160

Ashtanga Yoga. *See* Raja Yoga

asteya (do not steal), 298

astral chakra (svadhisthana), 246-247

astrology, calculating your karma, 292-293

At the Eleventh Hour, 256

atmosphere, creating for yoga sessions, 183

attentive relaxation, 29-30
 Child's Posture, 32-33
 Corpse Posture, 35-37
 Crocodile Posture, 34-35
 Knees-to-Chest Posture, 34
 Mountain Posture, 31-32

attentive state, intermediate level yoga postures, 131-132

Auspicious Posture (Swastikasana), 196-197

Autobiography of a Yogi, 5

awareness
 directing subtle bodies, 8-9
 inner awareness texts, 325-326
 kundalini, 241-242

Ayam Atma Brahma, 224

Ayurveda (science of longevity), 278-279
 balance, 280
 Kapha people, 279
 Pitta people, 279
 Vata people, 279

B

Back Bending Monkey Posture (Banarasana), 140-142

Back Care Basics: A Doctor's Gentle Yoga Program for Back and Neck Pain Relief, 176

backward-bending poses, 63
 Arch Posture, 72-73
 Boat Posture, 68-70
 Bow Posture, 70-71
 Bridge Posture, 73, 75
 Cobra Posture, 64-66
 Half Fish Posture, 71
 Locust Posture, 66-68
 recognizing limits, 75

Baddha Konasana (Butterfly Posture), 102

balance, 42-43
Tip Toe Stretch, 43-44
Tree Posture, 44-45
Balance Pose (Utthita Hastapadasana), 125-127
Balasana (Child's Posture), 32
Ballentine, Martha, 272
Ballentine, Rudolph, M.D., 24
Banarasana (Back Bending Monkey Posture), 140-142
bare feet, 17
Be Here Now, 6
Bellows Breath, 57
bending postures, 91
Butterfly Posture, 102
Churn Posture, 99
mental attentiveness, 104
Sitting Forward Bend, 97-99
Standing Backward Bend, 93-95
Standing Forward Bend, 95-96
Standing Side Bend, 92
Symbol of Yoga Posture, 100-102
Bhagavad Gita, 240, 325
Bhakti Yoga, 311
empowering your practice, 311-313
expressing emotions, 313
Bhastrika, 57
Bhujangasana (Cobra Posture), 64-66

Bihar School of Yoga, 242
biofeedback equipment, 184
Boat Posture (Naukasana), 68-70
bodies, subtle bodies, 8-11
directing awareness, 8-9
visualization, 10
Bow Posture (Dhanurasana), 70-71
brahmacharya (do not overindulge), 298
brain center (sahasrara chakra), 251-252
breath pillows, 51, 184
Breath, Mind, and Consciousness, 59
breathing, 48
Channel Purification, 52-56
Complete Breath exercise, 51-52
diaphragmatic breathing, 49-51
link between body and mind, 47-48
meditation, 204-207
safety tips, 18
vigorous breathing techniques, 56
Bellows Breath, 57
Glowing Face Breath, 56-57
Humming Breath, 57-58
safety, 58-59
Breathing Book, The, 54

Bridge Posture (Setu Bandhasana), 73-75
Brunton, Dr. Paul, 316
buddha, 327
buddhi, 282
as function of the mind, 283-284
intuition operations, 283
dhi, 283
prajna, 283-284
pratibha, 283-284
Butterfly Posture (Baddha Konasana), 102

C

Camel Pose (Ustrasana), 134-135
carpal tunnel syndrome, cautions when doing poses, 86
Cat Stretch, 24-26
cervical vertebrae, head roll, 19-20
Chair Posture (Maitri Asana), 200-201
chakras, 242-252
ajna chakra, 250
anahata chakra, 248
astral chakra, 246-247
guru chakra, 251
jnana chakra, 252
manipura chakra, 247
root chakra, 245-246

sahasrara chakra, 251-252

soma chakra, 252

vishuddha chakra, 249

Chakras: Energy Centers of Transformation, 245

Chakrasana (Wheel Posture), 155-156

Channel Purification, 52-56

chanting mantras (meditation), 208

Charaka Samhita, 278

Chernin, Dennis, M.D., 206

Child's Posture (Balasana), 32-33

Chin Lock (Jalandhara Bandha), 122

chitta, as function of the mind, 282-285

Choosing a Path, 310

Churn Posture, 99

classes, 185-186
    Gentle Yoga classes, 6

Classical Indian Hatha Yoga, 6

cleanliness, 275
    nasal wash, 275-277
    saucha niyama (keep clean), 299-300
    stomach wash, 277-278

clothing, 185

Cobra Posture (Bhujangasana), 64-66

codes of life, 295-301
    ahimsa (do not harm anyone), 297
    aparigraha (do not be greedy), 299
    asteya (do not steal), 298
    brahmacharya (do not overindulge), 298
    Ishvara pranidhana (surrender to a higher force), 301
    santosha (contentment), 300
    satya (do not lie), 297
    saucha (keep clean), 299-300
    svadhyaya (study yourself), 301
    tapas (be self-disciplined), 300

colon, 120

commitments (codes of life), 295-301
    ahimsa (do not harm anyone), 297
    aparigraha (do not be greedy), 299
    asteya (do not steal), 298
    brahmacharya (do not overindulge), 298
    Ishvara pranidhana (surrender to a higher force), 301
    santosha (contentment), 300

satya (do not lie), 297

saucha (keep clean), 299-300

svadhyaya (study yourself), 301

tapas (be self-disciplined), 300

Complete Breath exercise, 51-52

Complete Idiot's Guide to Hinduism, The, 14

Complete Illustrated Book of Yoga, The, 132

concentration, connecting with Higher Self, 12-13

connecting with your inner guidance, meditation, 226-227

consciousness
    kundalini, 240-242
        awareness, 241-242
        chakras, 242-252
    living consciously, 327-328

contemplate (Manana), second step to enlightenment, 314

contemplation
    dharana, 203
    meditation, 224

contentment, santosha niyama (stay content), 300

Corpse Posture (Shavasana), 35-37

cosmic patterns, visualizations, 222-223

Coulter, H. David, Ph.D., 71

craving (as obstacle to success in meditation), 232-233

creating atmosphere, designing yoga sessions, 183

Crocodile Posture (Makarasana), 34-35

Crow Posture (Kakasana), 150-152

cushions (meditation), 195-196

D

dahl recipe, 273

Dandamis, 4

Dandasana (Staff Posture), 77-79

Dass, Ram, 6

deep meditative absorption (samadhi), 253

delusion (as obstacle to success in meditation), 232

designing yoga sessions, 175-183

    Advanced routine, 182-183

    creating atmosphere, 183

    First Beginning routine, 179

    Gentle Hatha Yoga routine, 177-178

    Intermediate routine, 181-182

    Second Beginning routine, 180-181

Desikachar, T.K.V., 7, 324

Desk Pose. *See* Arch Posture

Devananda, Swami Vishnu, 325

Dhanurasana (Bow Posture), 70-71

Dharana (Raja Yoga limb), 308

dharana (contemplation), 203

dharma (ethical standards), 295-301

    ahimsa (do not harm anyone), 297

    aparigraha (do not be greedy), 299

    asteya (do not steal), 298

    brahmacharya (do not overindulge), 298

    Ishvara pranidhana (surrender to a higher force), 301

    santosha (contentment), 300

    satya (do not lie), 297

    saucha (keep clean), 299-300

    svadhyaya (study yourself), 301

    tapas (be self-disciplined), 300

dhi field of knowledge, 283

Dhyana (Raja Yoga limb), 308

dhyana (meditation), 204

diaphragmatic breathing, 49-51

diet of a yogi, recipes, 270-275

    dahl, 273

    ghee, 271

    paneer, 272

    subzi, 274

directing awareness, subtle bodies, 8-9

disciple-guru relationship, 302

    levels of enlightenment, 304

    recognizing the guru, 303

    testing the teacher, 305-306

distractions (as obstacle to success in meditation), 236

diurnal biorhythms, 177

Divine Romance, The, 298

Dolphin Posture (Matsyabhedasana), 144-146

Double Leg Lift (Utthita Dvipadasana), 124

doubt (as obstacle to success in meditation), 231

Down Facing Dog Posture (Adho Mukha Svanasana), 85-86

dressing for movement, 17

Dvipada Pitham (Arch Posture), 72-73

E

Eagle Posture (Garudasana), 135-136

Easy Posture (Sukhasana), 194-196

eating, practicing on an empty stomach, 17

emotional expression, Bhakti Yoga, 313

endocrine system, 83

energy
  kinetic energy, 32
  kundalini, 240-242
    awareness, 241-242
    chakras, 242-252
  potential energy, 32
  three energy states, 11

enlightenment, 304
  becoming an awakened person, 326-327
  Jnana Yoga, 314-315

Enneads, 5

equipment, 184
  biofeedback, 184
  clothing, 185
  mats, 184
  meditation cushions, 195-196
  props, 184
  sandbags/breath pillows, 184

erasing bad karma with upayas, 290-291

ESP (extrasensory perception), 253-254

ethics, 295-296
  ahimsa (do not harm anyone), 297
  aparigraha (do not be greedy), 299
  asteya (do not steal), 298
  brahmacharya (do not overindulge), 298
  Ishvara pranidhana (surrender to a higher force), 301
  santosha (contentment), 300
  satya (do not lie), 297
  saucha (keep clean), 299-300
  svadhyaya (study yourself), 301
  tapas (be self-disciplined), 300

events, 185-186

evolution of yoga, 3-4
  influential teachers, 5-6
  movement to the West, 4-5
  styles, 6-7

extrasensory perception. *See* ESP

eyebrow center (ajna chakra), 250

F

failure (as obstacle to success in meditation), 234

Farhi, Donna, 54, 85

fear (as obstacle to success in meditation), 236

Feuerstein, George, Ph.D., 67

finding your inner core, meditation, 224-225

First Beginning routine, designing your session, 179

First Lessons in Sanskrit Grammar and Reading, 138

five levels of being, subtle bodies, 8-11
  directing awareness, 8-9
  visualization, 10

floor postures, 77
  Down Facing Dog Posture, 85-86
  Pigeon Pose, 83
  Plow Pose, 81-83
  Shoulder Stand, 79-81
  Staff Posture, 77-79

flowing postures, Sun Salutation, 159-160
  Pose 1, 161-162
  Pose 2, 162-163
  Pose 3, 163-164
  Pose 4, 164-165
  Pose 5, 165-166
  Pose 6, 166-167
  Pose 7, 167
  Pose 8, 168
  Pose 9, 168-169
  Pose 10, 169
  Pose 11, 170
  Pose 12, 171-173

Folan, Lilias, 6

force, safety tips, 18

Friend, John, 7

From Death to Birth: Understanding Karma and Reincarnation, 286

Full Spinal Twist (Matsyendrasana), 153-154

functions of the mind
  ahankara, 285-286
  buddhi, 283-284
  chitta, 284-285
  manas, 282

G

Gajakarani (stomach wash), 277-278

Garudasana (Eagle Posture), 135-136

Gayatri mantra, 172, 226

genie control (meditation), 209-210

Gentle Hatha Yoga routine, designing your session, 177-178

Gentle Yoga classes, 6

ghee recipe, 271

Glowing Face Breath, 56-57

Gospel of Sri Ramakrishna, The, 311

Goswami, Shyam Sundar, 242

great sayings (maha vakyas), 224

group karma, 289

group meditation, 237-238

guidance versus garbage (meditation), 227

Gupta, Mahendranath, 311

guru chakra, 251

guru shakti, 303

gurus, 29
  guru-disciple relationship, 302
    "crazy wisdom," 304-305
    levels of enlightenment, 304
    recognizing the guru, 303
    testing the teacher, 305-306

H

Halasana (Plow Pose), 81-83

Half Fish Posture (Ardha Matsyasana), 71

Half Spinal Twist (Ardha Matsyendrasana), 112-113

Half Wheel. *See* Arch Posture

hand position (mudra), 54

Hatha Pradipika, 325

Hatha Yoga, 4-6
  abdominal poses, 120-121
    Balance Pose, 125-127
    Leg Lift, 124-125
    safety, 120-121
    Stomach Lift, 121-122
    Stomach Roll, 123
  advanced yoga postures, 143-144
    Crow Posture, 150-152
    Dolphin Posture, 144-146
    Full Spinal Twist, 153-154
    Headstand, 146-150
    Peacock Pose, 152
    Scorpion Posture, 156-157
    Wheel Posture, 155-156
  backward-bending poses, 63
    Arch Posture, 72-73
    Boat Posture, 68-70
    Bow Posture, 70-71
    Bridge Posture, 73-75
    Cobra Posture, 64-66
    Half Fish Posture, 71
    Locust Posture, 66-68
    recognizing limits, 75

bending postures, 91
  Butterfly Posture,
    102
  Churn Posture, 99
  mental attentive-
    ness, 104
  Sitting Forward
    Bend, 97-99
  Standing Backward
    Bend, 93-95
  Standing Forward
    Bend, 95-96
  Standing Side Bend,
    92
  Symbol of Yoga
    Posture, 100-102
designing sessions,
  175-183
  Advanced routine,
    182-183
  creating atmosphere,
    183
  First Beginning rou-
    tine, 179
  Gentle Hatha Yoga
    routine, 177-178
  Intermediate rou-
    tine, 181-182
  Second Beginning
    routine, 180-181
equipment, 184
  biofeedback, 184
  clothing, 185
  mats, 184
  props, 184
  sandbags/breath pil-
    lows, 184

floor postures, 77-86
  Down Facing Dog
    Posture, 85-86
  Pigeon Pose, 83
  Plow Pose, 81-83
  Shoulder Stand,
    79-81
  Staff Posture, 77-79
flowing postures, Sun
  Salutation, 159-173
identifying your inner
  body, subtle bodies,
  7-10
intermediate level yoga
  postures, 132-142
  Arch Posture,
    138-140
  Back Bending
    Monkey Posture,
    140-142
  Camel Pose,
    134-135
  Eagle Posture,
    135-136
  Inclined Plane
    Posture, 133-134
  King Dancer Pose,
    136-138
  remaining in an
    attentive state,
    131-132
meditation postures,
  192-201
  Accomplished
    Posture, 197-198
  Auspicious Posture,
    196-197
  Chair Posture,
    200-201
  Easy Posture,
    194-196

  Lotus Posture,
    199-200
  steady and comfort-
    able, 201-202
standing postures,
  86-89
  Horse Riding
    Posture, 88-89
  Warrior Posture,
    87-88
stretching postures,
  Rocking Chair Roll,
  116-117
twisting postures,
  105-116
  Angle Pose, 106-107
  Half Spinal Twist,
    112-113
  Reclining Twist,
    115-116
  Revolving Triangle
    Pose, 109-110
  Torso Twist, 111
  Triangle Pose,
    107-109
head roll, 19-20
Headstand (Shirshasana),
  146-150
heart center (anahata
  chakra), 248
Heart of Yoga: Developing a
  Personal Practice, The,
  324
Hellman, Sylvia, 152
Higher Self, connecting
  with, 12
  deep concentration,
    12-13
  role of spirit, 13

higher states of consciousness

  evaluating your progress, 265-266

  recognizing your presence, 264

  samadhi, 263-264

  turiya, 262-263

Himalayan Mountain Cookery, 272

Hinduism, 13

hip roll, 21-22

history

  evolution of yoga, 3-4

  influential teachers, 5-6

  movement to the West, 4-5

  styles of yoga, 6-7

Hittleman, Richard, 6

Horse Riding Posture (Utkatasana), 88-89

How to Know God, 234

How to Meditate Using Chakras, Mantras and Breath, 206

Humming Breath, 57-58

hypnagogic state, 257

I

ida (left nadi), 55

illness (as obstacle to success in meditation), 231

Inclined Plane Posture (Purvottanasana), 133-134

inconsistency (as obstacle to success in meditation), 234-235

Indian Hatha Yoga, 6

influential teachers, 5-6

inner body, subtle bodies, 7-10

  directing awareness, 8-9

  visualization, 10

inner messages, psychic powers, 255-257

Inner Quest: The Path of Spiritual Unfoldment, 299

inner sound (meditation), 211-212

Integral Yoga, 6

intermediate level yoga postures, 132-142

  Arch Posture, 138-140

  Back Bending Monkey Posture, 140-142

  Camel Pose, 134-135

  Eagle Posture, 135-136

  Inclined Plane Posture, 133-134

  King Dancer Pose, 136-138

  remaining in an attentive state, 131-132

Intermediate routine, designing your session, 181-182

intuition, 283

  dhi, 283

  prajna, 283-284

  pratibha, 283-284

invoking blessing force, Tantra Yoga, 320-322

inward journey stages (meditation), 203

  contemplation (dharana), 203

  meditation (dhyana), 204

  total mental absorption (samadhi), 204

Ishta Devata (personal God), 312

Ishvara (Supreme Being), 312

Ishvara pranidhana (surrender to a higher force), 301

Iyengar, B.K.S., 7

J

Jala Neti (nasal wash), 275-277

Jalandhara Bandha (Chin Lock), 122

japa, 215

Japa Kit, 213

Jathara Parivartanasana (Reclining Twist), 115-116

jivanmukta, 293

jnana chakra, 252

Jnana Yoga, 313

  experiencing truth, 315-316

  steps to enlightenment, 314-315

Johari, Harish, 59, 222

Joints and Glands Exercises, 24

Jois, K. Pattabhi, 7

Jyotir Vidya (astrology), 292

K

Kakasana (Crow Posture), 150-152

kama (sensual pleasure), 295-296

Kapalabhati, 56-57

Kapha people (Ayurveda), 279

Kapotasana (Pigeon Pose), 83

karma, 288

  agama, 288-289

  banishing negativity, 291-292

  erasing bad karma with upayas, 290-291

  group karma, 289

  kriyamana, 288

  moksha, 293-294

  prarabdha, 288-289

  purifying your mind, 289-290

  sanchita, 288

  yoga astrology, 292-293

Karma Yoga, 309-311

  seva (selfless service), 310-311

  working without worry, 309-310

karmashaya, 286

kinetic energy, 32

King Dancer Pose (Natarajasana), 136-138

knee roll, 22

Knees-to-Chest Posture (Apanasana), 34

Konasana (Angle Pose), 106-107

kriyamana karma, 288, 309

kundalini, 239-242

  awareness, 241-242

  chakras, 242-252

    ajna chakra, 250

    anahata chakra, 248

    astral chakra, 246-247

    guru chakra, 251

    jnana chakra, 252

    manipura chakra, 247

    root chakra, 245-246

    sahasrara chakra, 251-252

    soma chakra, 252

    vishuddha chakra, 249

Kundalini: The Arousal of the Inner Energy, 242

L

Lasater, Judith, 30

latent mental powers, 253

  cautions, 255

  ESP, 254

higher states of consciousness

  evaluating your progress, 265-266

  recognizing your presence, 264

  samadhi, 263-264

  turiya, 262-263

inner messages, 255-257

yoga nidra, 257-258

  lucid sleep, 258-261

  reducing need for sleep, 261-262

laws for the mental universe (Tantra Yoga), symbolism, 319-320

laziness (as obstacle to success in meditation), 231

Learn to Meditate, 221

Leg Lift (abdominal pose), 124-125

life force, vectors in the physical body, 59-60

lifestyle of a yogi, 269

  Ayurveda, 278-279

    balance, 280

    Kapha people, 279

    Pitta people, 279

    Vata people, 279

  cleanliness, 275

    nasal wash, 275-277

    stomach wash, 277-278

  nutrition, 269-270

    recipes, 271-275

    traditional diet, 270-271

limbs, Raja Yoga, 307-308
  asana, 308
  dharana, 308
  dhyana, 308
  niyama, 308
  pranayama, 308
  pratyahara, 308
  samadhi, 308
  yama, 308
linking body and mind through breathing, 47-48
  Channel Purification, 52-56
  Complete Breath exercise, 51-52
  diaphragmatic breathing, 49-51
  vigorous breathing techniques, 56-59
living consciously, 327-328
Living Goddess: Reclaiming the Tradition of the Mother of the Universe, The, 226
Locust Posture (Shalabhasana), 66-68
loosening up your body, 19
  ankle roll, 22-23
  head roll, 19-20
  hip roll, 21-22
  knee roll, 22
  shoulder roll, 20
  stretching poses, 23
    Cat Stretch, 24-26
    Lunge Stretch, 27-28
    Reclining Stretch, 23-24
    Standing Stretch, 23
  wrist roll, 21
Lotus Posture (Padmasana), 199-200
lucid sleep, 258-261
lumbar spine, 21
Lunge Stretch, 27-28

M

maha vakyas (great sayings), 224
Maharshi, Ramana, 316
mahat, 224
maintaining your center, 119
Maitri Asana (Chair Posture), 200-201
Makarasana (Crocodile Posture), 34
malas, 213-215
Manana (contemplate), second step to enlightenment, 314
manas, as function of the mind, 282
mandalas, 222
manipura chakra (navel center), 247
Mano Maya Kosha, 8
Mantra and Meditation, 249
Mantras (meditation), 208
  chanting, 208
  choosing, 210-211
  inner sound, 211-212
Maranatha, 312
mastering relaxation, 29-30
  Child's Posture, 32-33
  Corpse Posture, 35-37
  Crocodile Posture, 34-35
  Knees-to-Chest Posture, 34
  Mountain Posture, 31-32
mastering your mind (meditation), 212-213
  japa, 215
  malas, 213-215
mats, 184
Matsyabhedasana (Dolphin Posture), 144-146
Matsyendrasana (Full Spinal Twist), 153-154
Mayurasana (Peacock Pose), 152
medical benefits of meditation, 190
meditation
  breathing cycle, 204-206
  chanting mantras, 208
  choosing a mantra, 210-211
  connecting with your inner guidance, 226-227
  contemplation of an ideal, 224
  controlling the genie, 209-210
  cushions, 195-196
  establishing a routine, 218
    preparing to sit, 218-219
    sample session, 219-221

expanding your sense of self, 225-226

finding your inner core, 224-225

focusing on breathing, 206-207

group meditation, 237-238

guidance versus garbage, 227

inner sound, 211-212

inward journey stages, 203

   contemplation (dharana), 203

   meditation (dhyana), 204

   total mental absorption (samadhi), 204

mastering your mind, 212-213

   japa, 215

   malas, 213-215

medical benefits, 190

meditating on blessings (Tantra Yoga), 322-323

natural high, 191-192

obstacles to success, 229-230

   craving, 232-233

   delusion, 232

   doubt, 231

   failure, 234

   illness, 231

   inconsistency, 234-235

   laziness, 231

   misunderstanding instructions, 233-234

   Western concerns, 235-236

postures, 192-194

   Accomplished Posture, 197-198

   Auspicious Posture, 196-197

   Chair Posture, 200-201

   Easy Posture, 194-196

   Lotus Posture, 199-200

   steady and comfortable, 201-202

psychological benefits, 191

regulating your nervous system, 208

versus mood- and mind-altering drugs, 192

visualization, 221

   cosmic patterns, 222-223

   meditating on an image, 221

Meditation and Its Practice, 190

Meditation and Mantras, 325

memory, chitta, 284-285

mental powers, 253

   cautions, 255

   ESP, 254

   higher states of consciousness

      evaluating your progress, 265-266

      recognizing your presence, 264

      samadhi, 263-264

      turiya, 262-263

   inner messages, 255-257

   yoga nidra, 257-258

      lucid sleep, 258-261

      reducing need for sleep, 261-262

Milarepa (Tibetan yogi), 304

mind mastering (meditation), 212-213

   japa, 215

   malas, 213-215

mind-altering drugs versus meditation, 192

misunderstanding instructions (as obstacle to success in meditation), 233-234

moksha (spiritual liberation), 293-295

Monkey Posture (Banarasana), 140-142

mood-altering drugs versus meditation, 192

Mookerjee, Adjit, 242

Moon signs (astrology), 292

Mountain Posture (Tadasana), 31-32

mudra (hand position), 54

Muktananda, Swami, 305

muladhara (root chakra), 245-246

mysticism (Tantra Yoga), 318-319
  invoking blessing force, 320-322
  laws for the mental universe, 319-320
  meditating on blessings, 322-323

N

Nadi Shodhana, 52-56

nasal wash (Jala Neti), 275-277

Natarajasana (King Dancer Pose), 136-138

Nath, Gorakh, 4

Nath, Matsyendra, 4

natural high of meditation, 191-192

Naukasana (Boat Posture), 68-70

Nauli (Stomach Roll), 123

navel center (manipura chakra), 247

nervous system, regulating through meditation, 208

neti pots, 275

Nididhyasana (realize), third step to enlightenment, 314

niyamas (Raja Yoga), 296-308
  Ishvara pranidhana (surrender to a higher force), 301
  santosha (contentment), 300
  saucha (keep clean), 299-300
  svadhyaya (study yourself), 301
  tapas (be self-disciplined), 300

nonviolence (ahimsa), 297

nostril breathing, Channel Purification, 52-56

nutrition, 269-270
  recipes, 271-275
    dahl, 273
    ghee, 271
    paneer, 272
    subzi, 274
  traditional diet, 270-271

O

O'Brien, Justin, 167

obstacles to success in meditation, 229-230
  craving, 232-233
  delusion, 232
  doubt, 231

failure, 234
illness, 231
inconsistency, 234-235
laziness, 231
misunderstanding instructions, 233-234
Western concerns, 235
  distractions, 236
  fear, 236

P

Padahastasana (Standing Forward Bend), 95-96

padas, 214

Padmasana (Lotus Posture), 199-200

paneer recipe, 272

Paramahansa, Ramakrishna, 311

Parivritta Trikonasana (Revolving Triangle Pose), 109-110

Parshvottanasana (Angle Pose), 106-107

Paschimottanasana (Sitting Forward Bend), 97-99

Patanjali, ethical standards, 295-301, 307
  ahimsa (do not harm anyone), 297
  aparigraha (do not be greedy), 299
  asteya (do not steal), 298
  brahmacharya (do not overindulge), 298

Ishvara pranidhana (surrender to a higher force), 301

santosha (contentment), 300

satya (do not lie), 297

saucha (keep clean), 299-300

svadhyaya (study yourself), 301

tapas (be self-disciplined), 300

Path of Fire and Light, 144

Peacock Pose (Mayurasana), 152

physician approval, 16

Pigeon Pose (Kapotasana), 83

pingala (right nadi), 55

Pitta people (Ayurveda), 279

Play of Consciousness, The, 305

Plotinus, 5

Plow Pose (Halasana), 81-83

poses/postures

abdominal poses, 120-121

Balance Pose, 125-127

Leg Lift, 124-125

safety, 120-121

Stomach Lift, 121-122

Stomach Roll, 123

advanced yoga postures, 143-157

Crow Posture, 150-152

Dolphin Posture, 144-146

Full Spinal Twist, 153-154

Headstand, 146-150

Peacock Pose, 152

Scorpion Posture, 156-157

Wheel Posture, 155-156

backward-bending poses, 63

Arch Posture, 72-73

Boat Posture, 68-70

Bow Posture, 70-71

Bridge Posture, 73-75

Cobra Posture, 64-66

Half Fish Posture, 71

Locust Posture, 66-68

recognizing limits, 75

bending postures, 91-104

Butterfly Posture, 102

Churn Posture, 99

mental attentiveness, 104

Sitting Forward Bend, 97-99

Standing Backward Bend, 93-95

Standing Forward Bend, 95-96

Standing Side Bend, 92

Symbol of Yoga Posture, 100-102

floor postures, 77-86

Down Facing Dog Posture, 85-86

Pigeon Pose, 83

Plow Pose, 81-83

Shoulder Stand, 79-81

Staff Posture, 77-79

flowing postures, Sun Salutation, 159-173

Intermediate Level yoga postures, 131-142

Arch Posture, 138-140

Back Bending Monkey Posture, 140-142

Camel Pose, 134-135

Eagle Posture, 135-136

Inclined Plane Posture, 133-134

King Dancer Pose, 136-138

remaining in an attentive state, 131-132

meditation, 192-202

Accomplished Posture, 197-198

Auspicious Posture, 196-197

Chair Posture, 200-201

Easy Posture, 194-196

Lotus Posture, 199-200

steady and comfortable, 201-202

standing postures, 86

Horse Riding Posture, 88-89

Warrior Posture, 87-88

stretching poses, 23

Cat Stretch, 24-26

Lunge Stretch, 27-28

Reclining Stretch, 23-24

Standing Stretch, 23

stretching postures, Rocking Chair Roll, 116-117

twisting postures, 105-116

Angle Pose, 106-107

Half Spinal Twist, 112-113

Reclining Twist, 115-116

Revolving Triangle Pose, 109-110

Torso Twist, 111

Triangle Pose, 107-109

postures. *See* poses/ postures

potential energy, 32

Power of Mantra and the Mystery of Initiation, The, 219

Power of Now: A Guide to Spiritual Enlightenment, The, 238

Power Yoga, 7

prajna field of knowledge, 283-284

Prajnanam Brahma, 224

prakriti, 13

prana (life force/vital energy), 9, 59

vectors in the physical body, 59-60

Pranayama (Raja Yoga limb), 49, 308

prarabdha karma, 288-289

pratibha field of knowledge, 283-284

Pratyahara (Raja Yoga limb), 308

pregnancy, safety tips, 17, 121

preparing to do yoga

loosening up your body, 19

ankle roll, 22-23

head roll, 19-20

hip roll, 21-22

knee roll, 22

shoulder roll, 20

wrist roll, 21

stretching poses, 23

Cat Stretch, 24-26

Lunge Stretch, 27-28

Reclining Stretch, 23-24

Standing Stretch, 23

props, 184

psychic abilities, 253

cautions, 255

ESP, 254

inner messages, 255-257

psychological benefits of meditation, 191

psychology, 281-282

karma, 288

agama, 288-289

banishing negativity, 291-292

erasing bad karma with upayas, 290-291

group karma, 289

kriyamana, 288

moksha, 293-294

prarabdha, 288-289

purifying your mind, 289-290

sanchita, 288

yoga astrology, 292-293

reincarnation, 286

understanding yourself, functions of the mind, 282-286

purascharanas, 226

purifying your mind, karma, 289-290

purusha (soul/Higher Self), connecting with, 9-12
  deep concentration, 12-13
  role of spirit, 13
Purvottanasana (Inclined Plane Posture), 133-134
Pyrrho, 4

Q–R

Radha: Diary of a Woman's Search, 152
Raja Yoga limbs, 307-308
  asana, 308
  dharana, 308
  dhyana, 308
  niyama, 308
  pranayama, 308
  pratyahara, 308
  samadhi, 308
  yama, 308
Rajas (energy state), 11-13, 231
Rama, Swami, 5
Rao, K. N., 293
realize (Nididhyasana), third step to enlightenment, 314
recipes, 271-275
  dahl, 273
  ghee, 271
  paneer, 272
  subzi, 274

Reclining Stretch, 23-24
Reclining Twist (Jathara Parivartanasana), 115-116
reincarnation, 286
Relax and Renew: Restful Yoga for Stressful Times, 30
relaxation, 29-30
  Child's Posture, 32-33
  Corpse Posture, 35-37
  Crocodile Posture, 34-35
  Knees-to-Chest Posture, 34
  Mountain Posture, 31-32
religious traditions, 13-14
resources, 323-324
  Bhagavad Gita, 325
  Hatha Pradipika, 325
  inner awareness texts, 325-326
  Yoga Sutras, 324-325
retreat centers, 185-186
Revolving Triangle Pose (Parivritta Trikonasana), 109-110
Rig Veda, 3, 226
Rocking Chair Roll, 116-117
rolls, loosening up your body, 19
  ankle roll, 22-23
  head roll, 19-20
  hip roll, 21-22
  knee roll, 22
  shoulder roll, 20
  wrist roll, 21

root chakra (muladhara), 245-246
rosaries. *See* malas
routine, establishing a meditation routine, 218
  preparing to sit, 218-219
  sample session, 219-221
Royal Path. *See* Raja Yoga
Royal Path: Practical Lessons on Yoga, 6
rules for women, 16-17

S

sacral center (root chakra), 245-246
sacrum, 109
sadhana (spiritual practice), 307
safety
  abdominal poses, 120-121
  avoiding force, 18
  breathing, 18
  dressing for movement, 17
  gaining physician approval, 16
  practicing on an empty stomach, 17
  rules for women, 16-17
  vigorous breathing techniques, 58-59

sahaja samadhi, 264

sahasrara chakra (brain center), 251-252

Sakti Sadhana: Steps to Samadhi, 326

samadhi (deep meditative absorption), 204, 253, 263-264, 308

samana, 59

samskara, 285

sanchita karma, 288, 309

sandbags, 184

Sanskrit, 138

santosha (contentment), 300

Saraswati, Swami Satyananda, 242

Saraswati, Swami Satyasangananda, 257

Sarvangasana (Shoulder Stand), 79-81

Satchidananda, Swami, 6

satsang, 235

sattva (energy state), 11-13, 231

satya (do not lie), 297

saucha (keep clean), 299-300

Schatz, Mary Pullig, M.D., 176

Science of Breath: A Practical Guide, 48

Scorpion Posture (Vrishchikasana), 156-157

Search in Secret India, A, 316

Second Beginning routine, designing your session, 180-181

Self Realization Fellowship, 298

self-discipline, tapas niyama (be self-disciplined), 300

self-identity (ahankara), 285-286

self-review, taking stock of the day, 302

self-study, svadhyaya niyama (study yourself), 301

selfless service (seva), 310-311

sense of balance, 42-43
    Tip Toe Stretch, 43-44
    Tree Posture, 44-45

sense of self, meditation, 225-226

Serpent Power, The, 251

sessions
    designing, 175-183
        Advanced routine, 182-183
        creating atmosphere, 183
        First Beginning routine, 179
        Gentle Hatha Yoga routine, 177-178
        Intermediate routine, 181-182
        Second Beginning routine, 180-181

equipment, 184
    biofeedback, 184
    clothing, 185
    mats, 184
    props, 184
    sandbags/breath pillows, 184

Setu Bandhasana (Bridge Posture), 73-75

seva (selfless service), 309-311

sex center (astral chakra), 246-247

shaktipat, 303

Shalabhasana (Locust Posture), 66-68

Shavasana (Corpse Posture), 35

Shirshasana (Headstand), 146-150

shoulder roll, 20

Shoulder Stand (Sarvangasana), 79-81

Shravana (study), first step to enlightenment, 314

siddhas, 4

Siddhasana (Accomplished Posture), 197-198

siddhis, 253

Single Leg Lift (Utthita Ekapadasana), 124-125

Sitting Forward Bend (Paschimottanasana), 97-99

Sivananda Companion to Yoga, The, 132

Sivananda Yoga Vedanta Center, 95

small intestine, 120

soma chakra, 252

soul (purusha), 9

Sovik, Rolf, Psy.D., 79, 221

special yogic abilities, 253
  cautions, 255
  ESP, 254
  higher states of consciousness
    evaluating your progress, 265-266
    recognizing your presence, 264
    samadhi, 263-264
    turiya, 262-263
  inner messages, 255-257
  yoga nidra, 257-258
    lucid sleep, 258-261
    reducing need for sleep, 261-262

spine
  massaging, Rocking Chair Roll, 116-117
  posture, 117-118

spirit, connecting with Higher Self, 13

spiritual practice (sadhana), 307

Sri Yantra, 223

Staff Posture (Dandasana), 77-79

Standing Backward Bend, 93-95

Standing Forward Bend (Padahastasana), 95-96

standing postures, 86
  Horse Riding Posture, 88-89
  Warrior Posture, 87-88

Standing Side Bend, 92

Standing Stretch, 23

states of energy, 11
  kinetic energy, 32
  potential energy, 32

Stiles, Mukunda, 110

stomach exercises, 120-121
  Balance Pose, 125-127
  Leg Lift, 124-125
  safety, 120-121
  Stomach Lift, 121-122
  Stomach Roll, 123

Stomach Lift (Uddiyana Bandha), 121-122

Stomach Roll (Nauli), 123

stomach wash (Gajakarani), 277-278

stretching poses, 23
  Cat Stretch, 24-26
  Lunge Stretch, 27-28
  Reclining Stretch, 23-24
  Rocking Chair Roll, 116-117
  Standing Stretch, 23

string cleaning (Sutra Neti), 277

Structural Yoga Therapy: Adapting to the Individual, 110

study (Shravana), first step to enlightenment, 314

styles of yoga, 6-7
  Bhakti, 311
    empowering your practice, 311-313
    expressing emotions, 313
  Jnana, 313
    experiencing truth, 315-316
    steps to enlightenment, 314-315
  Karma, 309
    seva (selfless service), 310-311
    working without worry, 309-310
  Raja, 307-308
    limbs, 308

subtle bodies, 8-11
  directing awareness, 8-9
  visualization, 10

subzi recipe, 274

Sukhasana (Easy Posture), 194-196

Sun Salutation poses (Surya Namaskar), 159-173
  Pose 1, 161-162
  Pose 2, 162-163
  Pose 3, 163-164
  Pose 4, 164-165
  Pose 5, 165-166
  Pose 6, 166-167
  Pose 7, 167
  Pose 8, 168

Pose 9, 168-169
Pose 10, 169
Pose 11, 170
Pose 12, 171-173
Sun signs (astrology), 292
superconscious stage (turiya), 262-263
superconsciousness perspective, 224
supernormal powers, 254
Supreme Being (Ishvara), 312
surrender, Ishvara pranidhana niyama (surrender to a higher force), 301
Surya Namaskar (Sun Salutation poses), 159-173
Pose 1, 161-162
Pose 2, 162-163
Pose 3, 163-164
Pose 4, 164-165
Pose 5, 165-166
Pose 6, 166-167
Pose 7, 167
Pose 8, 168
Pose 9, 168-169
Pose 10, 169
Pose 11, 170
Pose 12, 171-173
sushumna, 55, 206
Sutra Neti (string cleaning), 277
svadhisthana (astral chakra), 246-247

svadhyaya (study yourself), 301
Svatmarama (*Hatha Pradipika*), 325
Svoboda, Robert E., 286
Swastikasana (Auspicious Posture), 196-197
Symbol of Yoga Posture (Yoga Mudra), 100-102
symbolism (Tantra Yoga), 320

T

Tadasana (Mountain Posture), 31
Tadasana Parshvabhangi (Torso Twist), 111
tamas (energy state), 11-13, 231
Tantra Yoga, 318-323
invoking blessing force, 320-322
laws for the mental universe, 319-320
symbolism, 320
meditating on blessings, 322-323
tapas (be self-disciplined), 300
Tat Tvam Asi, 224
teachers, 5-6
texts, 323-324
Bhagavad Gita, 325
Hatha Pradipika, 325

inner awareness texts, 325-326
Yoga Sutras, 324-325
throat center (vishuddha chakra), 249
Tigunait, Pandit Rajmani, 219, 256, 286, 299
Tip Toe Stretch, mastering balance, 43-44
Tolle, Eckhart, 238
Tools for Tantra, 222
Torso Twist (Tadasana Parshvabhangi), 111
total mental absorption (samadhi), 204
touring your body, 37
31 Points exercise, 38, 40-41
61 Points exercise, 38, 41-42
Tree Posture, mastering balance, 44-45
Triangle Pose (Trikonasana), 107-109
Tripura Rahasya, 326
truth, experiencing Jnana Yoga, 315-316
truthfulness (satya), 297
turiya (superconscious state), 262-263
twisting postures, 105-116
Angle Pose, 106-107
Half Spinal Twist, 112
Reclining Twist, 115-116
Revolving Triangle Pose, 109-110
Torso Twist, 111
Triangle Pose, 107-109

Tyberg, Judith M., 138
types of yoga
 Bhakti Yoga, 311
  empowering your
   practice, 311-313
  expressing emotions,
   313
 Jnana Yoga, 313
  experiencing truth,
   315-316
  steps to enlighten-
   ment, 314-315
 Karma Yoga, 309
  seva (selfless ser-
   vice), 310-311
  working without
   worry, 309-310
 Raja Yoga limbs,
  307-308

U

udana, 59
Uddiyana Bandha
 (Stomach Lift), 121-122
Ujjayi, 57-58
understanding yourself
 (yoga psychology), func-
 tions of the mind
 ahankara, 285-286
 buddhi, 283-284
 chitta, 284-285
 manas, 282
upayas, erasing bad karma,
 290-291

Upper Wash. *See* stomach
 wash
Ustrasana (Camel Pose),
 134-135
Utkatasana (Horse Riding
 Posture), 88-89
Utthita Dvipadasana
 (Double Leg Lift), 124
Utthita Ekapadasana
 (Single Leg Lift),
 124-125
Utthita Hastapadasana
 (Balance Pose), 125-127

V

value of desire, 232
Vata people (Ayurveda),
 279
vegetarians, 269-270
vigorous breathing tech-
 niques, 56-59
 Bellows Breath, 57
 Glowing Face Breath,
  56-57
 Humming Breath,
  57-58
 safety, 58-59
Vijnana Maya Kosha, 8
Vimanasana, 69
Viniyoga, 7
Virabhadrasana (Warrior
 Posture), 87-88
Vishnu-Devananda,
 Swami, 132

vishuddha chakra (throat
 center), 249
visualization, meditation,
 221
 cosmic patterns,
  222-223
 meditating on an
  image, 221
vital energy, vectors in the
 physical body, 59-60
viveka, 232
Vivekananda, Swami, 5
Vrikshasana, 44
Vrishchikasana (Scorpion
 Posture), 156-157
vyana, 59
Vyasa, Veda, 325

W

*Walking with a Himalayan
 Master,* 167
Warrior Posture
 (Virabhadrasana), 87-88
Wellness Tree, The, 191
Western movement, 4-5
Wheel Posture
 (Chakrasana), 155-156
women, safety rules, 16-17
Woodroffe, Sir John, 251
wrist roll, 21

X–Y–Z

Yama (Raja Yoga limb), 308

yamas, 296
  ahimsa (do not harm anyone), 297
  aparigraha (do not be greedy), 299
  asteya (do not steal), 298
  brahmacharya (do not overindulge), 298
  satya (do not lie), 297

yantras, 223

Yin Yoga, 7

yoga asleep. *See* yoga nidra

yoga astrology, 292-293

Yoga International, 6, 70

Yoga Journal, 6

yoga lifestyle, 269
  Ayurveda, 278-279
    balance, 280
    Kapha people, 279
    Pitta people, 279
    Vata people, 279
  cleanliness, 275
    nasal wash, 275-277
    stomach wash, 277-278
  nutrition, 269-270
    recipes, 271-275
    traditional diet, 270-271

Yoga Mind and Body, 95

Yoga Mind, Body and Spirit: A Return to Wholeness, 85

Yoga Mudra (Symbol of Yoga Posture), 100-102

yoga nidra, 253, 257-258
  lucid sleep, 258-261
  reducing need for sleep, 261-262

Yoga Nidra, 257

Yoga Philosophy of Patanjali, 234

yoga psychology, 281-282
  karma, 288
    agama, 288-289
    banishing negativity, 291-292
    erasing bad karma with upayas, 290-291
    group karma, 289
    kriyamana, 288
    moksha, 293-294
    prarabdha, 288-289
    purifying your mind, 289-290
    sanchita, 288
    yoga astrology, 292-293
  reincarnation, 286
  understanding yourself, functions of the mind, 282-286

Yoga Research Center in California, 67

Yoga Sutras, 255, 307, 324-325

Yoga Tradition: Its History, Literature, Philosophy and Practice, The, 67

Yoga Vasishtha, 326

Yoga: Mastering the Basics, 79

yogafinder.com, 16

Yogananda, Paramahansa, 5, 298

Yogi, Maharishi Mahesh, 6

Zen-style zafu cushions, 195